4.75

Scientific
Foundations
of Nursing

Scientific Foundations of Nursing

Madelyn T. Nordmark, R.N., B.S., M.S. (N.E.)
Formerly Research Assistant Professor, School of Nursing
University of Washington

Anne W. Rohweder, R.N., B.S., M.N.
Nursing Instructor, San Joaquin Delta College, Stockton, California;
Formerly Research Assistant Professor, School of Nursing
University of Washington

Foreword by **Mary S. Tschudin**
Dean, School of Nursing, University of Washington

SECOND EDITION

J. B. LIPPINCOTT COMPANY

Philadelphia   **Toronto**

Second Edition

Copyright © 1967, by J. B. Lippincott Company

Science Principles Applied to Nursing
First edition, by Madelyn Titus Nordmark and Anne W. Rohweder
Copyright © 1959
By J. B. Lippincott Company

Distributed in Great Britain by
Blackwell Scientific Publications,
Oxford, London, and Edinburgh

ISBN-0-397-54065-5

Library of Congress Catalog Card No. 67-17440

Printed in the United Stated of America

9   11   10   8

PREFACE TO SECOND EDITION

This book was conceived originally as a guide for teachers of nursing students. Since publication seven years ago, however, the book has been used increasingly by nursing students in both basic and graduate nursing programs. Comments and suggestions that filtered back to the authors seemed to indicate interest in a revision that would (1) increase the science content and the nursing applications, and (2) present the material in a form that might be more useful to students.

This current edition represents an amalgamation of the data from the original study done at the University of Washington, along with new material to expand both the science and the related nursing. The methods used for compiling the additional material are described in Part I.

The original Chapter II, "Potential Usefulness of the Principles for Nursing Education," which was specifically geared toward teacher use, has been revised as Part IV. In its place we have added a chapter to orient students and graduates to possible uses of the science and nursing sections. An index—an addition most frequently suggested by student users of the original text—follows Part IV.

We are grateful to Dean Mary S. Tschudin and Mrs. Louise Mansfield of the University of Washington School of Nursing for their cooperation and support during this year of revision. We also wish to take this opportunity to thank Mr. David T. Miller of the J. B. Lippincott Company, who has been a source of encouragement and assistance throughout the preparation of the revision.

Madelyn T. Nordmark
Anne W. Rohweder

FOREWORD TO FIRST EDITION

THE importance of the social, physical and biological sciences in nursing education has been emphasized repeatedly. The student is expected to draw upon all the science knowledge she possesses and to apply this knowledge in a variety of nursing situations. She is expected to see the relationships between many facts, principles and concepts and their relevance to particular problems in nursing, and, from this background, to make sound decisions for her nursing actions.

With the rapid expansion of scientific knowledge relevant to nursing care, the task of helping the student to achieve this level of performance becomes a major challenge for nursing educators. There is need to promote continued learning of the sciences throughout the educational program and to extend the meaningfulness of this knowledge for effective patient care.

This book presents the results of an extensive study of the application of social and natural science principles in nursing which was conducted at the University of Washington. A major portion of the material, which has been organized to facilitate its use by teachers, is devoted to the presentation of principles from psychology, sociology and anthropology, and from chemistry, physics, anatomy, physiology and microbiology, all of which are important to nursing. Accompanying each group of principles are the related statements of nursing care. Suggestions are offered to show how students may be helped to develop a greater understanding of the relevance of science to effective nursing care.

It is hoped that as teachers use the materials presented in this book, they will be stimulated to identify additional principles from the social and natural sciences and their implications for nursing practice.

Mary S. Tschudin, Dean
School of Nursing
University of Washington
Seattle, Washington

ACKNOWLEDGEMENTS TO FIRST EDITION

FOR many years nurse educators have shown a growing appreciation of the contributions of the basic sciences to nursing. This appreciation has led to the recognition of the need to delineate specifically the application of sciences to nursing practice. In addition, there has been an intensification of the felt need in the nursing profession for the formulation of a fundamental core of nursing knowledge. These two needs stimulated the study which is reported in this publication—an investigation that was supported by The Commonwealth Fund and carried out in the University of Washington School of Nursing.

A study of this kind cannot be accomplished without the cooperation and sustained efforts of many people. The authors wish to acknowledge, first of all, the members of the Natural and Social Science Committees of the University of Washington School of Nursing, who faithfully gave their time and energies during the five-year period. Members of the Natural Science Committee included: Helen Anderson, Helen Belcher, Lucy Enos, Shirley Frederickson, Julie Hanson, Stella Hay, Priscilla Normark, Bessie Robinson and Vesta Franz Skeins. Members of the Social Science Committee included: Viola Brown, Dorothy Burke, Marguerite Cobb, Betty Jane Ely, Betty Hart, Edith Heineman, Charity Kerby, Dolores Little, Mary O'Brien, Betty Olsen Ames, Maxine Patrick, Eleanor Perdelwitz, Lorraine Phillips, Patricia Rose, Patricia VanderLeest, Harriet Ulrich and Frances Zaleski.

The task of identifying important principles from the natural sciences was greatly aided by the major contributions of several of the teachers of science at the University of Washington. Dr. Julia Skahen, Assistant Professor of Physiology, Biophysics and Anatomy, devoted innumerable hours of her time to the study. Also of great assistance were Dr. B. S. Henry, Professor of Microbiology, Dr. S. G. Powell, Professor of Chemistry, and Dr. L. A. Sanderman, Associate Professor of Physics.

The following medical specialists were most gracious and helpful in reviewing and criticizing the nursing care principles related to the natural sciences: Doctors Robert M. Paine, Fred Casserd, Alexander P. Greer, Louis N. Hungerford, Jr., Hugh Jones, John F. Le Cocq,

Edward H. Morgan, Gerald Nowlis, Robert Pommerening, William J. Steenrod, Jr. and Heston L. Wilson.

For the collection of data for the social science portion of the study, the efforts of the nursing personnel in the five participating hospitals are particularly appreciated: King County Hospital, Northern State Hospital, Swedish Hospital, Seattle Veterans' Administration Hospital and Virginia Mason Hospital.

Special thanks go to Doctors Ivar Lovaas and James Taylor of the University of Washington Department of Psychology for reviewing and criticizing the social science data.

The authors are grateful to the members of both juries who evaluated the total data.

Much of the study was more easily facilitated by the secretarial assistance of Miss Doris Kelly, Mrs. Lois Martin and Mrs. Carolyn Miller.

The support and encouragements which the authors received from the entire faculty of the University of Washington School of Nursing were invaluable. Last, but by no means least, special thanks go to Dean Mary S. Tschudin and Assistant Dean Katherine Hoffman for their consistent support.

Anne W. Rohweder
Madelyn T. Nordmark
Seattle, Washington
December 25, 1958

Contents

xii   **Contents**

Part I

Orientation

INTRODUCTION

The nurse is constantly called upon to make independent decisions in the solution of such problems as those concerned with patient care, safety for herself and others, and interpersonal relationships. Increasingly, she is expected not only to make wise decisions for herself, but to guide auxiliary personnel who perform nursing care functions. In the process of executing nursing activities, the nurse cannot always find a policy, a "rule of thumb," or a person in authority to assist her when a problem arises. Even if comprehensive sets of rules were available, the habitual use of such rules would be potentially dangerous, in that they could very likely lead to unthinking and harmful actions because the nurse failed to understand the reasons behind the rule. As demands for nursing services increase, the professional nurse will become more and more the diagnostician of nursing care problems, expected to devise creative nursing interventions; less and less will she function primarily as a follower of medical orders and an overseer of routine procedures. It would seem vital, then, that the professional nurse be equipped to solve problems in a wise and resourceful manner.

The successful use of problem-solving methods—which, hopefully, the nurse will employ in making her decisions—implies that the problem-solver has in her possession or at her disposal the facts and understanding necessary for the analysis and solution of problems. This implication leads to two significant questions:

What knowledge is it important for a professional nurse to possess?

How can this knowledge and its use in solving nursing problems be learned most effectively?

Recognition of the significance of these questions led the original planners of the five-year curriculum study in basic nursing education (at the University of Washington School of Nursing[1]) to select as one area for investigation the relationship between the general and the professional education of nursing students. The Commonwealth Fund first supported this separate study within the framework of the total curriculum study, and the objective of the project was to find better ways to relate basic sciences and clinical nursing.

[1] Sand, Ole: Curriculum Study in Basic Nursing Education. New York, Putnam, 1955.

1

The basic sciences were considered to include the social and the natural sciences. The former were defined as psychology, sociology and anthropology. The natural sciences were defined as the biological sciences of anatomy, physiology (including biochemistry) and microbiology, as well as the physical sciences of chemistry and physics.

During the first three years of the study, primary emphasis was placed on the development of methods for (1) teaching students how to apply basic science knowledge in solving nursing problems, and (2) evaluating students' abilities to apply basic science knowledge in solving nursing problems. When the Commonwealth Fund extended its financial support for an additional two years, the emphasis of the investigation shifted to the critical problem of identifying the basic science content that is applicable to nursing.

Fundamental differences between the natural and the social sciences and their application to nursing influenced the methods of approach in identifying important science content. The methods used in the original study will be described briefly.

1

Methods Used in Original Study for Identification

The selection of methods amenable to the identification of science facts and principles important in nursing was somewhat problematic. The sheer bulk of natural science material alone, plus the wide variety of nursing practices dependent upon the application of natural science knowledge, presented a formidable barrier to the identification of specific facts and principles. The social sciences, although possessing a bulk of material, do not characteristically lend themselves to statements of science that can be directly applied. Much of social science knowledge is still in the stage of conceptualization and untested hypotheses. Nursing itself is not clearly defined, nor is nursing knowledge systematically organized; how then to pursue the task of identifying basic science content applicable to nursing?

NATURAL SCIENCES

Early in the study it was suggested that the science content generally taught to nursing students in the various science courses be examined in terms of possible applications to nursing. Although this was a feasible approach, it seemed that to work in exactly the opposite fashion might prove to be easier and somewhat more practical. By the "opposite fashion" is meant the examination of nursing itself to determine the related science content.

It was this latter approach that led to experimentation with the analysis of common nursing activities; such as, for example, measurement of blood pressure and catheterization. These procedures were examined in terms of facts from the natural sciences that when applied would result in procedures safely and effectively performed. Although these analyses proved useful for day-to-day teaching, this method was discontinued. The specific procedures represented a limited part of total nursing care, and the analyses completed showed—not surprisingly—too much repetition of some of the science content. For example, the fact that cleanliness inhibits the growth of microorganisms was repeated in each analysis.

At this point it was decided that a much broader view of nursing care should be considered in developing a methodology. It seemed that if the nursing care designed to meet expected physical and medical needs of patients with particular types of physiological problems were analyzed, the resulting science content would be more comprehensive and less repetitive. This method necessitated the development of nursing care plans for hypothetical patients with problems involving the different structures and functions of the body. Many faculty members contributed to the development of these care plans and the combining and condensing of the nursing care once identified. These activities proved to be highly valuable for teaching; however, when some of the completed sections of nursing care were analyzed for the related science content, the amount of science identified grew to such an extent that working with all the material in its interrelated and unorganized state was utterly impractical. It was obvious that some method of study had to be devised that could provide for organization of the science content. Surely, one way to provide some organization was to direct attention to one area of science at a time.

A review of the science already identified revealed that most of the science content came from anatomy and physiology. Moreover, it was notable that the statements concerned with physiology tended to fall into some broad categories—categories that involved such processes as blood circulation, fluid balance and nutrition. These two observations resulted in the use of the concept of physiological homeostasis as a basis for the determination of which content from anatomy and physiology is important in nursing. If the physical nursing care of patients is directed toward either the maintenance or the restoration of homeostasis, this concept should be an excellent organizing factor in the identification of basic science applicable to nursing.

Ten factors involved in the maintenance of a constant internal environment of an individual were identified. These included such things as oxygen, blood pressure, nutrition and electrolyte balance. Seven additional factors were then identified as being necessary for effective and independent functioning of the human organism (though not essential to homeostasis). These factors included locomotion, sensory processes and certain protective mechanisms.

After each of these factors had been identified and incorporated in a general statement that provided some indication of how this particular factor is important to the total functioning of the human organism, each factor was studied in terms of its embodiment of major facts from anatomy and physiology and the application of these facts in nursing. The process required two associated activities. Nursing care related to each of the factors had to be identified and then analyzed for related science content. Practically simultaneously, anatomy and physiology content related to the specific factor under consideration had to be reviewed and facts that seemed to be applicable to patient care had to be selected. One activity supplemented the other.

As the material was developed, no attempt was made to associate any specific science statements with any statements of specific nursing care. Instead, the material was prepared in sections; statements of nursing care related to each factor were made, and these were followed by selected facts from anatomy and physiology that were believed to underlie that nursing care. Because the human body is a whole functioning unit, the placement of the facts about structure and function into separate sections proved a difficult and perhaps impossible task. Repetition was purposely avoided, however, and this was achieved primarily through the use of many cross-references.

There were variations in the degree of specificity of the science statements. An attempt was made to keep the levels of the statements somewhat similar all the way through, but it seemed most important to state the science content in such a way that it could have meaning to a nurse and really serve as a guide to action. All the many details that are sometimes involved in a brief statement of scientific fact were not included, and, hopefully, generalizations were not made to the extent that nursing applications would be a puzzle or be so vague as to be of little practical use.

Elements of pathology were occasionally included along with the anatomy and physiology. The amount of pathology was kept to a minimum, but there were times when certain aspects of disease were important in the application of some of the content from physiology.

When each of the sections of nursing care and related science had been completed, the nursing care was reviewed and criticized by both a medical specialist and a committee of clinical nursing instructors. The science statements were reviewed and criticized by a physiologist. Changes were made as recommended by these people.

After the identification of the anatomy and physiology content had been completed, the nursing care was analyzed for the purpose of identifying any science aspects from the fields of physics and chemistry. Some of the chemistry identified, though not directly applicable in nursing, was thought to contribute to the intelligent application of some of the physiology content, and was thus included. Clinical nursing instructors and professors of chemistry and physics criticized the physics and chemistry statements, and changes were made as recommended. These statements were then added to each of the seventeen sections.

Nursing care concerned with the protection of patients from microbial injury provided the basis for the identification of important facts and principles from the field of microbiology. Again, nursing care was identified along with applicable science content. Clinical nursing instructors and a pathologist reviewed and criticized the nursing section, and a medical microbiologist criticized the science statements. Changes were made as recommended.

After the eighteen sections of nursing care and related science had been completed, the total material was given to a jury for evaluation. The jury was composed of six nurse educators in different parts of the United States who were known to have particular interest in one or more of the natural science areas. The jury members were asked to review and criticize all eighteen sections of nursing and science, and to evaluate the relatedness of the nursing and science in each. Their responses were used to reorganize, delete and correct the material.

THE SOCIAL SCIENCES

Since the social sciences are concerned with human behavior without respect to specific physiological illness, treatment, or nursing procedures, it did not seem expedient in the original study to analyze nursing care plans or nursing procedures to determine social science principles. Such plans and procedures are usually oriented toward physical care, toward maintaining physiological homeostasis, or toward the mechanics of carrying out a procedure. Any psychosocial aspects of care that might be appended to such plans or procedures would have had to be stated in broad, relatively meaningless terms, such as "provide reassurance" or "avoid embarrassment."

The possibility of analyzing social science texts, outlines or other reference material was also ruled out as a possible methodology. It would have been difficult to arrive at defensible criteria for the selection and/or ruling out of concepts and principles (as found in current textbooks) that would have particular relevance to nursing. It also would have been extremely difficult to develop a framework from which to review the diverse theories and approaches expounded in contemporary sociological literature. One finds a wide variety of theoretical approaches to man's individual and collective behavior, and not all theories are mutually compatible. This lack of agreement was especially crucial to the original study when choices had to be made regarding terminology. The problem of terminology is discussed later with particular reference to some of the concepts and principles included in Part III.

Eventually the author settled on an analysis of actual patient-nurse situations as a most profitable initial approach. Such a method could provide information about the kinds of psychosocial problems that patients actually encounter in the course of illness and hospitalization, irrespective of the presenting complaint, physiological illness or the resulting care and treatment. Material collected in this way also might help to circumvent one of the major complaints about the use of social science concepts in teaching nursing students—the difficulty in arriving at specific principles to guide the nurse's behavior.

With these considerations in mind, an adaptation of Flanagan's[2] "Critical Incident Technique" was chosen as the primary means of collecting source material for the original study. This method provided for the collection of descriptions of patient and nurse behavior in operationally defined critical situations. Critical incidents were defined as nurse-patient situations in which patients were either helped (a positive situation) or harmed (a negative situation) by some action of a nursing team member. The benefit or harm to the patient was described in terms of the patient's observable reaction to the situation.

Descriptions of nurse-patient situations were collected from nurses who were involved in giving patient care or in supervising patient care on medical, surgical and obstetrical[3] services of four large general hospitals. The nurses were asked to describe incidents in which they had recently been involved or which they had recently observed. These incidents then were analyzed in terms of the social science principles that seemed to be inherent in the situation. The collection and analysis of situations represented an attempt to arrive at some of the factors that influence the human being's psychosocial equilibrium while he is in a situation requiring nursing care.

The author was assisted in the process of screening and analyzing incidents by a group of faculty members from the University of Washington School of Nursing, who were representative of all clinical areas in nursing. Throughout the entire period of study, this committee functioned both as an informal jury to guide the decisions of the author and as a work group to analyze situations and formulate statements of principal. After preliminary work-up, the material was critically reviewed by two members of the University of Washington Department of Psychology.

The final draft of the material was submitted to a group of six additional social scientists for review. This group included one psychologist, two sociologists and three anthropologists. With the exception of the anthropologists, all of the reviewers had had some experience in the health science fields. They were asked to consider the principles and hypotheses from the standpoint of: (1) the truth of the statements, (2) the relevance of sub-statements to major statements, and (3) the relevance of the nursing section to the science sections. The responses of

2 Flanagan, John C.: The Critical Incident Technique. Psychological Bulletin, Vol. 51, No. 4, pp. 327-358, July 1954.

3 Since one of the hospitals did not have an obstetrical unit, material in this area was supplemented by a study using similar methods for the same purpose:
Rose, Patricia: The Identification of Psychiatric Principles Inherent in the Nursing Care of a Selected Group of Maternity Patients. (Unpublished Masters thesis. Univ. Washington, 1958.)

the reviewers were used to reorganize, delete and correct the material for publication.

Expansion of the Original Nursing and Science Sections

The original data and basic organizational pattern have been maintained in this revision. Additional sciences and nursing content have been added, using the original format as a guide. Consequently, neither the direction nor the intent of the original book has been changed. To provide for consistency in the presentation of the natural and the social science material, the sequence of science and nursing in the natural science section has been changed.

The science sections have been expanded by the addition of material abstracted from current science references, research data, and medical and nursing textbooks. The pathology has been increased and given a separate sub-section in each chapter of the natural sciences. The nursing sections have been expanded as possible nursing applications of the new science material were identified and added. Occasionally, as nursing applications were added, it became apparent that additional science background facts were involved. In these instances the pertinent and specific scientific facts were identified and inserted into the science section.

2

Suggestions for Students and Nurse Practitioners

SUMMARY OF THE NURSE'S ROLE

The two major areas of action of the professional nurse may be roughly defined as: (1) direct patient care, and (2) interaction with other health workers on behalf of the patient. Although the skills and abilities required for successful performance in both areas may overlap or be interdependent, it is still fruitful to examine them separately. The patient seeks assistance in solving his health problems because of some dysfunction that constitutes disequilibrium or a threat to the integrity of the very intricately balanced, interlocking systems that keep him functioning as a healthy individual within his particular environment. When the nurse becomes a part of the patient's means of problem-solving, certain kinds of skilled assistance are expected of her.

Provision for Normal Needs. When a patient is hospitalized, he surrenders to the hospital the responsibility for organizing environmental forces in such a way as to preserve normal function in areas not directly affected by his illness. Hopefully, he will not have to suffer total discontinuity in life style while temporary dysfunctions are being corrected, or while he is learning adaptations necessitated by permanent functional changes. For example, the agency in which the patient is in residence accepts responsibility for maintaining a comfortable environmental temperature; providing for normal nutritional and fluid balance needs; providing facilities to maintain cleanliness, safety and comfort; and promoting normal social interaction. Although responsibility is delegated to the institution as a whole, and departments are created to provide some of the necessary services (e.g., housekeeping and dietary departments), it is the nurse, in direct contact with the patient 24 hours a day, who observes, supervises and manipulates this environment to the best interests of the individual patient. To continue with the previous example, the nurse observes and regulates the physical environment of the room; transfers from doctor to dietary department the order for a

9

"regular diet," and supervises the distribution and intake of food and fluid; she supervises or participates in cleanliness and comfort procedures; she regulates social interaction; facilitates continuity of the patient's religious practices, and so forth. Except in unusual circumstances it is not necessary for the doctor to "order" nursing care of the variety described above. Such activities constitute the bulk of nursing services routinely offered to patients, with the unwritten assumption that they are nursing responsibilities.

Provision for Therapeutic Needs. Above and beyond continuity of normal practices, the patient has special needs occasioned by his illness. In this area, his doctor is immediately responsible for the diagnosis of problems and the orders for therapeutic procedures. But again, it is the responsibility of the nursing service to see that therapeutic procedures are effectively integrated into the total plan of care. This may mean that the nurse, under doctor's orders, manipulates special temperature-regulating and humidifying equipment because of the patient's problem with regulation of body temperature; she may, under doctor's orders, carry out special nutritional and fluid balance procedures such as gavage feeding or intravenous therapy; she may have to carry out or supervise adaptations of normal cleanliness and comfort procedures to adjust for immobility; she may have to engage in special interpersonal techniques if psychological disequilibrium is severe, and so forth. Regardless of the patient's particular health problem, the nurse must concern herself with the totality of care—the integration of care to meet both normal and therapeutic needs. It is assumed that the nurse has the intelligence and preparation to function without specifically written orders from a doctor regarding just how to go about bathing a patient with painful arthritis, just how to prevent skin breakdown of a comatose patient, or just what psychological techniques to employ when the doctor is difficult to work with.

Interaction With Others: Planning and Coordination. In all of the examples given, the nurse may take direct action herself or she may serve as a leader in nursing care programming. With the increasing demand for nursing services of both an in- and out-patient nature, she is more likely to serve as a supervisor, teacher and coordinator of a corps of auxiliary nursing personnel. Inescapably, she is required to coordinate the activities of nursing personnel and personnel from other departments in the hospital. In the future there will be an enormous increase in the cooperative contacts between nurses and community health agencies.

In all of these health personnel interactions, the nurse's attention must be directed toward maintaining the health of a social environment set up specifically with patient care as its goal. She assumes "wellness" on the part of health co-workers and is concerned primarily with knowing how to keep the environment functioning at optimal levels. Skills involved in this aspect of nursing are associated with such areas as communication, teaching and learning, leader and team interactions, counselling, guidance and motivation, group problem solving and change agent functions.

No matter what the specific nursing intervention required, the nurse cannot function as a consistently effective member of the health team unless her decisions for action are based on sound scientific knowledge of human physiological and psychosocial function. No matter how creative a problem solver she might potentially be, her solutions will be only as good as the mental data she has at her command to apply to practical situations.

PRACTICAL APPLICATIONS OF SCIENCE CONTENT AND NURSING APPLICATIONS

The material in this book was not meant to be used as a substitute "short course" for fullscale study of basic sciences. The professional nurse needs to study the sciences in depth and scope *before* she can organize and systematically use selected science concepts. Without such study, material as organized and presented here may be only vague and half-understood, therefore not maximally usable in immediate, acute and practical situations. For example, a conceptual statement such as "perception of a situation is unique to each individual in the situation," summarizes literally volumes of supporting evidence and detailed subconcepts or principles. The nurse does not need to have at her mental fingertips all of the supporting evidence from scientific studies, nor all the detailed sub-statements that construct or illuminate a concept—her full comprehension of the summarizing statement and its implications for nursing are limited without the initial encounter with such data that is obtained in collegiate basic science courses. If this book is not a capsule course in basic sciences, how can the nursing student and the graduate practicing nurse use the material to best advantage?

Organization of Knowledge. Perhaps one of the most useful functions of the material in Parts II and III is as a guide to the organization of knowledge from basic science and nursing courses. In the example of perception used previously, reference was made to the bulk of material studied in order to fully understand a given concept. Since not all of the reading and experimentation the student goes through is necessarily pertinent to nursing action, the individual student must find a way to summarize related material, to cull out the pragmatically important from supporting or incidental data. Rote memorization of all the facts one encounters is sheer intellectual waste.

Unless the student is already provided with a study guide for the organization of learning, she may find this book helpful for that purpose. Taking anatomy and physiology as an example, while the student is studying the circulatory system, she can use the sections in Part II relative to circulating blood and oxygen supply as guides in selecting areas for concentrated study, and as summarizing statements of detailed course learning. In addition, she may find that her particular instructor and text books place insufficient emphasis on given units of study that she, the student, knows will be important to her as a nurse. She can use the information from this book to guide independent study to a greater depth in those neglected areas.

Transfer of Theory to Practice. Basic science courses are seldom taught concurrent with nursing courses that require the application of the particular science being studied. At best, correlation of science and nursing courses is imperfect. Unless a science instructor is teaching a course for nurses only, he makes no special effort to point out nursing applications of science data. Nursing instructors, on the other hand, often base their teaching on an assumption that the student will *recall* science concepts and principles when presented with nursing situations where they are applicable. Any student is well aware that recall of pertinent science data is not nearly so automatic and instantaneous as might be desired!

The method of organization of basic science and nursing applications in Parts II and III can be helpful to students in the transfer of knowledge in both basic science and nursing courses. Review of nursing applications, even if the student is not yet far along in the clinical field, can provide examples of nursing applications that will make science more meaningful and therefore more easily learned. Continuing with the example of the circulatory system—if the student reviews nursing actions concerning blood pressure, she is more likely to be motivated toward the development of an understanding of physiology related to the pressure of circulating blood. Later, when she is assigned to patients with circulatory problems, she can review both the science and the nursing applications as a basis for progression of learning in nursing theory and practice.

Review and Re-learning. In a sense, review of past learning is not separate from the two previous examples of possible uses for this book. Review and re-learning does deserve some special note, however, for the graduate who has been away from nursing for some time and for the nurse who has been working in one specialized area of practice and is transferring to another. Nurses who find themselves in these situations may use the science and nursing application sections either as straight review material or as a guide to help them determine particular basic science areas in which they need more extensive study. It may be, for example, that a nurse who has been away from bedside practice for some years discovers while reviewing that there are some serious gaps in her original learning; or that developments in science and nursing practice since she was a student indicate a need for special references or for particular learning experiences. She can then, unless educational opportunities are readily available, set up a self-directed learning program.

Evaluation of Nursing Care. The authors would particularly like to see students and graduates use the science and nursing application sections for evaluation of individual nursing care plans. This does not mean that the nurse should sit down with the book every time she writes a care plan! It does mean that once the reader is familiar with format and content, she can direct her thinking about patient needs in an organized manner. It does mean that she can look at care plans with a full awareness of what is meant by totality of care, and that she can check her plans to see if she has given full consideration to all aspects of that care. It means, for example, that if her plan includes teaching a patient some aspect of self-care, she can review the material on learning to be sure her plans are well formulated and consistent with the dynamics of human learning. It also means that if she is responsible for the supervision and teaching of auxiliary personnel in the use of body mechanics, she can review both the sections on learning and body mechanics in order to evaluate her own knowledge as well as her supervisory and teaching behavior. In addition, it means that she has a ready reference for checking out the validity of ideas and care plans when she is in doubt about their scientific soundness.

One of the most common uses of material in the first edition was as a reference for students in the writing of care plan analyses. These analyses required the student to state scientific principles that justified or led to the nursing intervention planned for the patient. Although the graduate has not time for such lengthy written plans, she *must* have the science in mind and be able to verbalize it when necessary to guide the work of auxiliary personnel.

Development of a Way of Thinking. Hopefully, nurses of the present and the future, with their increased store of background knowledge, will not be poor human counterparts of data-processing computers. With all of their awe-inspiring and labor-saving characteristics, computers still are capable of only one thing—a reliable, accurate and predictable response when the right buttons are pushed. They are not capable of original thinking—of devising unique applications of old and new scientific data to changing and increasingly complex nursing care problems. No human being can hope to compete with a machine when it comes to storing information, any more than this book can contain all of the scientific information a nurse will need for planning and implementing patient care. But it is hoped that the material the book does contain, together with the format in which it is presented, will foster habits of analytical thinking. The nurse, whether a student or a graduate, can help develop nursing care of the future if she learns to approach every patient care problem with such questions as:

(1) What does the patient require to maintain optimal function?
(2) What do we know about human structure and function that will help determine what he needs and how we can help him?

(3) What scientific reason do we have for continuing this particular nursing practice?

(4) Is there a better way, scientifically based, for solving this problem?

In short, she can use computers to her own ends rather than becoming a human part of a computer system. The nurse of the future must be able to outgrow this or any text as she develops her own thinking processes in the solution of patient care problems.

Part II

Natural Sciences and Nursing Applications

INTRODUCTION

Part II is divided into 20 chapters. Each chapter contains science sections and a nursing section. Chapters 1 through 10 are concerned with essentials of homeostasis; Chapter 11, with locomotion; Chapters 12 through 15, with protective structures and functions; Chapters 16 through 18, with sensory processes, mental processes and speech; Chapter 19, with reproductive functions, and Chapter 20, with prevention of microbial injury. All of the chapters have been written in outline form because this seems to provide the clearest presentation of extensive material.

All chapters (with the exception of Chap. 20) are presented in the same sequence. Each science section is preceded by a general statement which pertains to the particular structures, functions or requirements of the human organism being considered in that chapter. This is followed by statements of scientific facts and principles from anatomy and physiology (combined), pathology, physics and chemistry. The nursing sections following contain statements of nursing care that are based upon the preceding science. The nursing care is related to: (1) observation of patients, (2) maintenance of normal structure and function or protection from injury, and (3) meeting specific or general needs of patients who have problems that affect the particular structures, functions or requirements included in that chapter.

In the original study, pathology was not considered to be one of the basic "natural" sciences. However, as pointed out in the Introduction in Part I, elements of pathology had been included in the original science data when they seemed to be particularly relevant. Lists of observable signs and symptoms associated with physiologic dysfunctions had been included in the nursing sections. In this edition pathology has been included as a basic science that has applications for nursing. The elements of pathology in the original study have been retained and more pathology has been added. The two major sources of reference used in the development of the pathology content were Hopp's

Principles of Pathology,[1] and *Signs and Symptoms*, edited by Cyril Mitchell MacBryde.[2]

The addition of pathology not only increased the amount of science in each chapter, but also resulted in (1) additions to the original anatomy and physiology content as more facts pertaining to normal structure and function were found to be related to the pathology, and (2) additions to the nursing content as applications of the pathology were identified. Although the anatomy and physiology has remained very similar to the original data, the nursing sections have been reorganized and rewritten. Many nursing textbooks (fundamentals of nursing, medical-surgical nursing, geriatric nursing, pediatric nursing and maternity nursing) were found to be helpful in identifying: possible nursing applications of the science data, factually based nursing care, and principles from the natural sciences.

The nursing applications are both general and specific. In many instances the general nursing measures are followed by examples of specific nursing actions that can be taken to achieve the primary objective of the more generally stated nursing measure. When generalizations are made regarding kinds of dysfunctions having implications for nursing, they are usually followed by examples of specific disease conditions in which the particular dysfunctions are likely to occur.

We recognize that it is essential that all nursing measures comply with existing medical orders. Occasionally special attention is called to the fact that a particular nursing measure should be taken within medical orders only, or that a particular nursing measure should (or may) be taken only *until* medical orders are available. In some cases attention is called to the importance of following medical orders exactly. This is not meant to imply that medical orders should not be followed exactly at all times. What this *does* imply is that in these specific situations it is extremely important that everyone, including the patient, understand that there are no exceptions or extenuating circumstances—the medical orders are to be followed *exactly*. Examples of such situations include the administration of insulin to a diabetic patient, the control of fluid and usually salt intake when a patient has edema, or the limitations of physical activity when a patient has problems involving the internal structures of the eye.

A few comments must be made about observation of signs and symptoms. Many observable signs and symptoms are listed in the pathology section of each unit. It is doubtful that a nurse would be expected to be aware continually of all the signs and symptoms mentioned; this is especially true if the signs and symptoms are subtle.

---

[1] Hopps, Howard C.: Principles of Pathology, ed. 2. New York, Appleton-Century-Crofts, 1965.

[2] MacBryde, Cyril M. (ed.): Signs and Symptoms, ed. 4. Philadelphia, Lippincott, 1964.

However, the more intelligent observations a nurse is able to make, the more assistance she can be to patients and to physicians. Although the nurse is not called upon to evaluate her observations for the purpose of diagnosing disease conditions, she can use her observations to diagnose patient needs that she may well be able to meet with nursing measures. The nurse's knowledge of important signs and symptoms in relation to specific physiologic dysfunctions enables her to recognize those signs and symptoms that have particular significance for the physician, and that should be reported either immediately or within a short period of time. In emergency situations the nurse's observations and her prompt reactions to those observations may be critical.

The science section of Chapter 20 is devoted almost entirely to microbiology. The science content included is sometimes quite general and sometimes very specific; the nursing applications have been kept at a fairly general level. Specific facts about some of the microorganisms that cause disease in man were included because they have direct application in nursing. For example, precautions taken to prevent the spread of infectious diseases depend upon the characteristics of the microorganisms involved, how they gain entrance into the body and how they are able to leave the body. Many more pathogenic microorganisms might have been included in this section, but it is hoped that the ones that have been included are fairly representative. A few of the helminths have been considered briefly; although the adult worms are not microscopic in size, their eggs and some of their other forms are.

In conclusion, it should be understood by persons using the material in Part II that the science and related nursing information has been purposely developed in units. The particular chapters have been found to be useful for the analytic study of extensive scientific and nursing knowledge and for the elimination of repetition and duplication. It is important to remember that the chapters are interrelated, and that the nursing applications contained in each are almost exclusively applications of the science material in that chapter. Cross-references have been made in many instances when nursing or science in one chapter has particular relevance in another.

1

Volume and Pressure of Circulating Blood

The blood is a means of transport for substances to and from the cells, and the volume and pressure of circulating blood must be maintained within certain limits to provide for the changing demands of organs.

ANATOMY AND PHYSIOLOGY

Cardiovascular System

1. The cardiovascular system is composed of the heart and blood vessels. Blood is pumped from the ventricles of the heart into the major arteries, from which it is forced into smaller and smaller arteries, then into arterioles, and finally into capillaries where exchanges of substances (e.g., nutrients, gases, catabolites) take place. From the capillaries the blood passes into venules, then to larger and larger veins, and finally back to the atria of the heart.

2. The right side of the heart receives deoxygenated blood from the systemic circulation and pumps it into the pulmonary circulation. The left side of the heart receives oxygenated blood from the pulmonary system and pumps it into the systemic circulation.

3. The major artery coming from the left ventricle is the aorta, which passes down through the thorax and the abdominal cavity before bifurcating.

4. The walls of the arteries and arterioles contain varying amounts of smooth muscle. The larger arteries contain considerable elastic tissue. In the aging process there are varying degenerative changes in the blood vessels, including loss of elastic tissue.

5. Arteries lying over bone or firm tissue that are usually palpable include:

   A. The internal maxillary artery, in front of and slightly below the ear.

18

    B. The superficial temporal artery, in the temple region.

    C. The subclavian artery, behind the inner end of the clavicle against the first rib.

    D. The external carotid artery in the neck.

    E. The facial artery, about an inch forward of the angle of the jaw.

    F. The brachial artery, on the inner aspect of the upper arm, about halfway between the shoulder and the elbow.

    G. The radial artery which passes down the radial side of the front of the forearm.

    H. The femoral artery, in the mid-groin.

    I. The popliteal artery behind the knee.

    J. The dorsalis pedis artery, below the ankle on the dorsum of the foot.

6. The small blood vessels in the uterus are arranged between the smooth muscle fibers in such a way that the uterine muscle contractions can partially occlude these blood vessels.

    A. Smooth muscle of the uterus normally contracts with mechanical stimulation (e.g., massage of the fundus).

    B. Inteference with uterine contractions may be caused by the upward pressure against the uterus from a full urinary bladder.

7. Blood is drained from the brain through large venous sinuses, which also drain blood from the scalp, the face and the mastoid region.

8. Many of the body organs have relatively large blood supplies or storage spaces for blood. These organs include the spleen, the liver, the pregnant and postpartum uterus, the kidneys, the lungs, the muscles, and the skin.

9. Veins have thinner walls than arteries; their walls have little elastic or muscle tissue. Many of the veins in the lower extremities have valves which normally prevent the backflow of blood.

10. The heart muscle receives blood primarily through the coronary blood vessels, which comprise a complex and anastomotic system having an extraordinarily rich capillary network.

Blood Volume

1. The cardiovascular system is a closed system, and blood is not usually found outside of the system except as it is found in the uterus related to reproductive functions.

    A. Approximately 2 to 8 oz. of venous blood, mixed with mucus and endometrial tissue, are lost during a normal menstrual period. (Normally, menstrual blood does not clot.)

    B. For its life, a fetus depends upon the blood of the mother circulating through the placenta.

    C. Labor may be accompanied by a loss of blood-tinged mucus from the cervix.

D. A loss of more than 500 cc. of blood during delivery is above normal.

E. Following delivery there is a flow of uterine discharge from the vagina which may last 1 to 6 weeks. (The flow is similar to a heavy menstrual period with the discharge changing from bloody to serous to mucous.)

F. Following delivery involution of the uterus occurs.

    (1) The fundus of the uterus should be firm and well below the umbilicus immediately after delivery.

    (2) The fundus of the uterus normally returns into the pelvis at a rate of approximately one-half inch a day, starting about the level of the umbilicus the first postpartum day.

2. Blood volume varies with body weight and surface area. It is estimated to be about 3 L./sq. m. of body surface.

A. In infants and children the blood volume is somewhat less per kilogram of body weight and per square meter of body surface than in adults.

B. The average-sized adult has about 5 to 6 L. of blood.

C. The rapid loss of more than 30 per cent of the total blood volume is usually incompatible with life.

3. Blood volume may be affected by variations in fluid balance within the body. (See Chap. 4.)

4. Agglutination and/or hemolysis of red blood cells may occur as a result of mixing incompatible blood groups.

A. This involves a type of antigen-antibody reaction; the antigen is in the red blood cells and the antibody is in the serum.

B. In transfusions, a recipient's serum can agglutinate the donor's cells.

    (1) Type A blood agglutinates the cells of both Type B and Type AB.

    (2) Type B blood agglutinates the cells of both Type A and Type AB.

    (3) Type AB blood does not agglutinate cells of any other type of blood because there is no antibody in the serum.

    (4) Type O blood is not agglutinated by any other type of blood because there is no antigen in the blood cells.

5. The color of the skin and of the mucous membrane is affected by the amount and the kind of blood in the superficial blood vessels (e.g., pale, flushed, cyanotic).

6. Capillary bleeding is slow and oozing. Arterial bleeding is rapid and may come in spurts, and the blood is bright red. Venous bleeding is slow and steady, and the blood is a dark red.

7. The body's defences against exsanguination include:

A. Contraction of small blood vessels.

B. Formation of a primary clot (thrombus).

C. Organization of the thrombus by fibrous consolidation.

D. Decreased blood pressure.

Blood Clotting

1. The normal blood clotting mechanism helps to protect the body against blood loss. Essentially, injured thrombocytes and tissues release chemical substances which react with globulin factors in the plasma (in the presence of calcium ions) to produce thromboplastin. Thromboplastin allows prothrombin to become thrombin. The thrombin reacts with the fibrinogen in the serum to produce fibrin, which forms the network of the clot.

   A. Prothrombin and fibrinogen are produced in the liver. (Vitamin K, a fat-soluble vitamin produced by microbial action on certain kinds of food in the intestinal tract, is needed for the production of prothrombin.)

   B. The disintegration of blood platelets is a prerequisite for the production of thromboplastin.

      (1) The average platelet (thrombocyte) count is about 250,000/cu. mm. of blood.

      (2) Clots formed in blood deficient in platelets are soft and friable and do not retract normally.

      (3) Platelets form a mechanical barrier to the escape of blood in very small blood vessels.

2. Blood, after it is shed, normally clots within 3 to 5 minutes *(clotting time)*.

3. Bleeding from punctured skin capillaries normally ceases within 2 minutes *(bleeding time)*.

4. *Prothrombin time* measures the activity of prothrombin in the blood. The normal prothrombin time is 14 to 18 seconds (Quick Test). If the time is prolonged beyond 30 seconds there is a bleeding tendency.

Blood Pressure

1. Arterial blood pressure can be defined as the amount of pressure exerted by the blood against the walls of the arterial blood vessels.

2. Arterial blood pressure varies with:

   A. The stroke-volume of the ventricular contractions.

      (1) The greater the force, the higher the pressure.

      (2) The greater the volume, the higher the pressure.

   B. The caliber of the arterioles. (The smaller the caliber, the higher the pressure.)

   C. The elasticity of the blood vessel walls. (The more rigid the walls, the higher the pressure.)

   D. The viscosity of the blood.

      (1) The greater the viscosity, the higher the pressure.

(2) Blood is about 5 times more viscous than water.

3. Arterial blood pressure can be measured by equalizing external pressure applied against an artery with the pressure within the artery.

A. Systolic pressure is the pressure at the time of ventricular systole.

(1) The systolic measurement affords information about the cardiac output and the state of the peripheral blood vessels.

(2) Taken in the brachial artery, the average range (at rest) for an infant is 55 to 80 mm./Hg., and the average range for an adult is 90 to 145 mm./Hg.

B. Diastolic blood pressure is the pressure at the time of ventricular diastole.

(1) The diastolic measurement affords information about the basic pressure in the circulatory system.

(2) Taken in the brachial artery, the average range (at rest) for an infant is 40 to 50 mm./Hg., and the average range for an adult is 60 to 90 mm./Hg.

C. Arterial blood pressure can be determined in any extremity where a blood pressure cuff can be applied closely above a point where a pulse can be felt.

D. The blood pressures in opposite extremities may vary.

E. Visible strong pulsations of the carotid arteries indicate a high systolic pressure.

4. The pulse is the resultant throb in an artery caused by the rise and fall of the arterial pressure as the left ventricle contracts.

A. The pulse can be felt wherever a superficial artery can be held against firm tissue.

B. The strength of a pulse varies with the amount of systolic discharge and the elasticity of the arterial wall.

5. The pulse pressure is the difference between the systolic and the diastolic pressures.

A. The pulse pressure varies directly with the amount of blood ejected by the systolic discharges.

B. The average range of pulse pressure is 30 to 50 mm./Hg.

6. Postural changes affect arterial blood pressure.

A. A sudden change from a lying position to a sitting or a standing position can result in a sudden decrease in the supply of blood to the brain.

B. There is an immediate rise in blood pressure when the position is changed from lying to sitting to standing.

7. Strenuous physical exercise (or contemplation of it) has the greatest of all physiological effects in raising the blood pressure.

8. The amount of blood pumped from the ventricles into the arteries is determined by:

A. The stroke-volume of the ventricular contractions.

B. The integrity of the atrioventricular valves.

C. The patency of the semilunar valves.

9. The amount of blood that reaches the ventricular chambers is determined by:

A. The patency of the atrioventricular valves.

B. The amount of venous return.

(1) Venous return is determined, in part, by the rate of cardiac contraction—i.e., the more rapid the contractions, the less the venous return.

(2) Venous return from the pulmonary circulation varies with the rate of blood flow through the pulmonary circuit and with the volume and pressure of blood in the left ventricle.

(3) Venous return from the systemic circulation varies directly with the gravitational force, the arterial blood pressure and the movement of the voluntary muscles; it varies inversely with the intrathoracic and intra-abdominal pressures.

10. The work of the heart depends chiefly upon the amount of blood ejected per minute against the average pressure in the systemic and pulmonary circulation.

A. The force of cardiac muscle contractions varies directly with the degree to which the ventricular chambers are filled with blood. (A rapid increase in the circulating blood volume markedly increases the work load of the heart.)

B. The greater the blood pressure in the periphery and/or in the lungs, the greater the force required by ventricular contractions to maintain an adequate blood flow. (A rise in the intra-abdominal pressure against the great vessels increases the systemic blood pressure, and the work load of the heart is increased.)

C. The work load of the heart is increased when blood must be pumped against the force of gravity.

D. Cardiac output is increased when there is an increased need for oxygen.

E. Cardiac output is increased when body tissues require an increased amount of circulation (e.g., when skeletal muscles are exercised, or when an injury has been sustained).

11. In general, the heart rate bears an inverse relationship to:

A. The size of the individual (e.g., the average rate for the newborn is 130 to 140 beats per minute, while the average rate for an adult at rest is 70 to 80 beats per minute).

B. The blood pressure.

12. In general, the heart rate bears a direct relationship to the metabolic rate (e.g., an increased heart rate occurs during muscular exercise, during digestion, in hyperthyroidism and in fever).

13. The heart rate may be accelerated or depressed by:
    A. Neural mechanisms.
       (1) The cardiac accelerator center is located in the medulla, and operates through the thoracolumbar division of the autonomic nervous system.
       (2) The cardiac inhibitor center is located in the medulla; the vagus nerves carry inhibitory impulses to the sinoatrial node and the sinoventricular node.
    B. Hormonal influence.
       (1) Epinephrine causes an increased heart rate.
14. The coordination of sequence in heart action rhythmicity is a function of the conduction system. The conduction system lies within the cardiac muscle. It is composed of nodes and bundles which are primarily specialized muscle tissue. This specialized tissue transmits electrical impulses which cause contraction of the cardiac musculature.
15. The apical heartbeat can be heard best at the fifth intercostal space, slightly to the left of the sternum. There are two sounds: the first is caused by the closing of the atrioventricular valves; the second, by the closing of the semilunar valves.
16. The heartbeats of a fetus can generally be heard by the fifth month of pregnancy. The average rate of heartbeats is 120 to 160 beats per minute.
17. The walls of the arterioles contain smooth muscle under autonomic nervous control.
    A. The vasomotor centers are located in the medulla oblongata.
    B. Vasoconstriction results from sympathetic stimulation.
    C. Vasodilatation results from the inhibition of sympathetic stimulation.
18. Blood pressure is greatly affected by the emotional state of an individual through the relationship between the emotions and the autonomic nervous system.
19. Local vasodilatation may be caused by:
    A. The local application of heat.
    B. A limited application of cold.
    C. Localized tissue injury.
    D. The application of counterirritant substances (e.g., mustard).
    E. Histamine or histaminelike substances.
20. Generalized vasodilatation may be caused by:
    A. The failure of the vasomotor centers to function properly (e.g., due to an inadequate blood supply to the brain).
    B. The stimulation of the vasomotor centers by such factors as an increased internal temperature or certain chemical substances (e.g., histamine).

21. Local vasoconstriction may be caused by:
    A. The prolonged application of cold.
    B. Certain reflex mechanisms (e.g., vasoconstriction of nasal and pharyngeal mucosal vessels when cold air is directed at the back or the arms).
22. Generalized vasoconstriction may be caused by:
    A. A pressor principle called angiotonin (or hypertensin), which may be produced in the body as an indirect result of impaired kidney circulation.
    B. Nor-epinephrine.
23. The cerebrospinal and intraocular fluids, formed from the blood, are absorbed continuously into the venous system. Because there is a close relationship between the blood pressure and the pressure of fluids in other closed fluid systems connected with the cardiovascular system, sudden blood pressure changes are reflected in the pressures of the cerebrospinal fluid and the intraocular fluids.
24. When the circulatory rate is slowed beyond certain limits:
    A. The veins may become engorged with blood containing reduced hemoglobin.
    B. The walls of the veins may become weakened, with resultant varicosities.
    C. The valves in the veins may become incompetent.
    D. Edema may result.
25. A reduced arterial blood pressure resulting in reduced renal flow causes decreased glomerular filtration in the kidneys. A systolic pressure of more than 50 mm./Hg. is needed for glomerular filtration.

General Circulation

1. The horizontal body position provides the most effective systemic circulation with the least demands upon the cardiovascular system.
2. A decrease in the volume and the pressure of circulating blood in any tissue results in the decreased functioning of that tissue.
3. Under normal conditions the blood supply to specific tissues is increased when:
    A. There is an increase in the functioning of the tissues (e.g., the contractions of skeletal muscles during exercise causes an increase in the blood supply to the muscles involved).
    B. There is tissue injury. (See Chap. 14.)
    C. Heat is applied to the tissues.
4. Inadequate circulation to peripheral nerves causes tingling and burning sensations, and eventually loss of sensation.
5. Inadequate circulation to muscle tissue results in severe pain.

6. Following a localized injury to the body there is a brief local vaso-constriction followed by an active hyperemia; this in turn is followed by decreased blood flow to the affected part.

PHYSICS

1. Gravity is the force of attraction between two objects (e.g., the earth and an object on or near the earth).
2. The law of gravitation states that any two objects in the universe are attracted to each other with a force that is proportional to the product of their masses and inversely proportional to the square of the distance between them.
3. Weight is the attraction of the body by the earth.
4. Energy is the capacity for performing work—the moving of a mass of matter through space. The amount of energy required to move mass is dependent upon the resistance offered by opposing forces (e.g., weight of object, gravity, friction, atmospheric pressure).
5. Pressure is the force exerted on a unit area.
6. Liquids at rest exert pressure. The pressure exerted by a column of liquid in a container is equal to the height of the liquid times its weight per unit volume.
7. Fluids flow from an area of higher pressure to one of lower pressure and the rate of volume flow is directly related to the pressure gradient.
8. Viscosity (fluid friction) is the internal resistance of fluid in motion and retards flow.
9. Gases are relatively insoluble in liquids unless the temperature is decreased and/or the pressure is increased.

CHEMISTRY

1. Immiscible liquids are ones that will not dissolve in one another (e.g., oil and water).
2. Plaster of Paris powder combines with water to form a solid mass of large crystals of gypsum, which occupy a larger volume than the original powder and water.
3. Some plastic materials used in making casts shrink as they dry.
4. Hemoglobin is a conjugated protein made up of heme, the red pigment, and globin, a protein. Heme contains iron.
   A. Oxyhemoglobin is scarlet in color. Reduced hemoglobin is a darkish purple color.
   B. When hemoglobin undergoes chemical breakdown different colored pigments are formed, depending upon the extent of oxidation and reduction processes (e.g., red, green, brown, yellow).
   C. When hemoglobin undergoes chemical digestion, the heme portion forms a black pigment.

PATHOLOGY

Signs and Symptoms

Signs and symptoms of problems that may be related to the volume and pressure of circulating blood include:

1. Bleeding.
   A. Observable bleeding (except as associated with normal female reproductive functions).
      This includes bleeding:
      (1) From skin or mucous membrane (e.g., due to a surgical wound or a traumatic injury). Careful observations must be made under the patient, under clothing, around dressings or casts, and so forth.
      (2) Into skin or mucous membrane (e.g., petechiae, ecchymosis, hematomas, purpura).
      (3) From any body opening (e.g., epistaxis, hematemesis, hemoptysis, or from auditory canal, anus, vagina, urinary meatus).
         (a) Bleeding from the gastrointestinal tract may be observed as gross blood or as digested blood (coffee-ground vomitus or melena).
         (b) Vaginal bleeding (including blood clots) during pregnancy and during the postpartum period is abnormal.
         (c) Excessive bleeding during delivery is abnormal.
      (4) In any body fluids that are eliminated normally or drained artificially (e.g., in respiratory secretion, in urine, in gastric drainage).
   B. Internal bleeding (which may lead to hemorrhagic shock). This includes:
      (1) Abnormally low blood pressure or a progressive drop in blood pressure.
      (2) Weak, rapid pulse, or no pulse.
      (3) Pale, cold, clammy skin with cyanosis around lips and nail beds.
      (4) Thirst.
      (5) Oliguria or anuria.
      (6) Inappropriate fatigue.
      (7) Behavioral changes (e.g., apprehensiveness, excessive irritability, apathy, restlessness, confusion). Apprehensiveness may be indicated by a tense, anxious facial expression, excessive or restricted verbal communication, inability to concentrate, increasing blood pressure, pulse and respirations, general muscular tension, diarrhea, frequency of urination, headache, gastric distress, muscular tremors, dryness of mouth.

(8) Dizziness, visual blurring, tinnitus, loss of consciousness.
C. Nonobservable bleeding within specific body parts. This includes:
  (1) Hemarthrosis—painful, tender, swollen and hot joints.
  (2) Intramuscular bleeding—painful, tender, swollen and hot muscles.
  (3) Intrapleural bleeding—dyspnea and painful respiration, splinting of chest wall, changes in heart action.
  (4) Bleeding into the respiratory tract—dyspnea, choking, wet "gurgling" cough, cyanosis, frequent swallowing, apnea.
  (5) Intraperitoneal or retroperitoneal bleeding—discomfort, distention, rigidity of abdominal musculature.
  (6) Bleeding into the gastrointestinal tract—frequent and possibly difficult swallowing, discomfort and distention of section involved.
  (7) Bleeding into uterus (postpartum)—a soft, boggy uterus which can be palpated high in abdominal cavity.
  (8) Bleeding into cranial cavity—behavioral changes; loss of consciousness; neuromuscular disturbances; marked changes in vasomotor mechanisms, heart action, breathing, body temperature; blurring of vision; tinnitus.
2. Abnormally high or low blood pressure.
3. Abnormal pulse rhythm, rate or character, or an apical-radial pulse differential.
4. Discomfort.
  A. Substernal pain—may be a dull ache, a feeling of pressure, or acute, sharp and severe pain.
  B. Pain in either shoulder, radiating down the arms.
  C. Pounding heart, palpitations, feelings of breathlessness.
  D. Claudication, numbing, tingling in extremities, cramping of leg muscles (particularly at night following day's activities).
  E. Feeling of heaviness in lower extremities, especially at end of day or after standing still for period of time.
  F. Feeling of cramping and pressure in lower abdomen and back at onset of menstruation.
  G. General abdominal discomfort, possibly similar to indigestion.
5. Dyspnea, orthopnea, moist cough, change in character of breathing.
6. Changes in skin color (e.g., red, pale, mottled, cyanotic).
7. Changes in skin temperature (cold or hot).
8. Hypothermia or hyperthermia.
9. Behavioral changes (e.g., apathy, excessive irritability, appehension, confusion, disorientation, loss of memory).
10. Loss of consciousness.
11. Swelling of feet or ankles.

12. Large, tortuous, engorged veins (e.g., in neck or lower extremities).
13. Signs and symptoms associated with anaphylactic shock:
    A. Local edema in which contact with the allergen was made.
    B. Itching, sneezing, prickling feelings in throat.
    C. Generalized edema.
    D. Cyanosis, choking, wheezing, dyspnea.
    E. Weak, rapid pulse.
    F. Falling blood pressure.
    G. Convulsions.

Hemorrhage

1. Hemorrhage is the escape of blood from the vascular system.
   A. It may be internal or external.
   B. It may be classified according to site.
   C. It may be classified according to structure.
      (1) Petechiae are small, punctated hemorrhages.
      (2) An ecchymosis is larger and more diffuse (e.g., a bruise).
      (3) Purpura is a condition in which petechiae and ecchymoses are so extensive they become confluent.
      (4) A hematoma is a discreet, localized hemorrhage within tissue.
   D. It may be classified as due to a break in continuity or to diapedesis (an oozing through damaged capillaries).
2. Conditions that affect blood vessels and may cause hemorrhage include:
   A. Trauma.
      (1) The continuity of blood vessels may be destroyed directly by outside force or indirectly by bone splinters.
      (2) A blow to the skull can cause hemorrhage within the cranial cavity. This can affect the blood supply to the brain directly, or it can result in increasing intracranial pressure which causes abnormalities in brain function. The symptoms produced depend upon the location of the pressure and how rapid the accumulation of blood is.
   B. Chemical erosion (e.g., in gastric ulcer).
   C. An aneurysm, a sac-like dilatation due to structural weakness of the walls of a blood vessel, may rupture with undue strain or stress (frequently seen in the aorta).
   D. Arteriosclerosis can weaken the walls of a blood vessel so that it will rupture.
   E. Occlusion of an artery, resulting in infarction, injures blood vessels.
   F. Hypoxia causes capillary hemorrhages (frequently observed in newborn).
   G. Capillary fragility can result from a deficiency in the vitamin C complex.

3. Conditions that affect blood constituents and may cause hemorrhage include:
   A. Hemophilia, an hereditary, sex-linked disease in which there is prolonged clotting time.
   B. Thrombocytopenic purpura, a condition in which there is spontaneous hemorrhaging into the skin and mucous membranes. The bleeding time is prolonged due to an inadequate number of platelets (usually below 50,000/cu. mm. of blood).
   C. Purpura, which may occur as an allergic response, or as a response to septicemia or to certain chemicals.
4. Chronic blood loss (such as may occur in chronic menorrhagia, ulcerative colitis, peptic ulcer or bleeding hemorrhoids) can generally be compensated for by the body, but the sudden loss of 35 per cent of the blood volume is often fatal.
5. The site of bleeding is significant because of the possible effects of the pressure exerted by the accumulating blood.
6. The degree of possible vasoconstriction can be limited by arteriosclerosis.
7. The time required for the healing process (scar formation, resorption of blood from the tissues, etc.) varies with the extent and the location of the hemorrhage, the blood supply to the part, and any interference with normal healing processes. The fibrous consolidation of a thrombus may be interfered with by trauma, infection, and chemicals such as digestive juices.

Shock

1. "Shock" results from a disproportion between the volume of blood and the volume of blood vascular space, so that the blood pressure falls and circulation becomes inadequate (the heart fails and the smooth muscle of arteries loses tone). In irreversible shock, vital tissues are injured by lack of oxygen and by toxic catabolites.

Congestion

1. Hyperemia (or congestion) is a condition in which there is an excess of blood in the blood vessels because of the dilatation and engorgement of the vessels. It may be active (due to increased blood flow) or passive (due to decreased blood flow).
2. Local passive congestion may be caused by:
   A. Thrombosis (intravascular clotting).
   B. Pressure exerted on a vein from without (e.g., due to tumor, pregnancy, scar tissues).
   C. Back-pressure due to varicose veins (veins become dilated with blood; if valves are present at the varicosity, they become incompetent as venous return is diminished).

3. General passive congestion can result from reduced blood flow through the heart or through the lungs.
   A. Congestive heart failure may involve low cardiac output or increased venous pressure. Causes of congestive heart failure include:
   (1) Hypertension.
   (2) Atherosclerosis of the coronary arteries (decreasing blood supply to cardiac muscle).
   (3) Mechanical disorders of the valves due to congenital anomalies, valvular stenosis, valvular insufficiency. (A frequent cause of valvular stenosis is rheumatic fever.)
   B. A compensated heart is one in which hypertrophy of cardiac fibers has increased the contracting power of the fibers so that the heart is able to attain some degree of normal function.
   (1) The amount of blood supply to the hypertrophied heart does not increase proportionately.
   (2) Repeated episodes of over-exertion leads to progressive congestive failure.
   (3) The degree of compensation varies among individuals.

Thrombosis and Embolism

1. Thrombosis is the formation of blood clots within the vascular spaces. It may be due to:
   A. Injury to the endothelium (e.g., trauma, chemicals, toxins, bacterial infections, atherosclerosis).
   B. Decrease in rate of blood flow (most common in deep veins of legs and pelvis; favored by generalized passive congestion; more common in aged or debilitated).
   C. Changes in blood constituents (e.g., increase in number of platelets or erythrocytes):
   (1) There is an increase in the number of platelets in the circulating blood following surgery.
   (2) Polycythemia vera is a condition in which there is a great increase in the number of erythrocytes (e.g., 8,000,000 per cu. mm. of blood).
2. Thrombophlebitis is a condition in which venous thrombosis is associated with inflammation of the veins. The causative agent is usually bacterial and the thrombus is generally firmly attached. Venous sinuses of the brain may become the site of thrombophlebitis, as a consequence of mastoiditis, infections of the face, or deep infected scalp wounds.
3. Phlebothrombosis is a thrombus in a vein. It may show no effects or may cause hyperemia, edema and pain. It is often fairly loosely attached, so it can become dislodged rather easily.

4. The effects of thrombosis depend upon such factors as:
   A. Whether or not the thrombus completely occludes a blood vessel.
   B. Location, size and type of blood vessel involved.
   C. The extent of collateral circulation that already exists or develops.
   D. If the thrombus breaks loose.
   E. If the thrombus is infected or not.
5. The possible results of thrombosis include:
   A. No observable effects.
   B. Passive congestion; edema.
   C. Mechanical interference with cardiac function.
   D. Blood infection.
   E. Ischemia; infarction of tissues affected by occlusion.
   F. Sudden death due to occlusion of a major artery (e.g., coronary, pulmonary, cerebral).
6. Embolism is a process wherein there is an impaction somewhere in the cardiovascular system of material brought there by the circulation. The material is called an embolus; it may be a solid, an immiscible liquid, or bubbles of air.
   A. Solid emboli may be composed of such things as coagulated or agglutinated blood, tissue cells, or parasites.
   B. Liquid emboli may be injected intravenously by accident, or they may be introduced into the bloodstream during major surgery or extensive traumatic injuries.
   C. Air emboli may be introduced into the bloodstream accidentally during intravenous therapy, or during injury or surgery involving the neck and the chest.
   D. The effects of emboli depend upon the site of its impaction, and upon the size of the embolus compared to the caliber of the blood vessel.

Ischemia

1. Ischemia is a condition in which the blood supply to a part is decreased. The decrease may be absolute (such as a sudden complete occlusion of a blood vessel), or relative (such as occurs with hypotension or failure to meet increased demands of tissues). Causes of ischemia include:
   A. Hypotension (e.g., with shock following anesthesia).
   B. Demand of tissues for sudden increase in circulation (e.g., during exercise; strong emotional reaction following injury).
   C. Mechanical occlusion.
      (1) Destruction of capillaries (e.g., burns, freezing).
      (2) Restrictive devices (e.g., tourniquet).
      (3) Tumor masses.

(4) Volvulus (redundant loop of intestine), intussusception (telescoping of intestines), strangulated hernia (loop of intestine protruding through an opening and mechanically cut off from circulation).

(5) Pressure against blood vessels (e.g., weight of body over bony prominence, especially when there is decreased adipose padding).

D. Disease conditions of the arteries.

(1) Raynaud's disease is a condition in which there is arterial spasm, usually in the fingers and the hands.

(2) Thromboangiitis obliterans (Buerger's disease) is a condition in which there is inflammation of the lining of the arterial wall, often accompanied by thrombus formation. It occurs most frequently in the lower extremities.

(3) Atherosclerosis is both a degenerative process and an inflammatory reaction involving the arteries. There is a thickening of the intima, the cells of which are loaded with fat. Cholesterol crystals appear and combine with calcium salts to form plaques. Consequently, the lumen of the blood vessel is not only narrowed but roughened (which may lead to clot formation), and weakened (which may lead to aneurysm formation or hemorrhage). Atherosclerosis affects those arteries with predominantly elastic media—the aorta and its major branches, the coronary arteries, and the larger arteries of the brain. Atherosclerosis is frequently associated with diabetes mellitus and hypertensive disease. It tends to occur increasingly during the aging process.

(4) Arteriosclerosis is an inclusive term which means literally the hardening of the arteries. It includes atherosclerosis, medial sclerosis (which involves the calcification of the medial layer of arterial walls), and hyperplastic arteriosclerosis (which involves the thickening of the medial layer of arterioles and small arteries and results in marked narrowing of the lumens). Hyperplastic arteriosclerosis frequently involves the kidneys and occular fundi.

E. Injury of peripheral nerves or plexus (e.g., injury of the brachial plexus can result in ischemia of the arm and hand).

F. Poor venous return from an involved part (e.g., varicosities in lower extremities).

2. Possible consequences of ischemia include:

A. Atrophy of the part (e.g., skeletal muscles, brain).

B. Decreased functioning (e.g., heart failure, changes in mental abilities, decreased urine production, poor digestion, claudication).

C. Poor wound healing.

D. Infarction. This is a condition in which the blood supply to a part is decreased below the limits the tissue can tolerate (e.g., because of further reduction of blood supply or a sudden demand for increased circulation). The tissues become hypoxic; the blood vessels become atonic and congested with blood; the tissues die because of anoxia and chemical injury. Examples include:
   (1) Decubitus ulcers (over bony prominences).
   (2) Chronic skin ulcers (lower legs).
   (3) Gangrene (of digits, extremities, and intestines).
   (4) Cerebral hemorrhages.
   (5) Myocardial infarcts (which may result in cardiac arrest, or the rupture of the heart).

3. The healing of an infarct involves the removal of dead tissue, the fighting of any infection that may be present, and the regeneration of cells, commonly with fibrous tissue.
   A. The time required for healing varies with such factors as the blood supply to the part, the nutritional status of the patient, the presence of infection, and rest for the part involved.
   B. The infarct area is weak until regeneration of cells is well underway.
   C. Fibrous tissue cannot function as other tissues that may have been destroyed (e.g., nervous tissue, muscle tissue, epithelial tissue).

Hypertension

1. Hypertension is a condition wherein there is sustained constriction of arterioles throughout the body. It may be associated with a number of conditions, including certain kinds of kidney lesions, hyperthyroidism, adrenal cortical tumors and emotional tension. An increased blood pressure increases the work load of the heart; this generally results in an enlarged heart which, in turn, may result in congestive failure.

NURSING APPLICATIONS

Observation and Evaluation

1. Patients should be observed for signs and symptoms of circulatory problems; these should be evaluated, investigated, reported and/or treated with appropriate nursing measures. Observation is of particular importance when the patient:
   A. Has a pathologic condition affecting:
      (1) The heart.
      (2) The blood vessels.
      (3) Blood coagulation.
      (4) The brain (especially the medulla oblongata).
      (5) The kidneys.

B. Has sustained a traumatic injury (e.g., surgery), which involves or may involve:
 (1) The heart.
 (2) The blood vessels (especially major vessels).
 (3) An organ that has a relatively large blood supply (e.g., skin, liver, uterus during pregnancy).
 (4) The brain (especially the medulla oblongata).
C. Has bleeding (apart from normal female reproductive function).
D. Has a pathologic condition in which hemorrhage is a common complication (e.g., liver disease, peptic or duodenal ulcer, lung abscess, malignant tumor).
E. Has sustained an injury in which there is a rapid loss of plasma (e.g., extensive burns, a generalized allergic response).
F. Has a proportionately large amount of blood in the peripheral circulation (e.g., during hot bath or in hot, humid climate; when standing still for a long period of time).
G. Has sustained severe physical trauma (e.g., newborn after long and difficult labor; in case of an accident).
H. Is experiencing severe emotional stress (e.g., fear, grief).
I. Is pregnant, is in labor or delivering, or is within three weeks postpartum.
J. Is in utero.
K. Is at extremes of age (newborn and elderly).
L. Has a history of hypersensitivity.
M. Has been receiving or is receiving medications which affect:
 (1) Heart action (e.g., heart stimulants, cardiotonics, heart depressants).
 (2) Vasomotor mechanisms (e.g., vasodilators, vasoconstrictors, ganglionic blocking agents, sympatholytic drugs).
 (3) Blood-clotting mechanisms (e.g., "hemostatics," anticoagulants).
 (4) The brain (e.g., central nervous system stimulants or depressants).
N. Is receiving therapy that may cause allergic response (e.g., transfusion, sera, desensitizing drugs).
O. Has a constrictive, or potentially constrictive, device applied to a body part (e.g., tourniquet, drying cast, bandage, traction).
2. A patient's observable blood loss should be evaluated in relation to such factors as:
A. His general physical condition (e.g., appearance, vital signs).
B. His diagnosed disease condition (e.g., any bleeding in a hemophiliac is potentially serious).
C. The type and rate of bleeding (e.g., arterial, venous, capillary).

   D. The estimated amount of blood loss, especially as related to the
      size of the patient.
      (Whenever possible, estimation of the amount of bleeding should
      be made and reported. Total or partial specimens should be
      saved for further inspection.)
3. A patient's blood pressure and/or pulse should be taken and
   recorded whenever there are signs and symptoms that indicate a
   problem, or potential problem, involving the volume and the pressure of circulating blood (see Nursing Application No. 1).
   A. The frequency of these measurements depends upon the condi-
      tion of the patient and the particular problem or potential
      problem presented.
   B. The pulse should be counted over whichever artery is most con-
      venient and easiest to palpate.
   C. When the pulse is irregular or weak (e.g., in cardiac disease), or
      when an absolutely accurate count is necessary (e.g., when a
      digitalis preparation is administered), a stethoscope should be
      used to listen to the apical heartbeat.
   D. When a blood pressure measurement cannot be made over the
      brachial artery, the auscultatory and/or palpatory methods may
      be used with other arteries (e.g., radial, popliteal or dorsalis
      pedis).
   E. Careful observations should be made of the fetal heart tones
      during pregnancy, labor and delivery. This is of particular
      importance when the mother has problems involving the volume
      and the pressure of circulating blood, oxygen lack, or fluid and
      electrolyte imbalance.
4. A patient's blood pressure and pulse should be evaluated in relation
   to such factors as:
   A. His usual blood pressure and pulse.
   B. Age.
   C. The weight-height comparison.
   D. The posture or position or any abrupt change in position.
   E. Any physical activity.
   F. The emotional state.
   G. The diagnosed disease condition.
   H. Medications he is taking or has taken.
5. When there is head injury, a rise in blood pressure and a fall in
   pulse rate is very significant—as is an ensuing fall in blood pressure
   accompanied by a rapid, weak pulse.

Promoting Good Circulation

1. Good blood circulation to the various body parts can be promoted by:
   A. Positioning.
   B. Active or passive exercise.

C. Massage.
D. Preventing externally-applied pressure (especially prolonged pressure) against blood vessels or peripheral nerves.
   (1) Position changes should be made frequently.
   (2) Good body alignment should be maintained.
   (3) Air rings, special mattresses, cradles, footboards and pillows should be used as necessary.
   (4) In the back-lying position or in chair sitting, pressure against the popliteal areas should be avoided.
   (5) Restraints, tourniquets and blood pressure cuffs should be used with caution; when they are used, adequate circulation in the extremities should be provided.
   (6) Careful and frequent observations should be made of the circulation in an extremity when a cast (especially while drying), traction, a bandage, or any restrictive device has been applied (e.g., skin color and temperature, pulse, any discomfort).
   (7) A newly applied wet cast should be handled and positioned so as to prevent pressure against it that could cause changes in its shape (e.g., the cast should have a soft but firm and even support).
   (8) Umbilical cord prolapse may be prevented during labor by encouraging the patient, whose membranes have ruptured (but the presenting part is not engaged), to remain in a horizontal position.
   (9) When prolapse of the umbilical cord does occur:
       (a) This is a medical emergency.
       (b) The presenting part should be held back from the birth canal as much as possible (e.g., use of Trendelenburg positioning, the exertion of mild pressure against the presenting part).
E. Preventing the entrance into the cardiovascular system of anything that might cause the obstruction of normal blood flow.
   (1) Immiscible liquids (e.g., oils, waxes) must never be injected into the bloodstream.
   (2) Air should not be allowed to enter the bloodstream during intravenous therapy.
   (3) All blood used for transfusions must be positively identified before administration. (Blood-typing and cross-matching must precede a blood transfusion.)
   (4) If a patient receiving a blood transfusion suddenly complains of chest pains, or has a chill and fever, the transfusion should be stopped and the symptoms reported.
   (5) If a patient who has received, or is receiving, an intravenous injection shows signs or symptoms of an inflammatory

response around the site of the injection (e.g., pain, redness, edema), the observation should be reported promptly.

(6) If a patient known to have poor systemic circulation (e.g., the aged or the debilitated), or a patient ambulating following surgery, delivery or prolonged bed rest, complains of a localized discomfort (e.g., tenderness) in a lower extremity, especially in the calf of the leg:

  (a) He should be placed on complete bedrest in horizontal position.

  (b) The physician should be notified immediately.

  (c) The affected limb should be at rest and never massaged.

  (d) He should be observed for signs and symptoms of emboli (dependent upon location of a circulatory obstruction).

F. Using caution in the local applications of cold.

  (1) Applications should be discontinued if the area becomes blanched and remains so more than 5 to 10 minutes, or if there is marked discomfort.

G. Avoiding extremes of external temperature (e.g., excessively hot bath).

2. Circulation of blood to a part may be increased (within physiological limits) by:

A. Positioning.

  (1) If increased arterial flow is desired, the part should be level with or slightly lower than the heart.

  (2) If increased venous return is desired, the part should be level with or slightly elevated above the heart.

B. Active or passive exercise.

C. Massage.

D. Local application of heat or counterirritant substance (e.g., mustard).

E. Limiting loss of body heat (e.g., extra blanket or clothing).

3. When a patient has sustained a severe traumatic injury or emotional shock:

A. He should be placed in horizontal position.

B. Complete physical and emotional rest should be encouraged.

4. When there is a possibility of a large amount of blood pooling in the periphery and/or splanchnic region (e.g., following lumbar sympathectomy or during early postoperative ambulation), the patient should be protected from sudden hypotension by:

A. Allowing only gradual postural changes and observing his total response to each change (e.g., color, pulse, blood pressure).

B. Use of elastic stockings, ace bandages, abdominal binder or special belts (applied before sitting or standing).

Bleeding

1. When there is active bleeding or a danger of potential bleeding from injured blood vessels:
   A. Movement of the injured part may be restricted or limited (e.g., bed rest, splinting).
   B. Any wound care should be done with great gentleness (e.g., moistening adhered dressings before removal; using caution in cleansing).
   C. No tubes or other objects should be inserted into an orifice from which the blood has come or is coming, unless medical orders specify that this should be done; however, any insertion should be done with extreme care.
2. When the source of observable bleeding has been determined:
   A. Pressure should be applied over the bleeding point whenever this is practical (e.g., a pressure dressing).
      (1) Exceptions to pressure treatment include the eye, the ear, and the area over the larynx.
      (2) When epistaxis occurs:
         (a) The patient should be in an upright sitting position (if possible), or prone if a horizontal position is indicated.
         (b) Cold may be applied to the nose and/or to the back of the neck.
   B. If bleeding is in an extremity:
      (1) The affected part may be elevated above the heart, unless the need for immobilization supersedes the importance of stopping the bleeding.
      (2) Pressure may be applied over a major artery that supplies an injured part.
      (3) A tourniquet may be applied only when there is careful observation. The tourniquet, if applied for any length of time, should be loose enough to allow some venous return and to provide enough circulation of blood to prevent tissue damage.
3. When there is bleeding, or suspected bleeding, in the gastro-intestinal tract, food and fluids should be withheld until medical orders are obtained. (An exception to this is a relatively small amount of rectal bleeding.)
4. When there has been prostatic surgery and a hemostatic retention catheter is in place, the patency of the catheter must be maintained (e.g., irrigations as necessary and within medical orders).
5. When there is bleeding, or potential bleeding, in the pelvic region (e.g., uterine, bladder, rectal):
   A. The patient should not be on his feet, especially for extended periods of time.

B. Good venous return from the extremities should be encouraged (e.g., pressure against popliteal areas should be avoided; prolonged standing should be avoided; use of elastic stockings or ace bandages, effective leg exercises).

C. Straining at stool should be avoided (e.g., administration of laxatives as necessary and as ordered; encouraging good elimination).

D. The elimination of flatus should be promoted (see Chap. 7 on Elimination), but no rectal tube should be inserted without medical orders.

E. The urinary bladder should not be allowed to become distended (e.g., by maintaining patency of any retention catheters; by noting time and amount of any voiding; by checking for bladder distention; by catheterizing as necessary and within medical orders).

F. Any treatment involving the pelvic area should be performed with great care (e.g., catheterizations, catheter or bladder irrigations, return flow enemas, insertion of rectal tube, vaginal irrigations).

6. Following delivery, the uterus should be maintained in a contracted state by:
   A. Uterine massage.
   B. Preventing distention of the urinary bladder.
   C. Administration of oxytocic drugs as ordered.

7. When there is bleeding or potential bleeding within the cranial cavity (e.g., cerebral vascular accident, head injury, brain surgery):
   A. The patient should be in a horizontal position with the head elevated slightly, within medical orders.
   B. Physical and emotional rest should be encouraged.
   C. The blood pressure and the pulse must be observed and evaluated frequently.
      (1) Any marked change should be treated as a medical emergency.
      (2) A rise in the blood pressure and a fall in the pulse rate should be reported immediately; also, an ensuing fall in blood pressure accompanied by a rapid, weak pulse should be reported.

8. When a patient shows signs and symptoms of internal hemorrhage and/or peripheral circulatory failure:
   A. This is a medical emergency.
   B. He should be placed in horizontal or slight Trendelenburg position, unless contraindicated by another condition such as brain injury or respiratory distress.
   C. The rate of flow of any intravenous fluids being administered should be increased, consistent, however, with the need to

decrease bleeding and/or the capacity or effectiveness of the cardiovascular system.

D. Intravenous equipment—possibly equipment for a venous cut-down—and appropriate intravenous solutions (e.g., plasma or plasma substitute) should be ready for use. When blood for transfusion is already available, it should be ready for use.

E. Emergency drugs (e.g., vasoconstrictors, heart stimulants) and the means for their administration should be ready for use. When anaphylactic shock occurs, or may possibly occur, epinephrine should be ready for immediate administration.

F. The patient should be kept comfortably warm, without any local applications of heat.

G. Complete physical rest should be encouraged.

H. Emotional support should be provided.

I. The blood pressure, pulse and respiration should be measured and recorded frequently.

J. Appropriate steps may be taken to provide for emergency surgical intervention (as indicated).

9. A sensitivity test should be performed before the injection of any serum.

10. When sera or antigen solutions are administered, the patient should be observed closely for any allergic responses for 15 or 20 minutes.

11. When a patient is receiving an intravenous injection, the amount and the rate of the injection must be controlled carefully according to:
A. Any medical orders.
B. The size of the patient.
C. The condition of the patient's heart and arteries.
D. The patient's blood pressure.

12. When there is a known weakness of arterial walls (generally, as in arteriosclerosis, or locally, as with an aneurysm):
A. More than usual sleep and rest should be encouraged.
B. Stress-producing situations (physical or emotional) should be avoided or controlled.
C. Postural changes should be made gradually.
D. Minimal desirable body weight should be encouraged.
E. Straining at stool should be discouraged.
F. The use of drugs which stimulate the heart rate or vasoconstriction should be discouraged (e.g., nicotine, caffeine).

13. When there is a problem with a patient's blood clotting mechanism (e.g., as in hemophilia, acute leukemia, thrombocytopenic purpura, or with anticoagulant therapy) or a potential problem (e.g., with biliary disease):
A. Close observation for bleeding should be made and any bleeding should be handled as a medical emergency.

  B. Great care should be taken to prevent traumatic injury (e.g., in mouth and skin care; handling body parts; using oral route for medications wherever possible).
14. When a patient is receiving anticoagulant therapy, it is essential that laboratory blood tests (e.g., prothrombin activity, clotting time) be performed frequently.

Blood Pressure and Volume

1. When a patient has an abnormally elevated blood pressure (e.g., essential hypertension):
   A. More than usual sleep and rest should be encouraged.
   B. The head of the bed may be elevated when the patient is lying down.
   C. Stress producing situations (physical or emotional) should be avoided or controlled.
   D. The rate of flow of any intravenous infusion should be relatively slow (e.g., less than 60 drops/minute).
   E. Any marked increase over the patient's usual blood pressure should be reported promptly, and ordered medications (e.g., sedatives or vasodilators) should be administered promptly.
   F. Headaches should be reported.
   G. The patient should be observed closely for signs and symptoms of related circulatory problems (e.g., impaired heart action, visual disturbances, urinary suppression, or cerebral vascular accident).
   H. Minimal desirable body weight should be maintained.
   I. The use of substances that may cause vasoconstriction or heart stimulation should be discouraged (e.g., nicotine, caffeine).
   J. Observations should be made for any possible related emotional components (e.g., hostility, frustration).
2. When a patient has an abnormally high or low blood pressure, the administration of any drug that could be responsible (e.g., vasodilators or vasoconstrictors) should be changed (within medical orders) or withheld prior to prompt reporting of the blood pressure change.
3. When a patient has injured peripheral arterial circulation (e.g., due to arteriosclerosis or thromboangiitis obliterans):
   A. His positioning should provide the best possible circulation to the affected part. (See No. 7-A)
   B. Postural exercises (elevating and lowering a part) may be helpful, and, when ordered, should be done correctly. The oscillating bed, when ordered, should be used effectively.
   C. Exercise should be limited to prevent pain.
   D. Minimal desirable body weight should be maintained.

E. The use of substances that may cause vasoconstriction should be discouraged (e.g., nicotine).

4. When a patient has impaired coronary circulation (e.g., angina pectoris, myocardial infarction, or impaired heart action such as valvular incompetence, arrhythmias, cardiac decompensation):

A. It is a medical emergency:
   (1) When there are signs and symptoms of sudden coronary occlusion (e.g., severe substernal pain, signs of shock, collapse).
   (2) When there is cardiac arrest.
   (3) When there is cardiac insufficiency due to arrythmias.
   (4) When there are signs and symptoms of pulmonary edema.
B. The patient should be lying well-supported with the head elevation determined by his need for improved circulation and/or respiration.
C. Pain should be alleviated as promptly as possible with appropriate drugs as ordered (e.g., vasodilators, narcotics).
D. Consistent emotional support should be provided.
E. More than usual sleep and rest should be provided.
F. Stress producing situations—physical or emotional—should be avoided or controlled.
G. Physical activity should be limited both according to medical orders and according to the patient's total response to any activity.
H. Minimal desirable weight should be maintained.
I. Small, easily digested meals with low residue, nonfermentative, nonirritating foods should be provided, followed by a rest period.
J. Straining at the stool should be discouraged.
K. The use of substances that may cause cardiac stimulation or vasoconstriction (e.g., caffeine, nicotine) should be discouraged.

5. When a patient's heart rate (or fetal heart tones) become abnormally rapid or slow, any drug which might be responsible (e.g., cardiotonics, heart stimulants, sedatives) should be withheld prior to the prompt notification of the physician.

6. When fetal heart tones are abnormally rapid or slow and the fetus is past seven months gestation, the physician should be notified immediately and preparation may be made for an emergency delivery.

7. When a patient has cardiac arrest:
A. This is a medical emergency.
B. Resuscitation methods should be started immediately (e.g., closed heart massage).
C. Emergency drugs (e.g., cardiac stimulants) and the means for administering them should be ready.
D. All equipment necessary for an emergency thoracotomy and open heart massage should be ready.

8. When a patient has sustained a traumatic injury to the heart (e.g., cardiac surgery):

A. The vital signs must be measured and recorded very frequently, and significant changes must be reported promptly.

B. The blood pressure must be maintained within medically specified limits (e.g., by varying within medical orders the dosage of any vasopressor drug being administered).

C. Peripheral circulation should be evaluated frequently (e.g., pulse, skin color, temperature, sensation).

D. Behavioral changes or loss of consciousness must be reported promptly.

E. The patient should be kept flat in bed with no position changes during the first 48 hours, unless medically specified otherwise.
   (1) Medical orders must specify when the head can be elevated and to what degree.
   (2) When elevation is allowed, it must be done gradually and the blood pressure must be checked after each position change. (If the blood pressure doesn't return to normal within a few minutes, the original position should be resumed.)

F. Effective chest drainage must be maintained and any abnormalities of the drainage (e.g., amount or type) should be reported promptly.

G. Effective gastric suction, if used, must be maintained.

9. When a patient has impaired venous circulation (e.g., due to varicose veins, pregnancy, prolonged bed rest):

A. Prolonged standing or sitting with knees bent or legs crossed should be avoided.

B. Elastic stockings or ace bandages should be applied upon arising but before standing.

C. Frequent elevation of the affected part(s) should be encouraged.

D. No tight, restrictive clothing should be worn (e.g., round or tight garters, or girdles).

E. Leg exercises (active or passive) should be encouraged, unless there is evidence of possible thrombus formation.

2

Adequate Supply of Oxygen

All the cells of the body require an adequate supply of oxygen.

ANATOMY AND PHYSIOLOGY

The Respiratory System

1. The respiratory system provides for the exchange of oxygen and carbon dioxide between the atmosphere and the circulating blood.
2. The air passages include the nose, mouth, pharynx, larynx, trachea, bronchi and bronchioles.
3. The nose has two air passages separated by a cartilaginous septum. There are hairs in the nose that help to filter the incoming air. There are many small superficial blood vessels within the nares that help to warm the incoming air. The paranasal sinuses open into the nose.
4. The respiratory tract and the alimentary tract have a common passageway in the pharynx.
   A. Normally, swallowing and breathing do not occur simultaneously.
   B. During swallowing, the larynx is raised by action of pharyngeal muscles to meet the epiglottis, and the laryngeal orifice is closed by intrinsic muscle action.
   C. Normally, pressure in the oropharynx causes swallowing.
5. If the muscles that protrude the tongue are not functioning properly (e.g., when there is loss of consciousness or paralysis), the tongue falls back into the pharynx. The genioglossus muscle, arising from the mandible and inserting in the tongue, pulls the tongue forward.
6. The pharynx has lying within it masses of lymphoid tissue, the tonsils (palatine, lingual and pharyngeal). The function of the tonsils is to protect against infection. When these tissues become hyperactive, they become enlarged.

45

7. The larynx is cartilaginous and muscular; it forms the upper part of the trachea. It contains the vocal cords.
8. There is no cartilage support in the respiratory tree below the terminal bronchioles.
9. The walls of the bronchioles and the alveoli contain some elastic tissue that allows distention. During the aging process some elasticity may be lost, and there may be an increase of fibrous tissue in the walls.
10. The walls of the bronchioles contain smooth muscle that is under autonomic nervous control. Parasympathetic nerves cause bronchiolar constriction; sympathetic nerves allow relaxation.
11. The alveoli provide the respiratory surface for the exchange of gases. They are tiny sacs composed of a thin elastic tissue wall containing a network of capillaries and a thin layer of epithelial cells through which molecules of gas can diffuse.
12. The lining of the respiratory tract is continuous throughout, extending from the alveoli to the paranasal sinuses and up the Eustachian tubes. With the exception of the pharynx and the alveoli, the lining is ciliated mucous membrane. The mucus moistens the inhaled air and prevents the drying of the membrane. The membrane is able to absorb only extremely small amounts of aqueous solutions.
13. Sneezing and coughing are protective reflexes for the expulsion of foreign material from the respiratory tract.
    A. There are nerve centers in the medulla oblongata which are concerned with these functions.
    B. The cough reflex may be initiated by stimulation of afferent nerve endings in the tracheal bifurcation, the laryngeal mucosa and the lung tissue or pleura by such factors as dryness, pressure, cold, laughing or talking excessively, smoke or other irritant fumes.
    C. The sneeze reflex may be initiated by stimulation of sensory receptors in the nasal or nasopharyngeal mucosa.

The Process of Breathing

1. Air enters and leaves the respiratory tract because of the intermittent periodic production of pressure changes in the intrapulmonic cavity.
    A. The mechanical process of breathing is accomplished by movements of the chest wall and the diaphragm.
    B. During inspiration the diaphragm descends as it contracts, and the rib cage is lifted upward and outward by:
        (1) The external intercostal muscles (in quiet breathing).
        (2) The sternocleidomastoid muscles, the scalenes, the thoracohumeral and the thoracoscapular muscles (in forced breathing).

C. Relaxation of the abdominal muscles allows greater diaphragmatic contraction, as does the absence of abdominal distention.

D. During expiration the diaphragm ascends as it relaxes, and the rib cage is drawn downward and inward by:
   (1) The relaxation of the diaphragm and the external intercostal muscles (in quiet breathing).
   (2) The contraction of the internal intercostal muscles and the abdominal muscles (in forced breathing).

E. The visceral and parietal pleura are serous membranes which are kept slightly moist by serous fluid. The serous fluid helps to prevent friction during the respiratory movements, and it helps to provide surface tension between the two layers of pleura.

F. Subatmospheric pressure changes in the intrapleural space cause similar changes in the intrapulmonic pressures.

G. Collapse of lung tissue is prevented by the maintenance of an intrapleural pressure that is less than atmospheric pressure.

H. Vital capacity is the total amount of air that can be exhaled after a maximal inspiration. Factors that affect vital capacity include:
   (1) The structure of the chest wall.
   (2) The movement of the rib cage and the diaphragm.
   (3) The elasticity of the lung tissue.
   (4) The amount of space available for lung expansion.

2. The internal and the external intercostal muscles are innervated by spinal nerves arising from the thoracic spinal cord.

3. The diaphragm is innervated by the phrenic nerve which arises from the cervical level of the spinal cord.

4. The auxiliary respiratory muscles of the chest are innervated by spinal nerves that arise at the cervical and thoracic levels of the spinal cord.

5. The inspiratory and the expiratory nerve centers are located in the medulla oblongata; the pneumotaxic, in the pons varolii. The inspiratory center initiates inspiration; the expiratory, expiration; and the pneumotaxic acts as an inhibitor of inspiration.

6. The nervous control of the rate and the depth of respiration is influenced by chemical stimulation of the respiratory centers.

A. Inspired air that contains over 3 per cent but less than 10 per cent carbon dioxide causes an increase in the rate and the depth of respiration.

B. Inspired air that contains less than 0.4 per cent or more than 10 per cent carbon dioxide causes a decrease in rate and depth of respiration.

C. A fall in the pH of the blood (which may be due to the inadequate elimination of carbon dioxide from the body) usually causes a temporary increase in rate and depth of respiration.

    (1) At birth, the respiration of the newborn is normally initiated by this means.

    (2) Increased cellular metabolism (e.g., in voluntary muscles during exercise) results in the increased production of carbon dioxide.

  D. Following an initial stimulation of respiration, oxygen lack depresses the respiratory centers.

7. The respiratory rate and depth can be controlled to a limited extent by volition.

8. The respiratory rate and depth are affected by emotions (e.g., in hysteria, respiration becomes shallow and rapid).

9. The average respiratory rate of a person at rest varies with age:
   A. The average rate for the newborn is 30 to 50 respirations/minute.
   B. The average rate for an adult is 16 to 20 respirations/minute.

10. Depending to some extent upon the depth of the respirations, a respiratory rate of less than 8 respirations/minute may fail to provide an adequate supply of oxygen.

11. Because of the "dead air" space in the upper respiratory passages, shallow breathing does not provide an adequate supply of oxygen.

Transportation of Oxygen to the Tissues

1. The diffusion of oxygen from the alveoli into the capillary blood is dependent upon:
   A. The amount of available permeable membrane.
   B. The difference in pressure between the oxygen in the alveoli and the oxygen in the blood.

2. The functional circulation in the lungs is derived from the pulmonary arteries which arise directly from the right ventricle. The oxygenated blood returns through the pulmonary veins to the left atrium.

3. Most of the oxygen is carried to the body cells in combination with hemoglobin.
   A. The amount of oxygen that can be carried by a given volume of blood is dependent upon the amount of hemoglobin contained in the red blood cells in that volume of blood. Only very small amounts of oxygen can be dissolved in plasma under normal pressure and temperature conditions.
   B. As a normal red blood cell matures, it loses its nucleus and is able to contain a larger amount of hemoglobin. Erythroblasts and normoblasts are immature red blood cells and contain very little hemoglobin.
   C. The normal red blood cell count for adults is about 4,500,000 to 5,000,000/cu. mm. of blood. The count in newborns is approximately the same as an adult's. In early life, there is a slight decline in this number, which is gradually increased to the normal adult count by the age of 12 years.

D. The normal range of hemoglobin in the adult is 12 to 15 Gm.%. The newborn normally has between 15 and 18 Gm.%, but this amount decreases during early life; however, the amount of hemoglobin gradually increases to the normal adult level by the age of 12 years.

E. The average volume of red blood cells after the blood has been centrifuged is 40 per cent of the total volume.

F. The red blood cells of the majority of human beings contain a chemical substance called the Rh factor. The Rh factor acts as an antigen if introduced into the blood of a person who lacks this factor.

G. Under normal conditions hemoglobin is 97 per cent saturated with oxygen in the lung capillaries. Increasing the concentration of oxygen in the alveoli causes a very slight increase in the amount of oxygen that can combine with the hemoglobin.

H. An increase of reduced hemoglobin in the skin capillaries above 5 Gm.% usually gives the skin a grayish blue hue (cyanosis). Cyanosis is more clearly evident in regions where the skin is thin and unpigmented (e.g., around mouth, lips, in nail beds). In the newborn there may be cyanosis in the hands and feet prior to the development of good peripheral circulation, so that the face and trunk showing cyanosis is more indicative of respiratory problems in the newborn.

Use of Oxygen by the Cells

1. The oxygen requirements of the cells vary directly with their metabolic rates. Metabolic rates vary directly with the amount of thyroid hormone, the amount of cellular activity and the body temperature.

2. Cellular metabolism varies directly with available oxygen.
   A. Abnormalities in cellular function occur if there is insufficient oxygen.
   B. Striated muscle can build up some oxygen debt, but nerve tissue and cardiac tissue cannot.
   C. If the cells in the capillary walls do not have sufficient oxygen they may allow the blood to seep out of capillaries, resulting in petechiae.

3. An individual can live only a few minutes without oxygen.
   A. The cells of the cerebral cortex may be damaged after as little as 30 seconds without oxygen and are generally irreparably damaged after as long as 5 minutes without oxygen.
   B. The cells of the brain stem are generally irreparably damaged after 25 to 30 minutes without oxygen.

4. When an individual's supply of oxygen becomes inadequate, anxiety results with all associated symptoms.

PHYSICS

1. Atmospheric pressure is the pressure exerted by the "sea of air" above the earth and is approximately 14.7 lbs./sq. in. or 760 mm./ Hg. at sea level.
2. Fluids (or gases) flow from an area of higher pressure to one of lower pressure. The rate of volume flow of fluids (or gases) is directly related to the differences in pressure (or pressure gradient).
3. The pressure exerted by gas molecules within an enclosed area (e.g., the lungs) is reduced if the size of that area is increased (e.g., by enlargement of the thoracic cavity and resultant lung expansion).
4. Pressure is the force exerted on a unit area.
5. Gravity is the force of attraction between two objects (e.g., the earth and an object on or near the earth).
6. The law of gravitation states that any two objects in the universe are attracted to each other with a force that is proportional to the product of their masses and inversely proportional to the square of the distance between them.
7. Gases are relatively insoluble in liquids unless the temperature is decreased or the pressure is increased.
8. The size of molecules allowed to pass through a membrane depends upon the permeability of the membrane.

CHEMISTRY

1. The atmosphere at sea level contains approximately 20 per cent oxygen and 0.04 per cent carbon dioxide.
2. Hemoglobin is a conjugated protein made up of heme and globin. Heme contains iron. Hemoglobin and oxygen form a rather unstable compound, oxyhemoglobin, which is scarlet in color. Reduced hemoglobin is purple in color.
3. The oxidation of carbon and hydrogen in nutrients (e.g., glucose) is an energy-liberating chemical reaction. When oxidation is complete carbon dioxide and water are produced.
4. Carbon monoxide and hemoglobin combine to form carboxyhemoglobin which is a more stable compound than oxyhemoglobin. Disassociation of carboxyhemoglobin in the lung capillaries can be increased by increasing the oxygen tension in the alveoli.

PATHOLOGY

Signs and Symptoms

Signs and symptoms of problems that may be related to oxygen insufficiency include:
1. Abnormal respiration:
   A. Dyspnea, orthopnea, apnea.

(3) Production of inflammatory exudates—catarrhal, fibrinous, membranous, purulent, sanguineous (or hemorrhagic).

(4) Fibrosis, possibly calcification.

(5) Destruction of cells, tissues.

The exudates formed in the respiratory tract may be eliminated through the process of resolution. This process involves both absorption into the lymphatic system and the expulsion of material through sneezing and coughing, and by gravity drainage.

C. Pneumoconiosis is a condition caused by the inhalation of dust particles, frequently silicon, into the lungs. The resulting physical and chemical injury causes the formation of fibrotic nodules, usually associated with lymphatic tissue. The nodules interfere with the flow of blood and the diffusion of gases; they decrease vital capacity and predispose to pneumonia and emphysema.

D. Allergic responses that involve the respiratory tract include:

(1) Edema of the glottis (occurs in severe hypersensitivity and infections).

(2) Constriction of the bronchioles (occurs in bronchial asthma).

(3) Congestion, swelling and edema of the mucous membrane lining (occurs in hay fever, vasomotor rhinitis).

(4) Excessive production of mucus (occurs in vasomotor rhinitis).

(5) Production of catarrhal exudate (occurs in hay fever).

E. Many microorganisms can cause injury to the upper respiratory tract and associated structures. The body's responses to these infections vary, depending upon the causative organism, the number of organisms, the location of the inflammation, the duration of the inflammation and the resistance of the host. Possible responses to microbial injury include all those listed previously in Statement B.

F. The common cold is a communicable viral disease which may affect the paranasal sinuses, the nasal passages, the nasopharynx, the larynx, the trachea and the major bronchi. It causes congestion and edema, excessive mucus production, and the production of catarrhal and fibrous exudates. If the infection is complicated by other microorganisms (e.g., staphylococci), a purulent exudate may also be produced. If the infection is very severe the exudate may become sanguineous.

G. Diphtheria is a communicable disease caused by the *Corynebacterium diphtheriae*. It affects the mucous membrane of the upper respiratory tract, causing congestion, edema and the production of a membranous exudate. The swelling and the exudate obstruct the airway.

H. Pertussis is a communicable disease caused by the *Hemophilus pertussis*. Following catarrhal symptoms there is production of a fibrous exudate in the bronchi and the bronchioles. The exudate is very difficult to expel and there are severe paroxysms of coughing with typical "whooping."

I. Pneumonia (or pneumonitis) is a condition in which the alveoli of the lungs become filled with inflammatory exudate that becomes consolidated. The condition is generally caused by microorganisms (e.g., certain viruses, rickettsia, bacteria, fungi) but it may result from a chemical irritation (e.g., lipids). The inflammatory exudate is usually eliminated through the process of resolution.

J. Pulmonary tuberculosis is a communicable disease caused by the *Mycobacterium tuberculosis*. The invasion of lung tissue by these bacilli results in the formation of tubercles that are nodular masses of granular tissue surrounded by a dense fibrous capsule. The tubercles may have soft, cheesy centers or they may be dense and fibrous. They can become calcified or even ossified. The inflammatory process may result in cavity formation (because of necrosis), extensive fibrosis and, possibly, hemorrhage. The infection may predispose to pneumonia.

K. Bronchiectasis is a condition in which there is permanent dilatation of one or several bronchi. There may be a congenital weakness of the bronchial walls, but the condition is generally associated with chronic irritation of the tract (e.g., due to infections, or to irritation of smoke) which has resulted in an accumulation of exudates.

L. Pulmonary emphysema is a condition in which the alveoli do not empty with expiration but remain overdistended. The normal elasticity of the bronchioles is impaired. The blood supply may become inadequate, causing atrophy. Fibrosis may occur. The condition may be a result of the aging process or of chronic inflammation of the alveoli.

M. Inflammatory responses to injury involving the pleura include:
   (1) Congestion and edema.
   (2) Excessive production of serous fluid.
   (3) Production of inflammatory exudates (serous, fibrous, purulent, sanguineous).
   (4) Fibrosis.
   (5) Destruction of cells, tissue.

N. Pleurisy (or pleuritis) is a condition in which the pleural membranes have responded to injury (e.g., lung infection) by congestion, edema and the production of a fibrous exudate. This results in friction during the respiratory movements. Pain is usually severe.

O. Pleural effusion is a condition in which the pleural membranes have responded to injury (e.g., lung infection), not only as they do in pleurisy, but also with the excessive production of serous or serosanguineous exudate. The exudates accumulate in the thoracic cavity and interfere with the respiratory movements and lung expansion.

P. Pleural empyema is a condition in which the pleural membranes have responded to injury (e.g., infection) with the production of a purulent exudate that accumulates in the thoracic cavity and interferes with respiratory movements and lung expansion.

Q. Tetanus is a disease condition caused by the *Clostridium tetani*. The organisms produce a toxin which causes nervous tissue to become hypersensitive. The result is severe muscle spasm. If the respiratory muscles go into spasm, breathing is markedly impaired.

R. Rabies is a viral infection that affects the brain. It can cause severe laryngeal and pharyngeal muscle spasms.

S. Poliomyelitis is a communicable viral disease that affects the central nervous system. The viruses invade the anterior horn cells, and they may invade the medulla oblongata. The latter is called bulbar poliomyelitis, which may cause paralysis of the respiratory muscles and the pharyngeal muscles.

T. Encephalitis is a disease condition that may be caused by a specific virus, or it may be a complication of acute communicable diseases (e.g., measles). The brain is injured, and if areas involved in respiration are affected, respiratory difficulty will result.

U. Laryngospasm may be caused by severe laryngitis (e.g., in croup), by some drugs, or it may occur in tetanus and rabies. Such spasms obstruct the airway.

4. Conditions involving traumatic injuries:

A. The normal functioning of the muscles of respiration may be impaired because of:
   (1) Penetrating wounds of the chest wall that cause injury to muscle tissue and blood vessels.
   (2) Crushing wounds of the chest that may result in injury to muscle tissue; fractures of the ribs, the sternum, the clavicle, the thoracic vertebrae; and injury to blood vessels.
   (3) Traumatic injury to the brain (especially medulla oblongata, motor area and motor pathways).
   (4) Traumatic injury to the cervical spinal cord (e.g., fractured cervical vertebrae).
   (5) Traumatic injury to the spinal nerves that innervate the respiratory muscles.

B. If the intrapleural pressure is increased to atmospheric pressure (e.g., when there is a rupturing of lung tissue or a penetrating chest wound), the lung will collapse.

5. Conditions having emotional components. Emotional problems can affect, through the autonomic nervous system:
   A. The rate and depth of respirations.
   B. The blood supply to the various tissues (vasomotor mechanisms).
   C. The production of mucus.
   D. The diameter of the bronchioles.

Conditions Affecting the Oxygen-Carrying Capacity of the Blood

1. Anemia
   A. Anemia is a condition in which there is an abnormally low number of mature erythrocytes or a decreased concentration of hemoglobin in the circulating blood.
   B. Possible causes of anemia include:
      (1) Bleeding (acute or chronic).
      (2) Excessive hemolysis of red blood cells.
         (a) Infections involving the blood (e.g., bacteremias, malaria) frequently result in excessive hemolysis.
         (b) Hemolysis of red blood cells may result from immune reactions (e.g., the immune bodies produced by a pregnant mother who lacks the Rh factor in her blood in response to the Rh factor in the blood of the unborn child can cause excessive hemolysis of the child's red blood cells).
      (3) Failure of the bone marrow to produce and release an adequate number of mature erythrocytes (e.g., as occurs in hypoplastic anemia, or when the bone marrow function has been depressed by chemical injury or by chronic infections).
      (4) Nutritional deficiencies
         (a) The blood hemoglobin and the red cell count are reduced when there is a deficiency of iron in the diet.
         (b) Pernicious anemia is a condition in which there is a macrocytic anemia. The cause is a deficiency in Vitamin B_{12}, the basic problem being a defect in the gastric secretory function.
         (c) Other macrocytic anemias may result from a deficiency in folic acid, which may occur when there is gastric cancer or poor absorption of food from the small intestine.
2. Carbon monoxide poisoning, in which the carbon monoxide combines with the hemoglobin in the red blood cells, reduces the oxygen-carrying capacity of the blood.

NURSING APPLICATIONS

Observation and Evaluation

1. Patients should be observed for signs and symptoms of oxygen insufficiency; these should be evaluated, investigated, reported, and/or treated with appropriate nursing measures. This is of particular importance when the patient:
   A. Has a pathologic condition or has sustained an injury that involves or may involve:
      (1) The air passages.
      (2) The lungs.
      (3) The heart.
      (4) The pulmonary circulation.
      (5) The brain (especially the medulla oblongata).
      (6) The cervical vertebrae.
      (7) The effective functioning of the respiratory muscles (e.g., damage to spinal nerves, abdominal distention, fractured ribs).
      (8) The red blood cells (e.g., anemias, hemorrhage).
   B. Has or may have a mechanical obstruction in the respiratory tract.
   C. Is at the extremes of age (very young or elderly).
   D. Is receiving medications that are central nervous system depressants.
2. The respiratory rate can be counted most accurately if the patient is unaware of the counting.
3. A patient's respirations should be evaluated in relation to such factors as:
   A. His age.
   B. His usual respirations.
   C. His posture or position.
   D. Any physical activity.
   E. His emotional state.
   F. The diagnosed disease condition.
   G. Medications he is taking or has taken.
4. A patient's cough should be evaluated in terms of:
   A. Frequency.
   B. Time of occurrence.
   C. Sound.
   D. Sputum production.
5. A patient's sputum should be evaluated in terms of:
   A. Amount.
   B. Consistency.
   C. Appearance.

Promoting Good Respiration

1. Good respirations can be promoted by such measures as:
   A. Encouraging frequent periods of deep breathing exercises.
   B. Providing positioning that allows the best possible lung expansion (e.g., sitting position with arms supported).
   C. Providing periods of exercise (active or passive).
   D. Providing clear air passage (e.g., suctioning, nose drops, humidified air).
   E. Alleviating discomforts associated with breathing (e.g., by splinting chest, administering medications for cough or pain).
   F. Avoiding abdominal distention (e.g., giving small, easily digested meals).
   G. Avoiding restrictive external pressure against chest (e.g., restraints).
   H. Using caution when caring for chest drainage.
   I. Using caution when administering central nervous system depressants.
2. Injury to the respiratory tract should be prevented by such methods as:
   A. Discouraging the inhalation of tobacco smoke.
   B. Using special precautions when exposed to irritating substances that may be inhaled, such as sand, dusts, allergens, fumes.
   C. Using preventive means to avoid respiratory infection (e.g., maintaining good nutrition; avoiding fatigue or chilling; use of medical aseptic techniques).
   D. Discouraging use of potentially harmful drugs for nose and throat treatments (e.g., repeated use of antiseptics, inhalers).
   E. Preventing coughing when it is nontherapeutic.
   F. Preventing aspiration of food, fluids, vomitus, foreign objects.
   G. Not using an oily substance in treatment involving the nose and pharynx (e.g., lubricating tube, nose drops).
   H. Using safety measures in performing all nursing activities involving the respiratory tract (e.g., suctioning, passage of tubes, aerosol therapy, oxygen therapy, throat irrigations).
3. The prevention of injury to the respiratory tract is of particular importance when the patient:
   A. Is very young or elderly.
   B. Is debilitated.
   C. Has a respiratory problem already.
   D. Has cardiac disease.
   E. Is scheduled to have a general anesthetic.
4. Obstruction of the air passages should be prevented by such methods as:
   A. Preventing injury to the respiratory tract (see No. 2 above).

B. Preventing aspiration of such things as:
   (1) Fluids
       (a) No unconscious person should be given liquid by mouth.
       (b) Only *very* small amounts of physiological saline solution should be used in tracheotomy tubes when this is ordered.
       (c) Infants should be watched closely while being fed from a bottle.
   (2) Foods
       (a) Caution should be used when feeding anyone who has difficulty in swallowing (e.g., the elderly, patients with paralysis, and infants, especially those suffering from an unrepaired cleft palate).
       (b) Taking quick breaths (e.g., as in laughing or excitement) should be avoided when the mouth contains food.
   (3) Vomitus.
       (a) Food and fluids should be withheld prior to administration of a general anesthetic.
       (b) Food and fluids should be withheld when there is violent coughing (especially with children).
       (c) Food and, to some extent, fluids should be withheld when a woman is in active labor.
       (d) When there is a likelihood of vomiting in an unconscious or helpless person, he should be positioned so as to prevent aspiration (e.g., prone, side-lying position, slight Trendelenburg).
   (4) Respiratory secretions or blood
       (a) Unconscious or helpless patients should be positioned for adequate drainage of the respiratory tract.
       (b) Frequent changes of position should be made when a patient is unconscious or relatively inactive, or when his respirations are impaired (e.g., following thoracic surgery; the elderly).
       (c) Deep breathing and productive coughing should be encouraged when there may be excessive respiratory secretions, restricted activity, limited respiratory movement, and so forth.
       (d) Nasopharyngeal suctioning should be used promptly and effectively when necessary. (An exception would be when the bleeding is from an injured area in the nose or the nasopharynx and the suctioning might cause further injury.)
       (e) When there is gross bleeding into the respiratory tract (e.g., following a head injury, or a tonsillectomy, in advanced pulmonary tuberculosis), it is a medical emergency.

(5) Foreign objects
  (a) Dentures should be removed from the mouth prior to the administration of a general anesthetic.
  (b) Children should be protected from the danger inherent in putting small objects in their mouths (e.g., toys, gum, hard candy).
C. Use of an airway in the unconscious patient until pharyngeal reflexes return.
D. Preventing the swallowing of the tongue (e.g., by positioning the patient on his side or by holding the mandible up and forward).
E. Preventing hyperextension of the cervical spine.

Respiratory Disorders

1. When a patient has an irritated respiratory tract (as indicated by such symptoms as coughing, sneezing, excessive mucus production, hoarseness):
   A. This should be medically investigated.
   B. He may be encouraged to restrict smoking.
   C. Warmed, humidified air may be helpful.
   D. Coughing may be alleviated by such methods as administering cough syrups and hot fluids, avoiding cold air, sucking on hard candy or cough drops.
   E. Possible causes (e.g., allergens, infection, smoke) should be recognized and reported.
   F. The patient should be observed closely for signs and symptoms of respiratory distress.
2. When a patient has insufficient oxygen reaching the lungs because of an obstruction in the upper respiratory tract (e.g., croup, aspiration, laryngospasm as in tetany laryngoedema, as may occur with allergic response or following thyroid surgery):
   A. This is a medical emergency.
   B. Coughing may be helpful in dislodging an obstruction.
   C. A quick blow on the back may be helpful in dislodging an obstruction (e.g., food in the larynx).
   D. Positioning the patient to promote drainage may be helpful (e.g., holding a child up by his feet).
   E. Warm, humidified air may be helpful.
   F. Suctioning material from the air passage may be necessary.
   G. Equipment for performing a tracheotomy should be ready.
3. When a patient has a clear airway (upper respiratory tract), but an inadequate supply of oxygen reaching the capillaries that surround the alveoli of lungs (e.g., as in pneumonia, tuberculosis, emphysema, bronchiectasis, asthma, drowning, pulmonary edema):
   A. Oxygen should be administered as necessary, possibly by positive pressure, if ordered. (An exception to this is emphysema).

B. A hand-operated resuscitator should be used, or mouth-to-mouth breathing if necessary.

C. The patient should be positioned, within medical orders, so as to facilitate breathing.

D. Any discomfort associated with breathing should be alleviated as promptly as possible (e.g., giving medication for pain; splinting the chest wall).

E. Physical activity should be limited according to the patient's tolerance.

F. Emotional support should be consistent.

G. Small, easily digested meals should be provided, followed by rest periods.

H. Postural drainage, when ordered, should be carried out effectively (e.g., in bronchiectasis).

I. The patient should be encouraged to use the abdominal muscles to increase expiration (in emphysema).

J. Epinephrine and equipment for its administration should be ready, and it should be administered promptly as ordered when there is bronchiolar constriction.

4. When the pulmonary circulation is impaired and pulmonary edema occurs (in addition to No. 3):

A. This is a medical emergency.

B. Tourniquets should be ready for use (three for rotating).

C. Cardiac stimulants and equipment for administration should be ready for prompt administration.

D. Equipment for an emergency phlebotomy should be ready.

5. When the primary muscles of respiration are unable to provide adequate breathing (e.g., in the newborn, or due to injury to the brain, the cervical spinal cord, the spinal nerves, or the thorax itself):

A. This is a medical emergency.

B. A respirator or some means of administering oxygen with positive pressure should be ready and used promptly as ordered.

C. Mouth-to-mouth breathing or a hand-operated resuscitator may be used as necessary.

D. Respiratory stimulants and equipment for administration should be ready for prompt administration.

E. If the patient is newborn or an infant, the skin may be stimulated (e.g., contrast baths or slapping), or rectal stimulation may be helpful.

F. The patient may be encouraged to use accessory muscles of respiration (e.g., using upper thoracic muscles when in body cast, or increasing diaphragmatic breathing to aid expirations when there is emphysema).

(Injury to the thoracic cage is included in Chap. 12.)

6. When a patient shows signs and symptoms of an asthmatic attack, any possible emotional components preceding the attack should be noted and reported appropriately.

7. When there is abnormal intrathoracic pressure (e.g., when the intrapleural space has been opened to the outside, as with a penetrating wound, a spontaneous pneumothorax or a ruptured lung abscess, or when there is an accumulation of fluid within the chest cavity, as with empyema or as a result of the accidental entrance of fluids through chest drainage tubes):

   A. This is a medical emergency.
   B. Any object (e.g., a knife) which is still in an external wound should not be removed.
   C. Any open chest wound should be covered promptly with a covering as airtight as possible.
   D. If air or fluid is entering the chest cavity through drainage tubes, the tubes should be clamped off immediately.
   E. Any chest tubes that do not appear to be draining properly should be reported immediately.
   F. Oxygen should be ready for immediate administration as needed or ordered.
   G. The patient should be positioned to facilitate breathing (e.g., well-supported or in semi-sitting position).
   H. The patient must be kept completely quiet.
   I. Emotional support should be consistent.
   J. A thoracentesis set should be ready for use.
   K. The patient should be observed closely for signs and symptoms of increasing respiratory distress and for mediastinal shift.

8. When a patient has a diminished supply of oxygen reaching the tissues because of poor general circulation (e.g., in cardiac disease) or lack of hemoglobin (e.g., in anemias, carbon monoxide poisoning):

   A. Oxygen may be administered as needed (important in carbon monoxide poisoning).
   B. Positioning should facilitate breathing.
   C. Stress-producing situations, emotional and physical, should be avoided or controlled.
   D. More than usual sleep and rest should be provided.
   E. Physical activity should be adjusted according to the patient's tolerance of it.
   F. Meals should be small and easily digestible and followed by rest periods.
   G. Emotional support should be consistent.

9. When a patient is receiving drugs that depress the central nervous system, his respiratory rate should be observed closely; if it slows significantly (e.g., below 12/minute in an adult), further medication should be withheld prior to notification of the physician.

10. If symptoms of an asthmatic attack occur during the administration of a transfusion, the transfusion should be stopped.
11. When carbon dioxide (e.g., as carbogen) is administered, the procedure must be done with great caution and the patient must be watched closely for signs and symptoms of respiratory distress.
12. Women who are pregnant should be encouraged to seek medical attention early in their pregnancy (e.g., to have the Rh factor of their blood determined).

3

Nutrition

All the cells of the body require adequate nutrition.

ANATOMY AND PHYSIOLOGY

Nutritional Needs

1. Sufficient amounts of carbohydrates, fats, proteins, vitamins and minerals are necessary in the diet in order to provide for:
   A. The building and repair of tissues.
   B. The synthesis of essential substances (e.g., enzymes, hormones and antibodies).
   C. The production of energy.
2. A healthy nutritional state is maintained by the regular intake of a properly balanced diet which supplies all the essential nutrients in adequate amounts. The properly balanced diet contains foods from the milk group, the meat group, the vegetable-fruit group, and the bread-cereal group.
3. Carbohydrates are used mainly as a source of energy, but they are found in all protoplasm and in many important compounds of the body.
   A. Each gram of carbohydrate yields 4 calories.
   B. The energy requirement of the normal adult resting is about 1 calorie/Kg. of body weight/hour. Moderate activity increases the need by about one-half.
   C. Starch is the most abundant source of carbohydrates in the diet.
   D. Carbohydrates must be hydrolyzed to monosaccharides before they can be absorbed into the blood.
   E. Most of the glucose in the body is converted to glycogen by the liver before use, although glucose may be used directly without this conversion.
   F. Excess amounts of glucose may be:
      (1) Excreted through the kidneys (if the blood level is above 160 to 180 mg. per cent).
      (2) Stored as glycogen in the liver and muscles.
      (3) Converted to and stored as fat (adipose tissue).

G. Nerve cells can survive only for short periods without glucose.
4. Some of the fatty acids are essential constituents of protoplasm.
   A. Brain and nervous tissue are rich in lipids.
   B. Cholesterol is found in all cells.
   C. Lipids are important constituents of cellular membranes.
5. Fat provides the main store of reserve food supply. Each gram of fat yields 9 calories.
   A. The glycerol of fats may be converted to glucose in the body.
   B. Fatty acids may be converted, to a limited extent, to substances that can be utilized for energy.
6. Some oily substances are not true lipids, so they cannot be hydrolyzed and absorbed into the lymphatic system. These pass through the gastrointestinal tract and are eliminated with the feces.
7. Protein is essential for the building and repair of tissue and the synthesis of many essential compounds.
   A. The body does not store protein to any extent.
   B. The need for protein is relatively greater when growth is occurring and during convalescence.
   C. The state of protein nutrition is of great importance in general physical health.
   D. Proteins must be hydrolyzed to amino acids before they can be absorbed into the blood.
   E. Essential amino acids are those that the body is unable to synthesize.
8. There are many minerals that are important for efficient cellular functioning and for the production of essential compounds. These include:
   A. Calcium. (See Chap. 1, 5 and 11.)
   B. Phosphorus. (See Chap. 3 and 11.)
   C. Sodium. (See Chap. 4, 5 and 6.)
   D. Potassium. (See Chap. 4, 5 and 6.)
   E. Iodine. (See Chap. 8.)
   F. Iron. (See Chap. 1.)
   G. Traces of other minerals that are constituents of enzymes and enzyme activators, or that have to do with the inter-relationships of ions.
9. Vitamins are chemical substances that, if lacking in the diet, manifest their absence by abnormal body functions and by certain disease conditions.
   A. Vitamin A is probably synthesized in the intestines from foods that contain carotene. It is necessary for the formation of visual purple, and for the normal growth and functioning of epithelial tissues.
   B. Vitamin D is synthesized when ergosterol in the skin is acted upon by ultraviolet rays. It plays an important role in mineral

metabolism, and is involved in the absorption of calcium and phosphorus from the gastrointestinal tract.
C. Vitamin K is synthesized by bacterial flora of the intestinal tract. It is essential for the production of prothrombin.
D. Vitamin C is required for the normal formation and maintenance of intercellular substances that have a cementing function.
E. The B-complex vitamins are essential in various metabolic processes that occur in all living cells; they are involved in the oxidation of carbohydrate to produce energy.
  (1) Thiamine is important in the metabolism of carbohydrate.
  (2) Riboflavin is important in the functioning of certain enzymes, and it is essential in the metabolism of amino acids, fatty acids and carbohydrate.
  (3) Niacin is important in the synthesis of certain enzymes involved in the production of energy.
  (4) Folic acid is required for normal tissue growth, including the production of red and white blood cells by bone marrow.
  (5) Pyridoxine is concerned with some aspects of protein metabolism and with the synthesis within the body of some fatty acids.
  (6) Vitamin B_{12} is necessary for normal body growth; it is essential for the normal structure and functioning of many of the body tissues (e.g., bone marrow, gastrointestinal tract, nervous tissue).
10. The sensation of hunger is experienced when:
A. The stomach is empty and contracting.
B. There is hypoglycemia.
11. Appetite is a desire for food. Factors that may affect appetite include emotions and certain visceral sensations (e.g., nausea).

The Digestive Tract and Accessory Structures

1. Food is taken into the mouth, chewed as necessary and swallowed.
A. The chewing of food is accomplished by the action of the jaw and the teeth; it is facilitated by saliva and the tongue.
  (1) The muscles of mastication originate on the zygomatic arch on the skull and insert in the mandible.
  (2) There are three types of teeth: the incisors and the canines, which are designed for biting, and the molars, which are adapted for grinding.
  (3) The teeth appear in two sets—first the deciduous, and later the permanent teeth.
    (a) There are 20 deciduous teeth. These begin to erupt by the sixth to ninth month after birth, and usually have erupted by the end of the second year.

     (b) About the sixth year the 32 permanent teeth begin to erupt, and usually all the permanent teeth have erupted by the eighteenth year.

     (c) The teeth are composed of dentine (the exquisitely sensitive basis of the tooth), enamel (the white insensitive covering of the crown of the tooth), and the pulp (the fibrous material projecting up into the dentine that contains nerves and blood vessels). The enamel can be decayed by the prolonged action of various acids upon it (e.g., acid produced by the action of lactobacilli on food particles in the mouth).

  (4) The tongue is a muscular organ under voluntary control.

  (5) There are three pairs of salivary glands, all of which have ducts opening into the mouth. The parotid glands lie below and in front of the ears. Parasympathetic nerves stimulate the production of saliva.

  B. The esophagus is a muscular tube that extends behind the trachea and through the diaphragm, ending at the cardiac orifice of the stomach. The upper portion is skeletal muscle, but is not under voluntary control. The lower portion is smooth muscle under autonomic control. The cardiac valve is a sphincter muscle located at the cardiac orifice. Sympathetic stimulation causes constriction of the cardiac sphincter.

2. In the stomach, the food is broken down into smaller pieces, mixed with the gastric juices and partially digested.

  A. The stomach is a musculomembranous pouch located between the esophagus and the duodenum. It can be greatly distended. The pyloric sphincter controls the passage of chyme into the small intestine.

  B. Mucosal cells produce hydrochloric acid, mucin, and digestive enzymes.

  C. The mucin of saliva and mucin produced in the stomach normally protects the stomach wall from the digestive action of the acid and the enzymes.

3. Digestion is completed in the small intestine, and the end products are absorbed into the lymph and blood.

  A. The small intestine is the musculomembranous tube that extends from the pylorus to the ileocecal valve. The mucosa consists of a layer of simple columnar epithelium supported by a thin layer of connective tissue. Below this is a thin layer of smooth muscle. Each villi (formed from the mucosa) contains capillaries and a lacteal. Glands secrete succus entericus, which contains digestive enzymes. In the duodenum large amounts of mucus are secreted. This mucus normally serves as a protection against the highly acidic chyme that enters the duodenum.

B. The smooth muscle of the gastrointestinal tract is stimulated through the mesenteric plexus. A local reflex stimulation causing local secretion and peristalsis can result from localized irritation. Autonomic nerves cause changes in over-all secretion and peristalsis. Parasympathetic stimulation increases peristalsis and relaxes the pyloric and the ileocecal valves, whereas sympathetic stimulation decreases peristalsis and constricts the sphincters. Reverse peristalsis can occur when there is intestinal obstruction.

C. Bile, formed in the liver, is stored and concentrated in the gallbladder. The gallbladder, which lies underneath the liver, is a small sac with a smooth muscle wall lined with mucosa. The hepatic duct from the liver joins the cystic duct from the gallbladder, to become the common bile duct, which opens into the duodenum. Through hormonal action, the presence of fat in the duodenum causes contraction of the gallbladder, forcing bile down the cystic duct and into the common bile duct.

D. The pancreas is an exocrine and endocrine gland. Its exocrine secretions are necessary to complete digestion and to neutralize the hydrochloric acid in the chyme. The pancreatic juices empty into the duodenum.

4. During the aging process, several changes may take place to varying degrees. These include:

A. Changes in the mucous membrane of the mouth, which allow it to be traumatized more easily.

B. Decreased production of saliva.

C. Loss of teeth.

D. Achlorhydria.

E. General loss of smooth muscle tone and support of abdominal musculature.

Chewing and Swallowing of Food

1. In the process of mastication, food is broken down into smaller pieces that can be acted upon more easily by the digestive juices.

2. Chewing is accomplished by the up and down and lateral movements of the mandible. The tongue moves the food around in the mouth.

3. The salivary glands are stimulated to produce saliva by the presence of food in the mouth, and by seeing, smelling and thinking about food. Secretion is controlled by autonomic nerves. The saliva moistens the food, facilitates chewing and swallowing, and begins the digestion of starches.

4. Swallowing is accomplished by voluntary and involuntary actions. The tongue pushes food back to the pharynx. When food reaches the posterior pharynx it is carried to the stomach by both gravity

and the action of striated muscle, and then by the peristaltic movement of smooth muscle. A deglutition center is in the medulla.

5. The pressure of stomach contents against the cardiac sphincter can
   result in the regurgitation of food.

Digestion and Absorption of Food

1. Gastric movements mix the food with gastric juices and also cause
   the food to become semi-fluid, which allows more thorough enzymatic action in the small intestine. Gastric motility is first increased
   by distention and then decreased.

2. The rate at which food passes through the pyloric sphincter into the
   duodenum varies with:
   A. The size of the opening.
   B. The amount of gastric motility.
   C. The type of food. (Carbohydrates pass through most rapidly,
      then protein next; fatty foods take the longest time.)
   D. The consistency of the food. (The more liquid the food, the
      faster it passes through.)

3. The stomach is emptied 3½ to 4 hours after a normal-sized mixed
   meal.

4. Peristaltic movement causes the chyme to pass through the duodenum to the jejunum and to the ileum. The rate of the passage
   varies with:
   A. The motility of the tract.
   B. The opening of the ileocecal valve. (Emotional excitement and
      the swallowing of food increase the rate of opening.)

5. The time of digestion in the small intestine usually does not exceed
   2 to 4 hours.

6. Although the daily secretion of gastric juices varies greatly, the total
   amount of saliva, bile, pancreatic juice and gastric secretions produced by the adult totals about 3 L. in 24 hours. The total amount of
   intestinal secretions is also approximately 3 L. Most of these secretions are completely reabsorbed before they reach the large intestine.

7. The hydrolysis of carbohydrates is begun by the action of ptyalin in
   the saliva, but most of the hydrolysis of carbohydrates is accomplished by the action of enzymes in the pancreatic juice and the
   succus entericus.

8. The digestion of lipids is accomplished by the emulsification of fats
   by bile salts and the hydrolysis of fats, primarily by pancreatic
   lipase. The presence of food, especially fats, in the duodenum
   causes the secretion of a hormone that stimulates the gallbladder to
   contract.

9. The hydrolysis of proteins into amino acids is accomplished by the
   action of pepsin in the stomach, of proteolytic enzymes of the pan-

creatic juice, and of the succus entericus in the small intestine. Hydrochloric acid is essential for the activation of pepsin.

10. The blood supply to the digestive tract is increased during digestion and absorption. It is decreased during strenuous muscular activity and when certain emotions are experienced (e.g., fear).

11. Gagging can occur when there is nausea and as the result of mechanical stimulation of the pharynx or uvula. It can cause vomiting.

12. Vomiting is accomplished primarily by contractions of the abdominal muscles. Projectile vomiting is sudden and forceful and is not preceded by nausea. The vomiting of fecal material can occur when there is reverse peristalsis in the intestinal tract.

13. The vomiting center, located in the medulla, may be affected by such factors as:
   A. Afferent impulses from the stomach.
   B. Strong sensations (e.g., taste, smell, pain, or strong affective reactions such as rage).
   C. Afferent impulses from parts of the body concerned with equilibrium (e.g., eyes, cochlea or cerebellum).
   D. Pressure on the vomiting center itself.
   E. Some drugs.

Utilization of Nutrients by the Body

1. Metabolism is the sum of all the chemical reactions that occur in the body.
   A. Carbohydrate metabolism:
      (1) Carbohydrate metabolism is controlled by the interaction of a number of hormones (adrenal, anterior pituitary, thyroid and insulin).
      (2) The liver plays an important role in the metabolism of carbohydrates. Liver cells convert glucose to glycogen.
      (3) Although tissues primarily obtain energy from glucose, they are able to utilize, to a limited extent, amino acids and fatty acids for this purpose.
      (4) Excess glucose can be stored as fat in adipose tissue.
      (5) Glucose is an important constituent of many body tissues.
   B. Protein metabolism:
      (1) The proteins and the amino acids of the body are continually being interchanged, in the process of building and repairing cells, and in the formation of special substances such as enzymes, hormones and antibodies.
      (2) The adrenocortical hormones influence the utilization of amino acids throughout the body.
      (3) The plasma proteins are formed chiefly by the liver.
      (4) Amino acids cannot be stored to any extent; when they

are not utilized as such the body converts them to glucose and fat. The deaminization of the amino acids takes place in the liver.
   C. Fat metabolism:
      (1) Fatty acids and fats are utilized by the body in the formation of many of the body tissues (e.g., in brain and nervous tissue) and organic compounds (e.g., sterols), and as a source of energy (immediate and reserve).
      (2) The liver plays an important role in fat metabolism.
2. The metabolic rate is affected by such factors as:
   A. Muscular exercise.
   B. The body temperature.
   C. Epinephrine (limited).
   D. Thyroxine.

PHYSICS

1. Energy possessed by an object is the ability or capacity to do work. Heat is a form of energy.
2. A nutritional calorie is the amount of heat needed to raise the temperature of 1 Kg. of water (2.2 lbs.) 1° C.
3. Gravity is the force of attraction between two objects.

CHEMISTRY

1. Enzymes are organic catalysts.
2. The hydrolysis of food involves chemical breakdown into simpler substances by reaction with water.
3. Starch is a polysaccharide that can be hydrolyzed to the disaccharide, maltose.
4. Maltose, sucrose and lactose are disaccharides that can be hydrolyzed to monosaccharides.
   A. Maltose is hydrolyzed to glucose.
   B. Sucrose is hydrolyzed to glucose and fructose.
   C. Lactose is hydrolyzed to glucose and galactose.
5. Lipids are esters of fatty acids and glycerol or other alcohols. Simple lipids can be hydrolyzed to fatty acids and alcohols.
   A. The lowering of surface tension aids in the emulsification of lipids. The surface tension of water may be decreased by bile salts.
   B. Simple lipids include fats, oils and waxes.
   C. Compound lipids include phospholipids and glycolipids.
   D. Lipids are insoluble in water.
   E. Mineral oil is a hydrocarbon—not a lipid—and is not digestible.
6. Proteins are very complex molecules that always contain nitrogen; they may be hydrolyzed to polypeptides, to peptones and, finally, to amino acids.

7. Energy in the body is derived through complex biochemical reactions involving glucose, glycogen, and certain compounds containing phosphorus (adenosine triphosphate, adenosine diphosphate and phosphocreatine).

PATHOLOGY

Signs and Symptoms

Signs and symptoms of problems that may be related to nutrition include:

1. General indications:
   A. Unusual weight loss or gain.
   B. Weakness, inappropriate fatigue, faintness, apathy, loss of muscle tone.
   C. Anorexia, excessive hunger.
   D. Retarded growth, dental problems, poor wound healing.
   E. Nausea, vomiting, regurgitation, eructation.
   F. Abnormal stools (e.g., diarrhea, or stools containing undigested foodstuffs, blood, mucus, pus, fat).
   G. Jaundice.
   H. Excessive flatulence, abdominal distention, pot belly.
   I. Pain—epigastric distress, feeling of fullness, gnawing, burning, or aching pain, generalized abdominal tenderness, cramping.
   J. Lowered resistance to infection.
2. Specific indications:
   A. Vitamin deficiencies:
      (1) Vitamin A—dry, hardened epithelial tissue, night blindness, skin lesions.
      (2) Vitamin B—weakness, dizziness, nervousness, excessive irritability, mania, polyneuritis, muscle pain, lesions of skin or mucous membranes, abdominal discomfort, problems of anemia.
      (3) Vitamin C—bleeding tendency (e.g., gingivitis, ecchymosis), poor development of bones and teeth, poor wound healing.
      (4) Vitamin D—abnormal bone development.
      (5) Vitamin K—bleeding tendency.
   B. Mineral deficiencies:
      (1) Calcium—abnormal bone development, abnormal muscle contractions, bleeding tendency.
      (2) Sodium and potassium—signs and symptoms of electrolyte imbalance.
      (3) Iodine—signs and symptoms of hypothyroidism.
      (4) Iron—signs and symptoms of anemia.
   C. Lack of available glucose—headache, perspiration, pallor, faintness, muscular tremor, hunger, loss of consciousness.

D. Acute abdominal inflammation—generalized abdominal pain that may become localized, tense and tender abdominal musculature, possible nausea and vomiting, rapid pulse.

E. Perforation of gastrointestinal tract—sudden sharp pain, generalized pain and tenderness, tense abdominal muscles, rapid and shallow respirations, rapid and weak pulse, fall in blood pressure.

F. Obstruction of the intestinal tract—possibly vomiting (which may be projectile or may be fecal), acute pain, abdominal distention, constipation.

Malnutrition and Its Causes

1. Malnutrition is a highly complex condition in which the body's nutritional needs are not adequately met. Malnutrition may result from problems related to:
   A. The intake of food.
   B. The digestion and absorption of food.
   C. The utilization of food.
   D. The increased need for food.
   E. The loss of food from the body.
2. Problems related to the intake of food include:
   A. Dietary deficiencies:
      (1) Dietary deficiencies are related to the quantity and the quality of food eaten, and the times at which food is eaten.
      (2) Starvation is a condition of over-all deficiency of carbohydrates, proteins, fats, vitamins and minerals.
      (3) Kwashiorkor is a condition caused primarily by a deficiency of protein. It is manifested by such conditions as apathy, a general wasting, retarded growth, and cirrhosis of the liver.
      (4) Beri-beri is a condition caused primarily by a lack of thiamin chloride. It may be manifested by problems involving edema, or by neurological problems, which result from the degeneration of nerves.
      (5) Pellagra is a condition caused by a lack of B vitamins. It is manifested by problems involving the skin and mucous membranes, the digestive tract and the nervous system.
      (6) Scurvy is a condition caused by a lack of vitamin C. It is manifested by bleeding tendencies, usually appearing first in the gums.
      (7) Rickets is a condition caused by a lack of vitamin D. It is manifested by the abnormal calcification of osseous tissue.
   B. Obesity is a condition of overweight. The caloric intake is greater than the caloric requirement and the excess carbohydrate is stored as fat.

C. Anorexia and nausea:
  (1) Anorexia is a condition in which there is lack of desire for food. It may be caused by psychic problems, emotional upsets, the effect of drugs, the effects of certain disease conditions (frequently those associated with the gastrointestinal tract).
  (2) Nausea is a condition in which there is a feeling of revulsion toward food. It is usually associated with other symptoms, such as salivation, sweating and changes in heart rate. It may be caused by the same factors listed above for anorexia. Nausea may or may not precede vomiting; it can result from brain injury and from disturbances of equilibrium.
D. Difficulty in chewing and swallowing food:
  (1) Teeth may be painful because of dental caries. They may be lost because of various dental problems (e.g., periodontal disease, dental caries) or because of traumatic injury.
  (2) Stomatitis is an inflammation of the mouth that may be caused by such conditions as vitamin deficiencies, systemic diseases, local injury due to chemicals, excessive heat, and microorganisms (may be specific or opportunists). Vincent's angina is an ulceromembranous stomatitis caused by species of *Borrelia* and *Fusobacterium*.
  (3) Parotitis is an inflammation of the parotid glands that may result from inactivity (when one does not chew solid food), or by microorganisms (e.g., the virus of mumps or opportunists). There is a decreased production of saliva, swelling and discomfort. There may be a purulent exudate.
  (4) Cleft lip or cleft palate (or a combination) results from a failure of growth and union of the bony and soft tissue structures on one or both sides of the palate and upper jaw. It can cause feeding problems as well as problems of aspiration.
  (5) Inadequate chewing of food can result from abnormal growths within the mouth, traumatic injuries involving the jaw, or injury of nervous tissue innervating the muscles of the tongue and jaw.
  (6) Inadequate swallowing of food can result from injury to the muscles involved in swallowing, or injury to the nervous tissues that innervate these muscles (e.g., as in rabies, tetanus, paralysis). Lack of adequate saliva or inadequate chewing of food may also cause difficulty.
  (7) The normal passage of food through the esophagus and into the stomach may be prevented by such things as:
    (a) Spasms of the smooth muscle of the esophagus (may be due to nerve damage or emotional problems).
    (b) Abnormal growths within or without the esophagus.

    (c) Esophageal atresia (congenital), strictures (acquired through injury or inflammatory process), fistulas (congenital or acquired) or diverticuli (due to congenital weakness).

    (d) A diaphragmatic hernia.

3. Problems related to the digestion and absorption of food include:

A. Problems concerned with the functions of digestion and absorption.

    (1) Hyposecretion and/or abnormal peristalsis may result from emotional disturbances, inherited conditions, obstructions, injuries to the gastrointestinal tract, inadequate circulation, inadequate nutrition and abnormal growths.

    (2) The inflammatory response of the gastrointestinal tract to injury includes:

        (a) Active hyperemia, edema, congestion.

        (b) Decreased function or loss of function (secretion, peristalsis).

        (c) Increased peristalsis.

        (d) Production of inflammatory exudates (catarrhal, purulent, fibrous).

        (e) Destruction of tissue (erosion, ulceration).

    (3) Gastritis is an inflammation of the stomach lining. It may be caused by injury due to eating and drinking irritating foods, certain drugs, microorganisms or their toxins (e.g., the exotoxin of *Staphylococcus aureus*). Gastritis usually causes nausea and vomiting.

    (4) Peptic ulcer is a condition in which there is destruction of mucosa and possibly submucosa of the distal esophagus, the stomach or the duodenum. The gastric juices digest tissue that has been injured. The injury seems to be related to changes that have occurred in the blood supply and in the gastric secretions. These changes appear to be related to such things as emotional states, chemical injuries and traumatic injuries. The ulcer may be superficial or deep. If deep, it may cause bleeding (which may be severe) and perforation, spilling gastric contents into the abdominal cavity.

    (5) Pancreatitis is a condition in which the pancreas has been injured (e.g., by microorganisms); this results in the hyposecretion of pancreatic digestive juices.

    (6) Regional enteritis is a nonspecific inflammation of the small intestine in which there is ulceration and thickening of the walls with scar formation. This interferes with absorption and may result in perforation and the formation of fistulas and adhesions.

    (7) An inadequate supply of bile in the small intestine may be

the result of liver disease or obstruction of the bile ducts (e.g., because of calculi or inflammation). If the common bile duct is blocked, jaundice results. If the gallbladder is injured (e.g., due to the pressure of accumulating bile, infections or stones), there is congestion, swelling and possibly necrosis and perforation.

(8) Celiac disease is a chronic functional disorder which occurs early in childhood. It involves the inability to digest starch and to absorb fat. The etiology is questionable.

(9) An abnormal increase in peristalsis interferes with adequate digestion and absorption of food. An increase in peristalsis can result from injury to the intestinal tract (e.g., due to irritating chemicals, highly fibrous foods or microorganisms), or from excessive parasympathetic stimulation. Excessive nervous stimulation also causes relaxation of the pyloric valve, allowing chyme to enter the duodenum before gastric digestion has been completed. Poor absorption and diarrhea usually result.

   (a) Ulcerative colitis is an inflammatory disease of the colon in which there are ulcerations and the production of catarrhal, purulent and sanguinous exudates. It causes severe diarrhea, anorexia and sometimes vomiting. Perforation of the ulcers may occur. Possible causative factors include infections and emotional states.

   (b) Specific microorganisms invade the intestinal tract and often cause decreased absorption and diarrhea. These include species of *Salmonella* (food poisoning, paratyphoid fever and typhoid fever), species of *Shigella* (bacillary dysentery), *Vibrio comma* (cholera), *Entamoeba histolytica* (amebic dysentery) and viruses (intestinal influenza).

(10) The amount of absorption of the end products of digestion into the villi of the small intestines is limited by the condition of the mucosa. Any injury resulting in inflammatory response and possibly fibrosis interferes with absorption.

B. Problems concerned with obstructions within the gastrointestinal tract.

   (1) The passage of food from the stomach through the small intestine may be interfered with by such things as smooth muscle spasms, stenosis (congenital or acquired), decrease or absence of peristalsis, volvulus, intussusception, strangulated hernia or adhesions.

      (a) Pyloric stenosis is a condition that may be congenital or acquired through scarring. It generally causes projectile vomiting, and always interferes with the adequate digestion and absorption of food.

(b) Abnormal constriction of the pyloric valve may be caused by excessive sympathetic stimulation (e.g., as in fear).

(c) Smooth muscle spasms may be caused by injury to the intestinal tract and by excessive sympathetic stimulation.

(d) Peristalsis may be decreased or lacking due to such conditions as inadequate circulation (e.g., portal congestion, mesenteric thrombosis); pressure from abnormal growths or fluids in the abdominal cavity; marked distention due to the accumulation of undigested food or feces, or gases; injury to the mesenteric plexus; or injury to the intestines (e.g., abdominal surgery, peritonitis, intestinal inflammation). Intestinal obstruction may cause reverse peristalsis with fecal vomiting.

4. Problems related to the utilization of food include:

A. Liver disease.

(1) The metabolism of carbohydrates, fats and proteins, and the storage of some vitamins and minerals, as well as the production of bile, are affected by abnormal liver function. The liver may be injured by inadequate circulation, malnutrition, chemical injury, traumatic injury and microorganisms.

(2) Cirrhosis of the liver is a condition in which there is degeneration of liver cells. Injury to the liver has resulted in an increase in connective tissue and fibrosis—this interferes with the complex circulation of blood through the liver, which affects the liver cells and can cause portal venous congestion, with its many problems. When bile pigments are not eliminated in the bile they remain in the circulating blood and are distributed throughout the body in tissues and fluids (jaundice).

(3) Viral hepatitis is a liver infection that may be caused by different viruses. The viruses invade the liver cells, causing degeneration and possibly necrosis, fibrosis and atrophy.

(4) Liver abscesses result from infections or infestations caused by microorganisms that have found their way into the liver from the blood, abdominal organs or from traumatic injury. A frequent cause is the *Entamoeba histolytica*, which causes amebic dysentery.

B. Diabetes mellitus.

Diabetes mellitus is a metabolic disease involving the utilization of glucose (and subsequently protein and fat metabolism). The hormone, insulin, is involved. Heredity and obesity are predisposing factors. Because glucose cannot be metabolized properly, the tissues are deprived of glucose, which results in a breakdown of protein and fat as the body attempts to produce substances that it can use to produce energy. Because only small percentages of amino acids and fatty acids can be utilized to produce energy, the tissues still are deprived of an adequate source of energy.

5. Problems related to the increased need for food include:
   A. Fever (increased metabolic rate).
   B. Extensive tissue repair (e.g., with severe burns).
   C. Hyperthyroidism (increased metabolic rate).
6. Problems related to the loss of food from the body include:
   A. Vomiting.
      (1) Vomiting may occur as a result of emotional disturbances, an increase in intracranial pressure, the effect of drugs either on the brain or on the gastrointestinal tract, the effect of toxic substances produced by the body or by microorganisms, allergic response, obstructions in the gastrointestinal tract, gastric disorders, effects of pregnancy, and disturbances of equilibrium.
      (2) Hyperemesis gravidarum is a condition that occurs fairly early in pregnancy and involves pernicious vomiting. Emotional components appear to be involved.
   B. Diarrhea.
      Diarrhea may occur as a result of emotional disturbances, mechanical irritation, chemical irritation (e.g., drugs, foodstuffs), changes in the intestinal flora, allergic response, and specific intestinal diseases. The actual loss of food depends upon the cause of the problem, the part affected and the severity of the problem.

NURSING APPLICATIONS

Observation and Evaluation

1. All patients should be observed for signs and symptoms of inadequate nutrition; these should be evaluated, investigated, reported, and/or treated with appropriate nursing measures. This is of particular importance when the patient:
   A. Has a dietary intake that is inadequate to meet normal nutritional requirements.
   B. Has a condition in which there are increased nutritional requirements (e.g., pregnancy and lactation, extensive tissue repair, hyperthyroidism, fever).
   C. Has a condition that interferes with normal chewing and

swallowing of food (e.g., loss of consciousness, paralysis, loss of teeth).

D. Has a condition in which there is a continued loss of nutrients from the body (e.g., through vomiting, diarrhea, fistulas).

E. Has a disease condition or has sustained injury to tissues or organs involved with the digestion and absorption of food:
   (1) Salivary glands.
   (2) Stomach.
   (3) Small intestines.
   (4) Pancreas.
   (5) Liver and biliary system.

F. Has a condition in which there is inadequate utilization of food in the body (e.g., liver disease, diabetes mellitus and other endocrine disorders).

2. An individual's nutritional requirements should be evaluated in relation to such factors as:
   A. Age and normal growth patterns.
   B. Physical activity.
   C. Weight and body build.
   D. General physical condition.
   E. Pregnancy and lactation.
   F. Any diagnosed disease condition.

3. A patient's eating habits should be evaluated in relation to:
   A. The quality of food eaten.
   B. The *quantity* of the food eaten.
   C. Frequency of eating.
   D. Rate of eating.

4. Vomiting should be evaluated and reported in terms of:
   A. The characteristics of the vomiting:
      (1) Type (e.g., projectile, regurgitation).
      (2) Frequency.
      (3) Relation to ingestion of food, administration of drugs, emotional status.
   B. The characteristics of the vomitus:
      (1) Amount.
      (2) Color.
      (3) Consistency (e.g., watery, undigested food, bloody).
      (4) Odor.

5. Diarrhea should be evaluated and reported in terms of:
   A. Frequency of stools.
   B. Amount of stools.
   C. Consistency of stools (e.g., mucus, blood, undigested food, watery).
   D. Time of occurrence in relation to ingestion of food, drugs or emotional status.
   E. Associated discomforts (e.g., cramping).

Promoting Good Nutrition

Good nutrition can be promoted by:
1. Encouraging and providing (as possible) a well-balanced diet with a variety of properly prepared foods that are compatible with cultural and individual tastes.
2. Encouraging the proper chewing of food (e.g., providing good oral hygiene, adequate dental care).
3. Providing foods of appropriate consistency for chewing or swallowing abilities.
4. Feeding, by appropriate means, those who are unable to feed themselves.
5. Providing adequate time for eating.
6. Providing relaxation before, during and after meals.
7. Preventing (as possible) stress-producing situations (physical or emotional) at meal times.
8. Providing optimal positioning for comfort during and after eating (e.g., sitting position or right side).
9. Discouraging the intake of foods that are irritating (e.g., hot, spicy foods) or known to be upsetting to the individual.
10. Discouraging excessive smoking or drinking of alcoholic beverages.
11. Utilizing known methods for prevention of communicable enteric diseases, parasitic infections or "food poisoning."
12. Utilizing various methods for improving the appetite.
    A. A generally pleasant atmosphere and service of food may be helpful.
    B. The temperature and the seasoning of the food should be appropriate and according to individual tastes.
    C. Unpleasant sights, noises, odors should be eliminated.
    D. Physical discomforts should be alleviated as much as possible.
    E. The mouth should be as clean, moist and fresh-tasting as possible; this is particularly important when the patient:
       (1) Has been vomiting.
       (2) Has been raising sputum.
       (3) Has inflammation in the oral cavity.
       (4) Has decreased salivary secretions.
13. Avoiding prolonged intake of nonabsorbable oils (e.g., mineral oil) without medical supervision.

Combating Malnutrition

1. When a patient has avitaminosis (general or specific), foods containing the vitamins that are deficient should be encouraged (e.g., vitamin C for scurvey, B vitamins for beri-beri and pallagra). Exposure to ultraviolet rays should be provided when there is a deficiency of vitamin D.

2. When there are increased nutritional requirements (e.g., pregnancy, lactation, rapid physical growth, hyperthyroidism, fever, extensive tissue repair), the diet should include foods high in protein, calories, vitamins and minerals.
3. When a patient is underweight, an increased caloric intake should be encouraged; when overweight, the total caloric intake should be decreased.
4. If a patient has difficulty in chewing or swallowing (e.g., an infant, cleft palate, lack of teeth, oral inflammations, lack of saliva, esophageal strictures, oral surgery), or if these functions are impossible (e.g., unconsciousness, paralysis, fractured jaw, lack of esophagus) :
   A. The types and consistency of foods should be in keeping with chewing and swallowing abilities as well as with the condition of the mouth (e.g., acid foods should be avoided when there are open lesions).
   B. The mouth should be moist but free of abnormal or excessive secretions.
   C. Positioning should provide optimal swallowing (as possible).
   D. Appropriate dental care should be encouraged or provided.
   E. The quality of the food should be increased as the quantity is decreased.
   F. Special feeding methods may be used (e.g., bottle and nipple, medicine dropper, gavage, gastrostomy tube feedings).
5. Nausea, vomiting or regurgitation may be prevented or limited by:
   A. Controlling the cleanliness, type and amount of food or fluids ingested.
   B. Assisting the patient to belch air swallowed during feeding (e.g., through positioning and the pressure of stomach contents against the esophageal opening).
   C. Limiting physical activity, especially after eating.
   D. Avoiding motions conducive to nausea (e.g., rapid or frequent change of position).
   E. Avoiding contact with the uvula or posterior pharynx during treatments.
   F. Alleviating pain as much as possible.
   G. Avoiding exaggerated Trendelenburg position within 2 to 3 hours after meals (e.g., postural drainage).
   H. Discouraging or restricting the ingestion of food when there is unusual emotional or physical stress (e.g., pain, severe anxiety, labor).
   I. Restricting the ingestion of food or fluids when nausea or vomiting persists. (Small amounts of sweet, hot tea or carbonated beverages may be helpful).
   J. Eliminating unpleasant sights, sounds, odors or tastes.

K. Avoiding or limiting visual work (e.g., reading).

L. Being aware of possible emotional components and providing supportive care accordingly.

M. Administering anti-emetic or sedative drugs as indicated or ordered.

6. Diarrhea may be prevented or limited by:

    A. Controlling the cleanliness, type or amount of food or fluids ingested.

    B. Limiting physical activity, especially after meals.

    C. Avoiding mechanical stimulation of the rectum (e.g., taking oral temperature when diarrhea exists).

    D. Being aware of possible emotional components and giving supportive care accordingly.

    E. Administering anti-diarrheal or sedative drugs as indicated and ordered.

7. When chemical burns of the mouth and esophagus have been sustained (e.g., due to strong acids or alkalis):

    A. Immediate neutralization of the chemical should be attempted, if the appropriate neutralization agent is known and available.

    B. Large quantities of fluids should be swallowed (if swallowing is possible), and then vomiting should be induced (e.g., by tickling the uvula).

    C. Lavage equipment should be ready.

8. When there is interference with normal digestive and absorptive functions in the stomach and small intestines (e.g., gastritis, peptic ulcers, regional ileitis, fibrosis, ulcerative colitis, mesenteric thrombosis, pancreatitis, surgical removal of viscera and so forth):

    A. The diet, within medical orders, should be adapted to the individual's needs, tastes and tolerances.

        (1) When the lining of the tract is injured and inflamed,

            (a) Bland foods are desirable.

            (b) Foods or fluids that are excessively hot or cold, highly fibrous, chemically irritating (some spices, alcohol, coffee), or tend to stimulate the secretion of hydrochloric acid (e.g., acids, raw fruits) should be avoided.

            (c) Antacid preparations may be administered as needed and ordered.

        (2) Only gradual increases in the quantity, quality and consistency of foods should be made, according to toleration.

        (3) Foods known to contain a high content of nutrients that are especially important for the individual patient's disease condition should be encouraged (e.g., a diet high in calories, protein, vitamins and minerals when there is ulcerative colitis).

    B. Positioning should provide comfort.

C. More than usual sleep and rest should be encouraged.

D. Stress-producing situations (physical and emotional) should be prevented or controlled as possible.

E. Possible emotional components should be recognized and reported appropriately.

F. Emotional support should be consistent (e.g., this will be especially important when there is peptic ulcer, ulcerative colitis).

G. Smoking should be discouraged.

H. Close observations should be made for signs and symptoms of bleeding and perforation.

9. When signs and symptoms of perforation of the gastrointestinal tract occur (e.g., when there are ulcers or traumatic injury):

A. This is a medical emergency.

B. Food and fluids should be withheld.

C. Equipment for starting gastric suction should be ready.

D. The patient may be placed in low Fowler's position unless contraindicated by shock.

E. Emotional support should be consistent.

F. Arrangements may be begun for prompt surgical intervention.

10. When signs and symptoms of a mechanical obstruction within the intestinal tract occur (as in strangulated hernia, volvulus, pyloric stenosis, decreased or absent peristalsis):

A. This may be a medical emergency (depending upon degree of obstruction).

B. Food and fluids should be withheld prior to obtaining orders, after which diet orders should be followed specifically.

C. Equipment for starting gastric or intestinal suction should be ready.

D. Positioning should be determined by comfort or any respiratory distress.

E. Any bowel movements or sounds of peristalsis should be reported.

11. When there is interference with the production or storage of bile or with its transport into the small intestine (e.g., liver damage, inflamed gallbladder, obstructing stones):

A. The intake of fatty foods should be limited.

B. Close observations should be made for signs and symptoms of jaundice.

12. When there is a tube draining fluid from any part of the gastrointestinal tract or from accessory structures:

A. The amount and type of drainage should be reported and recorded appropriately.

B. Abnormal amounts or types of drainage should be reported promptly, and total or partial specimens saved.

C. The function of the tube should be maintained:

    (1) The tubing and amount of drainage should be checked frequently.

    (2) The tube should be irrigated (if ordered) with the appropriate amount and type of liquid as often as indicated and ordered.

D. If the tube becomes dislodged, it should be reported promptly. A gastric tube should not be manipulated or reinserted (if dislodged) following gastric or esophageal surgery.

E. If the tube is ordered closed for a period of time, it should be opened for drainage if untoward symptoms occur (e.g., distention, pain, nausea and vomiting), and this should be reported.

13. When there are signs and symptoms of hypoglycemia (e.g., in hyperinsulinism or lack of food) a ready source of glucose (e.g., corn syrup, orange juice, hard candies) should be given promptly. If oral administration is not possible, this is a medical emergency and equipment for the prompt administration of glucose should be ready.

14. When there is interference with normal carbohydrate metabolism, as in diabetes mellitus, medical supervision is essential and all orders pertaining to diet, urine testing and insulin (or insulin-like medications) must be followed carefully.

15. Injury to the liver may be prevented by such means as:

A. Encouraging a well-balanced diet (this is of particular importance when there is a problem of alcoholism).

B. Avoiding the inhalation of substances known to be injurious to the liver (e.g., certain solvents).

C. Discouraging the use of patent medicines without medical supervision.

16. When there is injury to the liver (e.g., cirrhosis):

A. The diet should be highly nutritional (protein, vitamins, minerals and low in fat).

B. More than usual sleep and rest should be provided.

4

Fluid Balance

Definite amounts of water are essential to maintain the fluid balance of the body.

ANATOMY AND PHYSIOLOGY

Fluid Balance in General

1. The adult body is about 60 per cent water; the newborn's about 75 per cent. About two thirds of this water is within the cells (intracellular) and one third is extracellular. Approximately one quarter of the extracellular water is found in the plasma (intravascular); the rest is in the interstitial fluid.
   A. Plasma is a complex mixture of water and many substances, including proteins, inorganic salts, lipids, glucose, waste products, vitamins, gases, enzymes, hormones and antibodies.
   B. With the exception of proteins, all these substances are able to diffuse through the capillary walls into the interstitial fluid freely, and from the interstitial fluid into the capillaries.
2. In health, water intake is balanced against water loss, and the many forces that influence the movement of water between compartments operate to maintain the amount of water necessary in each compartment.
3. Diffusion, dialysis and osmosis are important processes underlying the interchange of water and other substances between the cells and their environment, the regulation of blood volume and kidney function.
4. The amount of intravascular water and interstitial water can vary to a limited extent, but the amount of water required in the cells is definite and even minor changes can cause cell damage and impaired cellular activity.
5. The isotonicity of body fluids is maintained largely by the retention or the elimination of water and certain electrolytes (primarily sodium and potassium) and is regulated by kidney function.
   A. A loss of sodium is followed by a loss of water.
   B. The ingestion of sodium is followed by water retention.

6. The state of hydration of cells depends primarily upon the concentration of sodium ions in the extracellular fluid.
7. The amount of water in the interstitial fluid varies with:
    A. The filtration of water from the capillaries into the interstitial fluid. The filtration varies in relation to:
       (1) The rate of blood flow—an inverse relationship. (The slower the blood flow the greater the filtration.)
       (2) The pressure of blood in the capillaries—a direct relationship. (The higher the pressure the greater the filtration.)
       (3) Capillary dilatation—a direct relationship. (The greater the amount of blood in the capillaries the greater the filtration.)
       (4) The osmotic pressure of the blood, due to plasma proteins—an inverse relationship. (The lower the osmotic pressure the greater the filtration.)
       (5) The concentration of sodium ions in the interstitial fluid—a direct relationship. (The higher the concentration of sodium ions the greater the filtration.)
       (6) The concentration of proteins in the interstitial fluid—a direct relationship. (The higher the concentration of proteins the greater the filtration.)
    B. The return of water from the interstitial fluid to the blood. This return varies in relation to:
       (1) The drainage of interstitial fluid by the lymphatics—a direct relationship. (The less the flow of lymph, the less the return.)
       (2) The concentration of sodium ions in the plasma—an inverse relationship. (The lower the concentration of sodium in the plasma the less the return of water from the interstitial fluid into the plasma.)
       (3) The concentration of proteins in the plasma—an inverse relationship. (The lower the concentration of proteins in the plasma the less the return of water from the interstitial fluid into the plasma.)
8. The plasma proteins, albumin and globulin, serve to maintain the osmotic pressure of the blood.
    A. These proteins are produced mainly in the liver.
    B. Albumin exerts the greatest force.
    C. Because albumin has the smallest molecular weight, it is the first protein able to pass through a capillary that is injured or has become more permeable.
    D. The normal serum protein is between 6 to 8 Gm.%.
    E. The normal albumin/globulin ratio is 1.5:1 to 3:1.
9. Water is normally taken into the body by drinking liquids and eating foods (many of which are very high in water content). Some water is produced in the body as a by-product of biochemical reactions.

   A. Infants require at least 125 ml. of water/Kg. of body weight in 24 hours.

   B. Older children and adults may require from 1500 ml. to 3000 ml. every 24 hours.

   C. Thirst generally gives indication of the need to increase the intake of fluid.

10. The water in the gastrointestinal secretions is normally reabsorbed in the small intestines.

11. The primary function of the colon is the absorption of water from the intestinal contents.

12. Water is lost from the body through the lungs (vapor), the skin (sweat), the gastrointestinal tract (feces), and the kidneys (urine).

13. The older child or adult may lose somewhere between 1500 ml. and 3500 ml. of water in 24 hours.

   A. In a temperate climate and with moderate exercise and a normal fluid intake, the fluid loss would probably be about:

     (1) 1500 ml. of urine.

     (2) 500 to 1000 ml. of observable sweat and insensible perspiration.

     (3) 400 ml. of vapor from the lungs.

     (4) 150 ml. in the feces.

   B. The amount of water lost through the kidneys varies inversely with the amount lost through other routes.

   C. An increase in perspiration normally occurs when there is need of increased heat loss.

   D. No appreciable amount of interstitial fluid is lost through the normal skin, because of the continuous layers of keratinized epithelium.

The Production of Urine

1. The kidneys play a key role in fluid balance, electrolyte balance, acid-base balance and the excretion of wastes.

2. There are two kidneys; they lie in the posterior abdomen behind the peritoneum. They are held in place by pads of adipose tissue that surround them and by blood vessels that enter and leave the kidneys.

3. The nephron is the working unit of the kidney; it is composed of the renal corpuscle (glomerulus and Bowman's capsule) and the renal tubule. There are approximately one million nephrons in each kidney.

4. A difference in blood pressure between the afferent and efferent arterioles (leading into and away from the glomerulus) causes fluid to be forced from the glomerulus into the Bowman's capsule.

5. The resulting filtrate from the Bowman's capsule is essentially an aqueous solution of all the constituents of plasma, with the excep-

tion of the blood cells and the proteins. In the adult the filtrate amounts to about 200 L. in 24 hours. All but about 1½ L. are absorbed back into the blood by the renal tubules.

6. The walls of the renal tubules select those substances that the body needs from the glomerular filtrate; these are reabsorbed into the blood. The remainder is eliminated as urine.
   A. Passive reabsorption involves the simple diffusion of water and electrolytes.
   B. Active reabsorption requires work on the part of the tubules, and involves the reabsorption of substances from an area of a lesser concentration to one of a higher concentration.
   C. The tubular walls are also able to excrete small amounts of certain organic and inorganic substances which are in the blood (e.g., creatinine, potassium and some drugs) and ammonia.
7. The total volume of urine produced varies with the amount of glomerular filtration and the amount of tubular reabsorption.
   A. The amount of glomerular filtration varies directly with:
      (1) The amount of available filtering surface.
      (2) The blood pressure in the glomeruli.
      (3) The amount of renal blood flow.
      (4) The rate of tubular reabsorption.
   B. The amount of glomerular filtration varies inversely with the osmotic pressure exerted by the plasma proteins.
   C. The amount of tubular reabsorption of water varies directly with:
      (1) The amount of water in the blood.
      (2) The amount of antidiuretic factor secreted in the posterior lobe of the pituitary gland.
      (3) The amount of adrenocorticotropic hormone and/or adrenocortical hormone (associated with sodium loss and potassium retention).
   D. The amount of tubular reabsorption varies inversely with:
      (1) The rate of blood flow in the efferent capillaries.
      (2) The concentration of threshold substances in the tubules (e.g., glucose).
8. A definite amount of water is necessary for the excretion of nitrogenous waste products by the kidneys and for maintaining in solution various threshold substances (e.g., calcium may increase in amount when there are changes in bone metabolism).
9. The kidneys produce urine continuously at the average rate of 60 to 120 ml./hr. Variations from 25 to 500 ml./hr. may be considered just within safe limits. The newborn should start voiding within 24 to 36 hours after birth.
10. The volume of urine produced is influenced also by:
    A. The amount of fluid intake.
    B. The body temperature (the more perspiration, the less urine).

C. Emotional stress (changes in blood pressure affect urine production).

D. Pain (usually causes decrease in production).

E. Age. (Infants produce, for their weight, 3 to 4 times more urine than adults.)

F. Diuretics. (Some substances increase urine production by increasing the filtration rate or by decreasing tubular reabsorption. An example is caffeine.)

11. The urine produced in the nephrons collects in collecting tubules that lead to the calyces; it then empties into the pelvis of the kidney. The urine travels from the kidney pelvis to the urinary bladder through the ureters, both by gravity and by the peristaltic action of smooth muscle in the ureteral wall.

12. Urine, freshly voided, is usually pale yellow to light amber and clear with no sediment. Concentrated urine is dark and odorous.

13. The average range of specific gravity of urine is 1.010 to 1.030. Normally, the specific gravity goes down as the volume of urine increases.

14. In the aging process degenerative changes take place in the kidneys. Circulation may be impaired; the kidneys may become atrophied. Some of the nephrons may not function properly or at all. There may be fibrosis.

The Lymphatics

1. The lymphatic vessels transport lymph (interstitial fluid) from the interstitial spaces to the large veins of the neck. They originate as tiny capillaries and become larger and larger to eventually form two main vessels that empty directly into the circulating blood.

2. Lymph enters the lymphatic capillaries when the pressure of the interstitial fluid rises. Lymph flows through the lymphatic vessels by gravity, voluntary muscle contractions and the help of intrinsic valves.

Sweat

1. Sweat glands are distributed over the entire body. They produce sweat, a weak solution of sodium and other salts in water with small amounts of organic wastes (e.g., urea).

2. The secretion of sweat is primarily a heat-regulating mechanism, but it may occur as a result of emotional stress (e.g., anxiety states).

3. Sweat glands are under the control of autonomic nerves.

PHYSICS

1. Gravity is the force of attraction between two objects (e.g., the earth and an object on or near the earth).

2. Pressure is the force exerted on a unit area.

3. Liquids at rest exert pressure. The pressure exerted by a column of liquid in a container is equal to the height of the liquid times its weight per unit volume.
4. Fluids flow from an area of higher pressure to one of lower pressure, and the rate of volume flow is directly related to the pressure gradient.
5. Specific gravity is the weight of a substance compared with the weight of an equal volume of water. Specific gravity can be determined by dividing the weight of 1.0 ml. of fluid by the weight of 1.0 ml. of water—which is 1.0 Gm. A urinometer is used in determining the specific gravity of urine.

CHEMISTRY

1. A true solution is a liquid mixture of ions, atoms, or molecules of two or more substances in which there is apparent homogeneity.
   A. Water is by far the commonest and most useful solvent.
   B. The amounts of constituents in a solution may vary within certain limits.
2. Diffusion is a process in which, because of molecular motion, two or more substances (gases, liquids, or solids) become perfectly mixed.
3. Osmosis is the process whereby the molecules of a solvent pass through a semi-permeable membrane from the area of lesser to greater concentration of the solute.
   A. A semi-permeable membrane is one that shows selective action with regard to the passage of different substances through it.
   B. Solvent molecules pass through the semi-permeable membrane, because of osmosis, until the pressure exerted on the side of the formerly stronger solution is great enough to establish a state of equilibrium. The amount of pressure necessary to prevent the flow of solvent molecules across the membrane is called the osmotic pressure of the solution. (The greater the difference between the concentrations of the solutions on either side of the membrane, the greater the osmotic pressure will be).
   C. An isotonic solution is one that exerts the same osmotic pressure as a solution on the other side of a semi-permeable membrane.
      (1) A hypotonic solution has less osmotic pressure, so the solvent passes through the membrane to the more concentrated solution on the opposite side.
      (2) A hypertonic solution has a higher osmotic pressure, so the solvent of the less concentrated solution passes through the membrane to the hypertonic side.
      (3) Physiological saline solution (isotonic with body fluids) is

approximately a 0.9 per cent aqueous solution of sodium chloride.
4. Dialysis is the process wherein simple molecules or ions pass through a permeable membrane. (The size of the molecules allowed to pass through depends upon the permeability of the membrane).

PATHOLOGY

Signs and Symptoms

Signs and symptoms of fluid imbalance include those related to dehydration and edema.
1. Signs and symptoms related to dehydration include:
   A. Thirst, dysphagia.
   B. Dry skin and mucous membranes, thick secretions.
   C. Constipation.
   D. Fever.
   E. Loss of weight.
   F. Oliguria with highly concentrated urine.
   G. Weakness, faintness, exhaustion and collapse.
   H. Fall in blood pressure accompanied by weak and rapid pulse.
2. Signs and symptoms related to edema include:
   A. Weight gain.
   B. Swelling of subcutaneous tissues (generalized, dependent, facial).
   C. Abdominal distention (ascites).
   D. Those related to laryngeal edema and pulmonary edema. (See Chap. 2).
   E. Those related to cerebral edema (increased intracranial pressure —headache, behavioral changes, convulsions, changes in vital signs).
   F. Those related to dehydration (if edema is severe).
3. Signs and symptoms of renal disease may include those of edema and/or dehydration, plus:
   A. Anorexia, nausea and vomiting.
   B. Weakness, pallor.
   C. Hematuria, pyuria, abnormal specific gravities of urine.
   D. Nocturia, oliguria and anuria.

Dehydration

Dehydration is a condition in which there is fluid imbalance involving the loss of water from plasma, interstitial fluid and/or cells.
1. Possible causes of dehydration include:
   A. Inadequate intake of fluid (e.g., because it is not available, inability to swallow or presence of nausea).
   B. Inadequate absorption of water from the intestinal tract (e.g., in certain intestinal disorders).

    C. Loss of fluid from the gastrointestinal tract (e.g., with vomiting, diarrhea, fistulas).

    D. Excessive perspiration.

    E. Loss of blood or plasma from wounds, burns, and so forth.

    F. Inadequate absorption of water or excessive excretion of water in kidneys (e.g., in electrolyte imbalance, hormonal imbalance, renal disease).

    G. Severe edema.

2. Specific problems involving excessive fluid loss include:

    A. Excessive perspiration.

    This may occur as a result of the body's attempt to increase heat loss (e.g., when there is high external temperature or fever) or when there is excessive stimulation of the sympathetic nervous system (e.g., in certain anxiety states).

    B. Third degree burns.

    Burns may be caused by such things as heat, radiation, electricity and certain chemicals (e.g., strong acids or alkalis). In a third degree burn all layers of the skin are destroyed; tissue fluid leaks into the injured area and plasma escapes from injured capillaries. If burns are extensive, large amounts of plasma may be lost from the blood, leading to hemoconcentration and hypotension.

    C. Diabetes insipidus.

    Diabetes insipidus is a condition in which a decreased production of anti-diuretic hormone by the posterior lobe of the pituitary gland results in marked diuresis.

    D. Uncontrolled diabetes mellitus.

    Diabetes mellitus can cause excessive loss of water through the kidneys. When there is glycosuria, water normally reabsorbed by the renal tubules is decreased; this causes greater dilution of the glucose in the urine.

    E. Decreased secretion of adrenocortical hormones or adrenocorticotropic hormone.

    A decrease in these hormones interferes with the normal reabsorption of water in the renal tubules.

Edema

Edema is the excessive accumulation of fluid in the interstitial spaces. It may be generalized or local; occurring in loose areolar tissue, the lungs, the brain, the abdominal cavity, and so forth. Dependent edema is seen as an effect of gravity. Edema helps to dilute toxins in the interstitial fluid and protects the cells from electrolyte imbalance. The bad effects of edema depend upon the extent of the fluid loss from the plasma, the location of the edema, and the amount of edema. Excessive interstitial fluid interferes with the transfer of substances between the blood and the cells.

1. Possible causes of edema include:
    A. Increased capillary permeability (e.g., due to anoxia, allergic response, inflammatory response, trauma, nutritional deficiencies).
    B. Decreased osmotic pressure of plasma due to decrease in plasma proteins (e.g., in burns, nutritional deficiency, liver disease or renal disease).
    C. Obstructions of lymphatic drainage (e.g., by abnormal growths, radical surgery, filariasis).
2. Specific problems involving the accumulation of interstitial fluid include:
    A. Heart failure.
        In congestive heart failure, increased venous pressure increases filtration pressure in the capillaries. Sodium retention is also a problem. Both cause the accumulation of interstitial fluid. The rate of accumulation is greater than that at which the lymphatics can carry it away. The resulting edema is generalized and dependent.
    B. Inflammations.
        When there is injury to the body (e.g., due to second degree burns, certain chemicals such as histamine in allergic response or microorganisms), capillaries may be damaged directly, allowing plasma proteins and blood cells to pass into the interstitial fluid. Inflammatory response results in increased capillary permeability, which allows the escape of plasma proteins. The resultant decrease in the osmotic pressure in the capillaries and the increase of filtration pressure due to hyperemia lead to edema. Reduction in the flow of lymph may be involved also. If the edema is extensive, hemoconcentration and hypotension can follow.
    C. Edema associated with starvation.
        Starvation edema generally involves the accumulation of tissue fluid in the abdominal cavity. Both protein deficiency and sodium retention seem to be causative factors.
    D. Ascites.
        Ascites, the accumulation of interstitial fluid in the abdominal cavity, may occur when there is generalized edema or as a direct result of conditions such as cirrhosis of the liver. When there is cirrhosis of the liver (see Chap. 3), the filtration pressure in the capillaries increases because of portal venous congestion. There is retention of sodium and water due to liver dysfunction and there is a decrease in the osmotic pressure because of a decrease in the production of plasma proteins by the liver.

E. Lymphedema.

Lymphedema involves the accumulation of lymph in the subcutaneous tissue because of obstruction of the lymphatic vessels. The obstruction is usually acquired and may be caused by abnormal growths, surgical procedures, inflammatory reactions that involve scarring, and parasites. Filariasis is a parasitic infestation in which the adult round worms present in lymph channels block the flow of lymph. When the worms die they become calcified and may cause permanent blockage. If the majority of lymph channels of the lower extremities are affected, elephantiasis may develop.

F. Myxedema.

Myxedema occurs when there is a long deficiency of thyroxine. Tissue metabolism is altered and an increase in the osmotic pressure of interstitial fluid results in a general shift of water from the plasma into the interstitial spaces. The resulting edema is usually not severe.

Water Intoxication

Water intoxication involves having an excessive amount of water in the body. It may occur when there is a loss of electrolytes from the body or when there is an intake of too much water (which dilutes the electrolytes). The ultimate result is an increase in intracellular fluid, which interferes with normal cellular function.

Renal Disease

Renal disease may cause not only fluid imbalance, but other problems related to inadequate kidney function (e.g., electrolyte imbalance, acid-base imbalance and uremia).

1. Fluid imbalance occurs as a result of increased capillary permeability, sodium retention, increased filtration pressure and hypoproteinemia.
2. Renal failure may be due to:
   A. Nephron damage caused by:
      (1) Infections.
      (2) Mechanical obstructions of ureters or renal pelvis.
      (3) Cyst formations.
      (4) Certain poisons, toxins (e.g., hemoglobin when incompatible blood transfusions are given).
      (5) Certain drugs that are excreted by the kidney.
   B. An inadequate blood supply caused by:
      (1) Nephrosclerosis.
      (2) Thrombi, emboli.
      (3) Hypotension.
      (4) Problems related to toxemias of pregnancy.

3. Glomerulo-nephritis is an inflammatory condition that involves the glomeruli. It is usually preceded by an upper respiratory infection involving *Streptococcus hemolyticus.* The onset may be sudden or slow. Damaged glomeruli allow blood cells and plasma proteins to enter the renal tubules and be excreted in the urine. Chronic nephritis is extremely serious and usually leads to renal failure.

4. Pyelitis and pyelonephritis are inflammatory processes usually caused by microorganisms (frequently *Streptococcus* and *Escherichia coli*). The inflammation can cause local congestion, swelling, production of exudates, tissue destruction and fibrosis.

5. Hydronephrosis is a condition in which there is dilatation of the kidney pelvis. It is caused by an obstruction in the upper urinary tract that causes an accumulation of urine in the kidney pelvis. Tissues are stretched and there is hyperperistalsis of the smooth muscle of the ureter. Obstructions may be caused by calculi, abnormal growths, ureteral constriction and nephroptosis.

6. Polycystic kidney is a familial disease in which there is multiple cyst formation in both kidneys. These interfere with kidney function and renal failure usually ensues.

7. Nephrosclerosis is a condition in which there is narrowing of the renal arterial blood vessels. The decrease in blood flow interferes with normal kidney functioning. When severe it results in necrosis and various degrees of renal failure.

8. The nephrotic syndrome is peculiar to young children. It is characterized by generalized and extensive edema, albuminuria and hypoproteinemia.

9. The toxemias of pregnancy are characterized by generalized and dependent edema. Several factors seem to be involved. These include:
   A. An increase in filtration pressure in the general circulation and in the pelvic area in particular.
   B. a decrease in plasma albumin and albuminuria.
   C. Renal retention of sodium (probably due to effect of hormones).

NURSING APPLICATIONS

Observation and Evaluation

1. Patients should be observed for signs and symptoms of fluid imbalance (dehydration and edema); these should be evaluated, investigated, reported and/or treated with appropriate nursing measures. This is of particular importance when the patient:
   A. Has a condition in which the pressure and volume of circulating blood is not within normal limits. (See Chap. 1.)

B. Has a condition in which there is an abnormal loss of fluid from the gastrointestinal tract or the skin.
C. Has renal disease.
D. Has liver disease.
E. Has a condition involving hormones that directly or indirectly affect fluid and/or electrolyte balance (e.g., pituitary hormones adrenocortical hormones, insulin, thyroxine).
F. Is pregnant.
G. Is at extremes of age.
2. A patient's fluid intake should be evaluated in relation to:
A. The urinary output.
B. Age.
C. Physical activity.
D. The type of diet.
E. Any unusual loss of fluid through the skin or from the gastro-intestinal tract.
F. The patient's state of hydration.
G. The diagnosed disease condition.
3. A patient's urinary output should be evaluated in relation to:
A. The amount of urine that the kidneys should excrete within a given period of time.
B. The fluid intake.
C. Age.
D. The patient's state of hydration.
E. The time of output in relation to the amount.
F. Any excessive loss of fluid (other than urine).
G. The environmental temperature.
H. The patient's emotional state.
I. Any diuretic drugs acting on the patient.
4. A patient's urine may be evaluated in relation to:
A. The amount.
B. The color and transparency.
C. The odor.
D. The presence of sediment.
E. The specific gravity.
F. The presence of abnormal substances (e.g., blood, pus).

Promoting Fluid Balance

Fluid balance may be promoted by:
1. Providing for oral fluid intake (according to individual needs) during waking hours.
2. Observing for and reporting appropriately any abnormalities in fluid intake or fluid loss.
3. Measuring and reporting accurately fluid intake and fluid loss when the patient has a potential fluid imbalance.

A. When a patient has a tube draining fluid from the body into a container, the drainage should be measured and reported appropriately.

B. Accurate measurements (whenever possible) and estimated descriptions (when necessary) of fluid loss (e.g., perspiration, vomitus, stools, fluids that have been aspirated or drained, or that have escaped from the body) should be made and reported appropriately.

4. Encouraging oral fluids when there has been or is excessive fluid loss (unless contraindicated by such conditions as nausea and vomiting or impared kidney or heart function).

5. Encouraging the additional intake of sodium chloride along with oral fluids when there has been or is excessive perspiration.

6. Discouraging the "forcing" of fluids beyond an amount specified by medical orders.

7. Encouraging women who are pregnant to have medical supervision throughout their pregnancies.

8. Discouraging the excessive use of saline cathartics.

Combating Fluid Imbalance

1. When there is a problem of fluid imbalance, the patient should be observed closely for signs and symptoms of electrolyte imbalance, acid-base imbalance and/or uremia. (See Chap. 5, 6, and 7.)

2. When there is a problem of dehydration (e.g., due to uncontrolled diabetes mellitus, extensive burns, excessive vomiting or diarrhea):

A. Accurate measurements of fluid intake and loss should be made and reported appropriately.

B. Oral fluids should be encouraged (unless contraindicated).

C. Equipment for the administration of parenteral fluids should be ready. Plasma or plasma expanders should be available when plasma proteins are lost.

D. Careful observations should be made for signs and symptoms of circulatory failure. (See Chap. 1.)

3. When there is a problem of edema (e.g., due to congestive heart failure, generalized allergic response or nephrotic syndrome):

A. Accurate measurements of fluid intake and loss should be made and reported appropriately.

B. Accurate measurements of daily weights may be indicated.

C. The intake of sodium may be restricted and, if so, the patient should follow any medical orders specifically.

D. Medical orders relative to the amount and type of fluid intake should be followed exactly.

E. The rate of flow of any parenteral fluids should be controlled within specified limits.

F. Careful observations should be made for signs and symptoms of cerebral edema, pulmonary edema, laryngeal edema, local infections and circulatory failure.

   (1) Cerebral edema represents a medical emergency, and equipment for the prompt administration of appropriate diuretic drugs should be ready.

Circulatory failure is included in Chap. 1; pulmonary edema and laryngeal edema, in Chap. 2; and infections, in Chap. 20.

4. Potential injury to the kidneys may be prevented by:
   A. Observing for, evaluating, reporting and treating appropriately hypotension that may accompany surgery, extensive burns, severe trauma or hemorrhage.
   B. Observing for, reporting and taking appropriate action relative to signs and symptoms of transfusion reactions (see Chap. 1).
   C. Encouraging adequate medical supervision when there are acute or repeated upper respiratory infections.
   D. Changing the position of a bedridden patient frequently.
   E. Encouraging and providing adequate fluid intake to meet individual needs.
   F. Providing regular exercise, active or passive, whenever possible when there is inactivity or immobilization of body parts.
   G. Providing for effective and safe catheter care (e.g., checking for and maintaining patency, maintaining adequate drainage, maintaining sterility or cleanliness as indicated).

5. When injury to the kidney has occurred (e.g., in acute glomerulonephritis, nephrotic syndrome, hydronephrosis, nephrosclerosis):
   A. Accurate measurements of fluid intake and loss should be made and reported appropriately.
   B. Medical orders relative to the amount, type and rate of fluid intake should be followed exactly.
   C. Dietary orders (e.g., regarding sodium restrictions or protein intake) should be followed exactly.
   D. Infections should be prevented.
   E. More than usual sleep and rest should be provided.
   F. Physical activity should be limited to avoid fatigue.
   G. The patient should be observed closely for signs and symptoms of electrolyte imbalance, acid-base imbalance and uremia. (See Chap. 5, 6 and 7.)

5

Electrolyte Balance

All the cells of the body require definite amounts of certain electrolytes for efficient functioning.

ANATOMY AND PHYSIOLOGY

1. Electrolytes play an essential role in metabolic processes. Electrolytes:
   A. Contribute to proper osmotic pressure relationships.
   B. Provide buffer systems and mechanisms for regulating acid-base balance.
   C. Provide proper ionic balance for normal tissue irritability and function.
   D. Often act as enzyme activators.
2. The body fluids normally maintain an osmotic pressure of about 0.9 per cent sodium chloride. Change of this osmotic pressure can result in overhydration or dehydration of the cells.
3. Electrolytes are distributed in all the body fluids.
   A. The primary cations are sodium, potassium, calcium and magnesium.
      (1) The primary extracellular cation is sodium.
      (2) The primary intracellular cation is potassium.
   B. The primary anions are chloride, bicarbonate, dihydrogen phosphate, sulfate and protein.
      (1) The primary extracellular anions are chloride and bicarbonate.
      (2) The primary intracellular anions are bicarbonate and proteins.
4. Proper concentrations of intracellular potassium and extracellular sodium are essential to fluid balance and acid-base balance.
5. Kidney function plays a key role in electrolyte balance through:
   A. The retention or elimination of water.
   B. The tubular reabsorption of electrolytes.
   C. The tubular excretion of potassium.
   D. The substitution of ammonium ion for sodium ion when sodium is needed by the body. (See Chap. 4.)

6. The tubular reabsorption of sodium, potassium and chlorides is influenced by adrenocortical hormones. (See Chap. 8.)
7. Electrolytes are lost normally through the urine, although fairly large amounts of sodium chloride can be lost if there is excessive sweat production.
8. The body normally requires a daily intake of sodium. An increase in sweat increases this requirement.
9. Proper concentration of calcium is essential to blood coagulation, bone metabolism, cardiac rhymthicity, normal neuromuscular irritability and membrane permeability.

CHEMISTRY

1. An ion is a charged atom or group of atoms, caused by gain or loss of electrons.
   A. Strongly electro-positive elements form positive ions (e.g., potassium, sodium, calcium, magnesium).
   B. Strongly electro-negative elements form negative ions (e.g., fluorine, oxygen, chlorine).
2. Electrolytes are electrovalent compounds that, in solution, form ions and conduct electricity.
   A. Positively-charged ions are attracted to the negative pole, or cathode, and are called cations.
   B. Negatively-charged ions are attracted to the positive pole, or anode, and are called anions.
3. Osmosis is the process whereby the molecules of a solvent pass through a semi-permeable membrane from the area of lesser to the area of greater concentration of the solute.
   A. A semi-permeable membrane is one that shows selective action with regard to the passage of different substances through it.
   B. Solvent molecules pass through the semi-permeable membrane, because of osmosis, until the pressure exerted on the side of the formerly stronger solution is great enough to establish a state of equilibrium. The amount of pressure necessary to prevent the flow of solvent molecules across the membrane is called the osmotic pressure of the solution. (The greater the difference between the concentrations of the solutions of either side of the membrane, the greater is the osmotic pressure.)
   C. An isotonic solution is one that exerts the same osmotic pressure as a solution on the other side of a semi-permeable membrane.
      (1) A hypotonic solution has less osmotic pressure, so the solvent passes through the membrane to the more concentrated solution on the opposite side.
      (2) A hypertonic solution has a higher osmotic pressure, so the solvent of the more dilute solution passes through the membrane to the hypertonic side.

(3) Physiological saline solution (isotonic with body fluids) is approximately a 0.9 per cent aqueous solution of sodium chloride.

PATHOLOGY

Signs and Symptoms

1. Signs and symptoms of sodium deficiency include:
   A. Weakness, hypotension, headache.
   B. Vomiting, diarrhea.
   C. Muscle cramping, spasms and convulsions.
   D. Peripheral vascular collapse.
   (Pathology related to excess sodium (edema) is included in Chap. 4.)
2. Signs and symptoms of potassium deficiency include:
   A. Apathy, mental confusion.
   B. Muscle weakness (which may involve respiratory muscles).
   C. Changes in cardiac action.
3. Signs and symptoms of excess potassium include:
   A. Weakness, muscle flaccidity.
   B. Mental confusion.
   C. Feeling of numbness in extremities.
   D. Peripheral muscular collapse.
4. Signs and symptoms of calcium deficiency include:
   A. Numbness in extremities.
   B. Excessive irritability.
   C. Muscle twitchings, tetany, convulsions.
   (Pathology related to chlorides and bicarbonates is included in Chap. 6.)

Electrolyte Imbalance and Its Causes

1. Fluid imbalance and electrolyte imbalance are interrelated.
   A. Because water in the body is in solution, shifts of water between fluid compartments or loss of water are accompanied by shifts or loss of electrolytes.
   B. Because electrolytes are in aqueous solution, shifts of electrolytes between fluid compartments or loss of electrolytes are accompanied by shifts or loss of water.
2. Sodium deficiency may occur when there is:
   A. Inadequate dietary intake to replace daily loss of sodium.
   B. Renal disease. (See Chap. 4.)
   C. Excessive loss of gastric juices or prolonged diarrhea. (See Chap. 3.)
   D. Acid-base imbalance. (See Chap. 6.)
   E. Adrenocortical hormone imbalance. (See Chap. 8.)

3. Low salt syndrome occurs when, during excessive sweating, the water loss is replaced by water intake but the salt loss is not replaced adequately.
4. Potassium deficiency may occur when there is:
    A. Inadequate dietary intake.
    B. Excessive tissue destruction.
    C. Fluid imbalance. (See Chap. 4.)
    D. Adrenocortical hormone imbalance. (See Chap. 8.)
    E. Sodium deficiency.
5. When there is excessive tissue destruction (e.g., severe burns), damaged cells lose potassium. Sodium enters the cells to replace the potassium and normal cellular metabolism is no longer possible.
6. When there is a deficiency of sodium in the interstitial fluid, potassium shifts from the intracellular to the interstitial fluid in an attempt to provide ionic balance on either side of the cell membrane.
7. Potassium excess may occur when there is:
    A. Renal disease. (See Chap. 4.)
    B. Adrenocortical hormone imbalance. (See Chap. 8.)
8. Calcium deficiency may occur when there is:
    A. Inadequate dietary intake (especially during pregnancy, lactation and periods of rapid bone growth).
    B. Abnormal bone metabolism, which may be due to such things as:
        (1) Prolonged physical inactivity. (See Chap. 11.)
        (2) Vitamin D deficiency. (See Chap. 3.)
        (3) Hypoparathyroidism. (See Chap. 8.)

NURSING APPLICATIONS

1. Patients should be observed for signs and symptoms of electrolyte imbalance; these should be evaluated, investigated, reported and/or treated with appropriate nursing measures. This is of particular importance when the patient:
    A. Has fluid imbalance or potential fluid imbalance. (See Chap. 4.)
    B. Has malnutrition. (See Chap. 3.)
    C. Has a condition involving:
        (1) Renal function. (See Chap. 4.)
        (2) Adrenocortical hormones. (See Chap. 8.)
        (3) Parathyroid hormone. (See Chap. 8.)
2. Electrolyte imbalance may be prevented by:
    A. Encouraging and providing for good nutrition. (See Chap. 3.)
    B. Promoting fluid balance. (See Chap. 4.)
    C. Taking action to prevent excessive vomiting and/or diarrhea. (See Chap. 3.)
    D. Restricting oral intake of fluid when gastric contents are being removed continuously by suction or by vomiting.

3. When a patient has electrolyte imbalance involving sodium and potassium (e.g., in severe burns, diabetic acidosis, malnutrition, lack of adrenocortical hormone):

   A. Medical orders relative to diet and fluid intake must be followed carefully.

   B. Accurate measurements (time and amount) of fluid intake and fluid loss must be made, evaluated and reported appropriately. (See Chap. 4.)

   C. Careful observations should be made for signs and symptoms of fluid imbalance, more advanced electrolyte imbalance and acid-base imbalance.

4. When a patient has potassium intoxication (e.g., in renal failure), any enemas or colonic irrigations used to interfere with potassium absorption in the intestines must be performed with the utmost effectiveness.

5. Direct injury to body cells can be prevented by the use of isotonic solutions when performing treatments (e.g., irrigations).

6

Acid-Base Balance

All the cells of the body require a definite pH environment.

ANATOMY AND PHYSIOLOGY

1. Normal cellular functioning requires an environment with a pH
   value of about 7.4.
   A. Variations of even a few tenths may be fatal.
   B. To maintain this nearly neutral pH, the basic and acid elements
      of the body fluids must balance.
2. The proper pH of body fluids is maintained by:
   A. The buffering action of various buffer systems, such as those
      composed of:
      (1) Phosphate.
      (2) Bicarbonate.
      (3) Protein.
   B. The elimination of carbon dioxide in the lungs.
   C. The elimination or retention of certain electrolytes by the kidneys.
3. The pH of the plasma depends upon the ratio between the amount
   of carbonic acid and the amount of sodium bicarbonate. Rapid
   adjustment of this ratio may be brought about by changes in the
   rate and depth of respiration, by certain compensatory chemical
   shifts in the blood, and by the elimination or retention of certain
   electrolytes (e.g., bicarbonate, chlorides) by the kidneys.
4. The alkali reserve represents the amount of base in the blood that is
   available for the neutralization of fixed acids (e.g., lactic acid,
   hydrochloric acid). Practically all estimations of acid-base balance
   are based upon the analysis of the bicarbonate buffer system.
5. Hydrochloric acid is produced by gastric glands.
6. The intestinal digestive juices (succus entericus, pancreatic juice
   and bile) are all highly alkaline.

PATHOLOGY

Signs and Symptoms

1. Signs and symptoms of a decrease in the alkaline reserve of the
   blood may include:

   A. Signs and symptoms of dehydration. (See Chap. 4.)

   B. Signs and symptoms of electrolyte imbalance. (See Chap. 5.)

   C. Deep and rapid respirations (forced breathing).

   D. Loss of consciousness.

   E. Odor of acetone in breath (when there is impaired carbohydrate metabolism).

2. Signs and symptoms of an increase in the alkaline reserve of the blood may include:

   A. Signs and symptoms of dehydration.

   B. Signs and symptoms of electrolyte imbalance.

   C. Loss of consciousness.

   D. Excessive neuromuscular irritability, muscle twitchings, convulsions (when there has been excessive loss of gastric secretions).

Decreased Alkaline Reserve

1. A decrease in the alkaline reserve of the blood is sometimes referred to as decreased alkalinity or as acidosis. In severe cases the pH of the blood actually does become lower and it may, in rare instances, fall just below 7.0. Such a variation in pH is almost without exception incompatible with life.

2. A decrease in the alkaline reserve of the blood may occur when there is:

   A. Excessive intake of highly acid foods or drugs.

   B. Inadequate intake of alkaline foods.

   C. An abnormal loss of bicarbonate from the body through loss of the intestinal digestive juices. (See Chap. 3.)

   D. Renal failure. (See Chap. 4.)

   E. Inadequate carbohydrate metabolism. (See Chap. 3.)

3. Problems that may cause inadequate carbohydrate metabolism include:

   A. Starvation (this includes low carbohydrate diets).

   B. Loss of food through vomiting, diarrhea, draining fistulas.

   C. Uncontrolled diabetes mellitus.

4. When it is necessary for fatty acids to be oxidized for energy (instead of glucose), acetoacetic acid, beta-hydroxybutyric acid and acetone are formed. The neutralization of these acids reduces the alkaline reserve. The more acids produced, the more depleted the alkaline reserve. Acetone is eliminated both in the urine and through the lungs.

5. When there is a decrease in the alkaline reserve of the blood:

   A. The urine becomes more acid (pH less than 5) as chlorides and other acid substances are eliminated.

   B. The amount of blood bicarbonate decreases as it is used to neutralize acidic substances; it is eliminated in urine.

   C. Sodium is lost in the urine. When there is renal failure, this happens more quickly because the kidney is unable to substitute ammonium ions for the sodium ions.

D. Diuresis occurs as a direct result of the increased requirements for elimination and the loss of sodium.

E. The changed ratio between carbonic acid and bicarbonate in the blood stimulates the respiratory center. Rapid, deep respirations result as the body attempts to rid itself of carbon dioxide and re-establish a balance between the carbonic acid and bicarbonate.

F. Loss of consciousness results when the decrease in blood alkalinity is marked enough to cause injury to the brain cells.

Increased Alkaline Reserve

1. An increase in the alkaline reserve of the blood is sometimes referred to as increased alkalinity or alkalosis. In severe cases the pH of the blood may actually rise as high as 7.8. Such a variation in pH is almost always incompatible with life.

2. An increase in the alkaline reserve of the blood may occur when there is:
   A. Excessive intake of highly alkaline foods or drugs.
   B. Inadequate intake of acid foods.
   C. An abnormal loss of chlorides from the body through loss of gastric juices. (See Chap. 3.)
   D. Renal failure. (See Chap. 4.)

3. When there is an increase in the alkaline reserve of the blood:
   A. The urine becomes more alkaline (pH more than 7.4) as the kidneys excrete more bicarbonate.
   B. The increased elimination of sodium results in diuresis.
   C. The changed ratio between carbonic acid and bicarbonate in the blood depresses the respiratory center and slow, shallow respirations result. There may be periods of apnea and then hyperpnea resulting first from the relative decrease and then the build-up of carbonic acid in the blood.
   D. Loss of consciousness results when the increase in blood alkalinity is marked enough to cause injury to the brain cells.

NURSING APPLICATIONS

1. Patients should be observed for signs and symptoms of acid-base imbalance; these should be evaluated, investigated, reported and/or treated with appropriate nursing measures. This is of particular importance when the patient:
   A. Has malnutrition. (See Chap. 3.)
   B. Has impaired carbohydrate metabolism. (See Chap. 3.)
   C. Has fluid and electrolyte imbalance. (See Chap. 4 and 5.)
   D. Has renal disease. (See Chap. 4.)

E. Has markedly impaired circulation. (See Chap. 1.)

F. Has markedly impaired respirations. (See Chap. 2.)

2. Acid-base imbalance may be prevented by such measures as:

A. Encouraging and providing for good nutrition. (See Chap. 3.)

B. Preventing fluid and electrolyte imbalance. (See Chap. 4 and 5.)

C. Discouraging rapid, shallow breathing that may occur when there is severe pain or emotional stress.

D. Discouraging the continued or excessive oral intake of highly acid or alkaline substances without medical supervision.

E. Observing for, evaluating and reporting appropriately signs and symptoms of diabetes mellitus. (See Chap. 8.)

F. Encouraging and providing medical supervision and appropriate patient care when there is diagnosed diabetes mellitus.

3. When there is acid-base imbalance:

A. This represents a medical emergency.

B. Equipment for the intravenous administration of appropriate parenteral fluids should be ready.

C. Accurate measurement of fluid intake and loss must be made and reported appropriately.

D. Medical orders relative to the amount and type of diet must be followed exactly.

E. Medical orders related to the amount and type of fluid intake must be followed exactly.

4. When a patient is in diabetic coma, in addition to the measures in No. 3:

A. Insulin must be available for immediate administration as ordered.

B. Equipment for urine testing (e.g., glucose, diacetic acid, acetone and pH) must be ready.

C. Any urine tests must be performed on time, with absolute accuracy and reported appropriately.

7

Elimination

Efficient body functioning requires that food residues and gases be eliminated from the gastrointestinal tract, that urine be eliminated and that toxic substances formed in the body be rendered harmless and/or eliminated.

ANATOMY AND PHYSIOLOGY

Elimination from the Gastrointestinal Tract

1. The large intestine is a musculomembranous tube that extends up the right side of the abdominal cavity (starting at the ileocecal valve), across the abdomen and down the left side, and ends with the anal canal.
   - A. The rectum, in the adult, is about 6 to 8 inches long. It extends from the sigmoid flexure to the anus.
   - B. The anal canal, approximately an inch in length, has two sphincter muscles. The internal sphincter is smooth muscle; the external, striated muscle.
2. Much of the water of the intestinal contents is absorbed into the capillaries of the large intestine.
   - A. If the body is dehydrated, water absorption in the colon increases.
   - B. Retention of feces leads to increased water absorption.
   - C. Increased intestinal motility decreases the amount of water absorption.
3. Peristaltic movements that propel the intestinal contents through the large intestine result from:
   - A. Stimulation by autonomic nerves. (Parasympathetic stimulation increases peristalsis; sympathetic stimulation decreases peristalsis.)
   - B. Local reflex stimulation caused by such factors as internal pressure, mechanical irritation or chemical irritation. (The effects of different foodstuffs upon motility varies with individuals.)
4. Some atony of the smooth muscle may occur:
   - A. When fecal bulk is retained.
   - B. In old age.
   - C. When the muscles have been stimulated excessively.

5. The feces normally contains bacteria, sloughed off epithelial cells, food residues, bile pigments, some mucus and some inorganic salts.
   A. The volume of feces is increased by indigestible matter (e.g., cellulose).
   B. Lack of food intake causes the bulk of feces to be greatly reduced.
   C. Bile pigments give a brown color to the feces.
   D. The color and consistency of feces varies to some extent with the type of food eaten.
   E. Although some food residues are evacuated within 24 hours after ingestion, the major portion is gradually disposed of over several days.
   F. The odor of feces is due primarily to gases formed in the large intestine by putrefaction.
6. Meconium is a greenish tarry substance in the intestines of the newborn. It is normally eliminated completely within 2 to 3 days following delivery.
7. The sudden passage of feces into the rectum initiates the defecatory reflex.
   A. Sensory impulses are relayed to the spinal cord, and peristalsis is stimulated by motor nerves.
   B. The internal sphincter is relaxed and (after voluntary control is developed) the external sphincter is relaxed voluntarily.
   C. The contraction of the levator ani muscles pulls the anal canal up over the feces.
   D. Downward pressure can be exerted by contracting the abdominal muscles and the diaphragm against the abdominal organs.
8. Eating stimulates peristalsis and the passage of feces into the rectum, especially if the stomach has been without food for some length of time (e.g., overnight).
9. The act of defecation can usually be inhibited by voluntarily constricting the external anal sphincter. A child usually has enough neuromuscular development by the age of two to be ready to learn to voluntarily control defecation. (This development may be earlier in some children, a little later in others.)
10. Bowel movements may occur normally as frequently as several times a day or as infrequently as once or twice a week.
11. Prolonged internal pressure against the walls of the rectum may cause headache and lethargy.
12. Sensory nerve endings for pain and pressure in the bowel wall are stimulated by smooth muscle spasms and by distention.
13. Gas in the intestinal tract is primarily swallowed air. Small amounts of other gases may be formed from intestinal putrefaction or fermentation.
14. Gases may be eliminated from the gastrointestinal tract by:
    A. Belching.
    B. Passing flatus rectally.

Elimination of Nitrogenous Wastes and Other Toxic Substances by the Kidneys

1. The kidneys eliminate most of the nitrogenous wastes of cellular metabolism.
   A. Nitrogenous wastes come from protein metabolism.
      (1) The organic compounds include urea, uric acid and creatinine. The liver plays a predominant role in the formation of urea.
      (2) The most abundant inorganic compound is ammonia, which is eliminated in ammonium salts.
   B. Kidney function normally keeps the blood urea nitrogen level below 20 mg.%.
   C. Solids must be in solution in order to be excreted by the kidneys.
2. Sweat normally contains small quantities of urea.

Elimination of Urine

1. The bladder is a muscular sac in which urine is stored before being eliminated from the body. The two ureters extend from the kidney pelvises to the bladder. The urethra extends from the bladder to the outside (the urinary meatus).
2. The bladder is located in the pelvic cavity. It is in front of the vagina in the female and in front of the rectum in the male.
3. Urine is released from the bladder by reflex or voluntary and reflex action.
4. The act of micturition involves the action of the detrusor reflex and the opening and closing of the internal and external sphincters.
   A. The bladder wall contains sensory receptors that respond to the rise in pressure exerted on them as the bladder fills. When the volume of urine reaches a point at which the pressure excites the stretch receptors, sensory stimuli travel to the spinal cord.
   B. Parasympathetic nerves cause contraction of the detrusor muscle and the opening of the internal sphincter (between the bladder and the urethra).
   C. The external sphincter can be powerfully closed by voluntary muscle contraction even when the detrusor muscle contracts.
   D. The spinal reflex responsible for detrusor contraction can be inhibited or facilitated by nerve inpulses from the higher centers.
5. Awareness of the need to void normally occurs in the adult when the bladder contains 300 to 500 ml. of urine. The desire to void may be increased markedly when external pressure is exerted on the bladder, or when the bladder or the urethra is irritated.
6. A distended bladder can be palpated above the symphysis pubis. Bladders can be greatly distended. Some adult bladders can hold up to 3,000 to 4,000 ml. of fluid before rupture occurs. Others can contain much less than this.

7. Continued stretching of the bladder wall by the accumulation of urine causes loss of bladder tone. Recovery of the tone may occur more readily if the internal pressure is decreased gradually.
8. An overflow of urine from the bladder may occur when the pressure caused by the accumulated urine is sufficient to overcome the normal tone of the sphincters. Dribbling continues until the pressure has been decreased enough for sphincter control to be resumed.
9. The prostate gland is a firm body located just below the internal urethral orifice and around the proximal portion of the urethra in the male. The gland produces secretions important in male reproductive function. It is fairly common for the gland to become enlarged during later life, causing difficulty in micturition.

Elimination of Bile Pigments and Detoxification by the Liver

1. The liver excretes bile continuously. About 1,000 ml. of bile are produced by the adult liver daily. The bile is stored and concentrated in the gallbladder.
2. Bile contains bile salts (important in fat emulsification), bile pigments, mucin, minerals and cholesterol. (The biliary tract is considered in Chap. 3.)
3. The liver detoxifies many injurious substances formed in the body (e.g., products of intestinal putrefaction and intermediate products of metabolism).

Elimination of Carbon Dioxide in the Lungs

1. Carbon dioxide, a waste product of carbohydrate metabolism, is carried to the lungs by the plasma and red blood cells as bicarbonate, as carbonic acid, and as a combined form with hemoglobin.
2. Under normal conditions the partial pressure of carbon dioxide in the alveoli of the lungs is less than that in the venous blood. The carbon dioxide is released from the various compounds and diffuses into the alveoli. It is exhaled during the expiratory phase of respiration.

PHYSICS

1. Pressure is the force exerted on a unit area.
2. Fluids flow from an area of higher pressure to one of lower pressure, and the rate of volume flow is directly related to the pressure gradient.

CHEMISTRY

1. The human digestive system does not have appropriate enzymes for the digestion of cellulose.
2. Fermentation is a chemical process in which carbohydrates are

decomposed by the action of microorganisms. Carbon dioxide and hydrogen are formed in the process.

3. Putrefaction is a chemical process in which proteins are decomposed by the action of microorganisms; several gaseous products are produced (e.g., hydrogen sulfide).

4. The chemical breakdown of hemoglobin in the formation of bile salts involves the breakdown of heme to bilirubin (red), which can be oxidized to biliverdin (green), which can, in turn, be reduced to sterobilin (brown). Sterobilin gives the normal brown color to feces.

PATHOLOGY

Elimination from the Gastrointestinal Tract

1. Signs and symptoms of inadequate elimination of gases and food residues from the gastrointestinal tract include:
   A. Headache, general malaise, anorexia.
   B. Abdominal pain, cramping (which may be severe).
   C. Feeling of rectal fullness.
   D. Abdominal distention.
   E. Small amounts of dry, hard stool.
   F. Stools of very narrow caliber.
   G. Small amounts of liquid stool.
   H. Stool retention.

2. Constipation may be caused by problems that involve:
   A. Nervous control of evacuation.
   B. Reflex peristalsis necessary for evacuation.
   C. Mechanical obstruction to normal evacuation.

3. Problems that involve nervous control of evacuation include:
   A. An imbalance between parasympathetic and sympathetic stimulation, which causes excessive tonus. This may result from emotional disturbances. The colon is sometimes referred to as "irritable".
   B. Certain psychic disturbances that result in the retention of feces (often related to bowel training in childhood).
   C. Interference with the normal conditioned reflexes because of time pressures of daily living.
   D. Interference with normal conditioned reflexes because of actual damage to afferent or efferent nerves (e.g., spinal cord tumors, or various degenerative conditions involving the brain, the spinal cord, or the peripheral nerves).
   E. Interference with normal conditioned reflexes because of pain associated with defecation (e.g., hemorrhoids, anal fissure, rectal surgery).

4. Problems that involve reflex peristalsis necessary for bowel evacuation include:
   A. Lack of sufficient food or bulk in the diet.
   B. Lack of tonus due to too much stimulation by irritating substances (e.g., laxatives, bran).
   C. Lack of bile in the intestines. (See Chap. 3).
   D. Inflammation of the abdominal or pelvic viscera, which results in decreased peristalsis.
5. Problems that involve mechanical obstruction include:
   A. Weakness of the smooth muscle of the intestinal tract which may be congenital or acquired. Acquired weakness may result from degenerative changes of aging or deficiencies in certain vitamins and minerals.
   B. Weakness of the voluntary muscles used in normal evacuation. Such weakness may accompany a generalized weak condition, obesity, pregnancy, acites, emphysema, or surgery involving the abdomen, pelvis or perineal area.
   C. Actual mechanical obstruction, which may be caused by compression, inflammatory edema of intestinal walls, abnormal growths, pockets of gas, strangulated hernias, fecal impactions, imperforate anus or rectoceles.
6. Hemorrhoids are dilated, congested and sometimes thrombosed hemorrhoidal veins. They may occur internally or externally. They may be a result of many factors, such as poor venous return (e.g., during pregnancy), straining at stool or congenital weakness of the veins. They may cause itching or rectal discomfort, and may be extremely painful.
7. An anal fissure is an ulceration of the anal wall. It is irritating, painful and often becomes infected, leading to abscess formation. This, in turn, may lead to the formation of an anal fistula.
8. A fecal impaction is a large hard mass of feces that fills and obstructs the rectal vault. Sometimes small amounts of liquid stool seep around the impaction and are expelled.
9. A rectocele is an outpouching of the rectum and vaginal wall into the vagina. It may be due to muscle injury which may occur during childbirth.

Elimination of Nitrogenous Wastes and Other Toxic Substances by the Kidneys

1. Signs and symptoms of renal failure and associated uremia include:
   A. Signs and symptoms of fluid, electrolyte and acid-base imbalance. (See Chap. 4, 5 and 6).
   B. Oliguria with low specific gravity.
   C. Anuria.
   D. Uremic "snow" and odor of urine on skin.

2. Uremia is a condition in which there is an increase of nitrogenous waste products (primarily urea) in the bloodstream. Uremia accompanies renal failure. The nitrogenous wastes are toxic to the body cells. An increased amount of urea is excreted in sweat, and this can sometimes be seen as tiny white particles on the skin.

Elimination of Urine

1. Signs and symptoms of urine retention include:
   A. Absence of voiding; voiding frequently in small amounts.
   B. Palpable bladder.
   C. Discomfort in pelvic area, possibly severe pain.
   D. Restlessness.
   E. Signs and symptoms of urinary infection (e.g., burning sensation during and after voiding, urgency, frequency, back pain).
2. Possible causes of urine retention include:
   A. Ureteral or urethral strictures (acquired or congenital).
   B. Calculi.
   C. Pressure against the tract from without (e.g., abnormal enlargement of the prostate gland, abnormal growths in the pelvic area).
   D. Inflammatory edema or abnormal growths within the tract.
   E. Local injuries affecting the bladder wall or muscles involved in micturition (e.g., cystocele).
   F. Injury to sensory and/or motor nerves that are involved with micturition (e.g., spinal cord injury).
3. Enlargement of the prostate gland may be the result of benign hypertrophy or may be due to tumor growth.
4. A cystocele is a downward displacement of the bladder and vaginal wall into the vagina. It may be caused by injuries related to childbirth.

Elimination of Bile Pigments and Detoxification by the Liver

1. Signs and symptoms of impaired liver function may include those related to:
   A. Inadequate nutrition. (See Chap. 3).
   B. Fluid and electrolyte imbalance. (See Chap. 4 and 5).
   C. Blood clotting. (See Chap. 1).
   D. Specific cellular damage due to injurious effects of toxic substances in the blood (e.g., brain damage).
   E. Jaundice.
2. Signs and symptoms of jaundice include:
   A. Yellowing of sclera, skin and mucous membranes.
   B. Clay-colored stools.
   C. Dark brown urine.
3. Jaudice is a condition in which bile pigments accumulate in body

tissues and fluids. This accumulation may be due to an excessive breakdown of erythrocytes or impaired excretion of bile pigment, or a combination of both.

A. Impaired excretion of bile pigment may be due to liver disease. (See Chap. 3).

B. Impaired excretion of bile pigment may be due to obstruction in the biliary system. Obstruction may be caused by gallstones, parasites, neoplasms, strictures, spasms, inflammatory edema or adhesions. The back pressure of bile in the liver can cause liver damage.

Elimination of Carbon Dioxide in the Lungs

1. Signs and symptoms of inadequate elimination of carbon dioxide include those related to a decrease in the alkaline reserve of the blood. (See Chap. 6).

2. Emphysema (considered in Chap. 2) is a respiratory condition in which inadequate expiration may lead to an excess of carbon dioxide in the blood. Any increased cellular metabolism (e.g., physical exercise) can result in a decrease in the alkaline reserve of the blood.

NURSING APPLICATIONS

Elimination from the Gastrointestinal Tract

1. Patients should be observed for signs and symptoms of inadequate elimination of food residues and gases from the gastrointestinal tract; these should be evaluated, investigated, reported and/or treated with appropriate nursing measures. This is of particular importance when the patient:

A. Is at extremes of age.

B. Is dependent upon others for physical care (e.g., because of loss of consciousness, psychic disorders or age).

C. Is dehydrated. (See Chap. 4).

D. Has renal failure. (See Chap. 4).

E. Has a condition that interferes with normal neuromuscular mechanisms necessary for bowel evacuation (e.g., paralysis, obstruction).

2. The elimination of feces should be evaluated in relation to:

A. The individual's usual pattern for bowel evacuation.

B. The amount and type of diet.

C. The state of fluid balance.

D. The presence of any signs and symptoms of possible constipation.

3. Observations should be made of the feces (e.g., color, odor, consistency, number, presence of abnormal constituents) and any abnor-

malities should be reported appropriately. Specimens of abnormal stools should be saved for medical inspection.

4. Good bowel elimination can be promoted by:
    A. Encouraging positive attitudes toward bowel training in early childhood.
    B. Encouraging and providing a well-balanced diet with adequate roughage.
    C. Encouraging and providing an adequate fluid intake.
    D. Encouraging and providing for regularity of bowel habits.
    E. Providing for bowel evacuation when the urge to defecate is felt.
    F. Providing adequate time for complete evacuation.
    G. Providing a posture as close to usual for defecation as is possible.
    H. Providing physical comfort. (See Chap. 15.)
    I. Providing emotional comfort.
    J. Providing physical exercise as possible.
    K. Discouraging the prolonged or excessive use of laxatives or enemas unless used under medical supervision.

5. When constipation does occur:
    A. Foods that tend to have a laxative effect for the individual may be encouraged (within dietary orders).
    B. Fluids should be encouraged (within medical orders).
    C. Possible emotional components should be recognized and reported appropriately.
    D. Enemas should be administered effectively as frequently as ordered and indicated.

6. When bowel elimination is contraindicated (e.g., following some surgeries and certain treatments), orders relative to diet must be followed exactly.

7. When a patient has a colostomy and irrigations are ordered:
    A. These should be done as close to the same time each day as possible.
    B. They should be effective in terms of providing for the emptying of the colon (e.g., amount of fluid used and time allowed for drainage).

8. Flatulence may be prevented by:
    A. Encouraging and providing a well-balanced diet, including adequate roughage.
    B. Restricting intake of food that is gas-forming (e.g., that which causes excessive fermentation or putrefaction).
    C. Discouraging excessive (or any) intake of carbonated beverages.
    D. Discouraging the swallowing of air (e.g., as may happen with sipping fluids or when there is a lot of belching).
    E. Helping an infant to bring up swallowed air during and after feeding.

9. Flatulence may be decreased by:
   A. Encouraging the voluntary expelling of gas through rectum unless contraindicated by certain kinds of surgeries or treatments involving the lower pelvic region).
   B. Providing an optimal position for expelling of gas (e.g., upright for belching, or knee-chest for rectal expulsion).
   C. Increasing physical activity (as possible).
   D. Changing positions frequently (as possible).
   E. The effective use of a rectal tube or enemas as ordered and indicated.

10. When gastric or intestinal suction is used:
    A. The appropriate suction must be maintained effectively (e.g., by ascertaining if equipment is in good working condition; checking patency of tubes; irrigating tube properly as ordered).
    B. The drainage must be observed carefully and any abnormalities reported promptly.
    C. Accurate measurement and recording of the drainage must be done daily.
    D. No food or fluids should be given by mouth unless specifically ordered. (The care of patients with intestinal obstruction is included in Chap. 3.)

Elimination of Nitrogenous Wastes and Other Toxic Substances by Kidneys

1. Patients should be observed for signs and symptoms of the inadequate elimination of wastes through the kidneys; these should be evaluated, investigated, reported and/or treated with appropriate nursing measures. This is of particular importance when the patient:
   A. Has renal disease. (See Chap. 4.)
   B. Has circulatory failure. (See Chap. 1.)
   C. Has dehydration. (See Chap. 4.)
   D. Is pregnant.

2. When a patient has uremia:
   A. He should be observed closely for signs and symptoms of both fluid and electrolyte imbalance, and these should be reported promptly.
   B. Fluid intake and fluid loss must be measured and recorded accurately. A decrease in fluid loss below minimal safe limits must be reported promptly.
   C. Protein foods may be limited.
   D. Medical orders relative to both diet and fluid intake must be followed exactly.
   E. Adequate bowel elimination should be promoted.

Elimination of Urine

1. Patients should be observed for signs and symptoms of urine retention; these should be evaluated, investigated, reported and/or
   treated with appropriate nursing measures. This is of particular
   importance when the patient:

   A. Is male and over fifty years of age.
   B. Depends upon others for care (e.g., due to unconsciousness,
      psychic disorders or age).
   C. Has sustained injury to the bladder, urethra, or local voluntary
      muscles that interferes with normal micturition (e.g., surgery
      that affects these tissues or parturition).
   D. Has a sensory or motor disturbance that interferes with normal
      micturition.
   E. Has an obstruction between the kidney and tubes leading to the
      outside (e.g., enlarged prostate gland, plugged catheters, calculi,
      edema in or around tubes).

2. Elimination of urine from the bladder may be facilitated by:

   A. Providing for as close to normal voiding position as possible.
   B. Providing physical comfort. (See Chap. 15.)
   C. Providing emotional comfort.
   D. Providing local warmth in peritoneal and lower abdominal
      regions (e.g., a Sitz bath if allowed).
   E. Providing for the sound of running water and/or the feel of
      warm water running over the external genitalia (e.g., taking a
      shower can be helpful if allowed).
   F. Catheterizing promptly and effectively as ordered and indicated.

3. A distended bladder should be emptied gradually.

4. When a tube is draining urine from the urinary tract:

   A. It must be maintained patent, and any problems should be
      reported promptly.
      (1) No catheter should be clamped without specific medical
          orders to do so. These orders should include the frequency
          and period of time the catheter can be clamped.
      (2) Ureteral catheters are never clamped.
      (3) The amount of urine drained should be checked frequently.
      (4) Tubes should not be kinked or compressed and their posi-
          tions should not interfere with drainage.
      (5) Patency of the tubes should be checked frequently.
      (6) Catheter irrigations, if ordered, must be performed effec-
          tively.
   B. The urinary output and fluid intake should be carefully mea-
      sured and recorded.

Elimination of Bile Pigments and Detoxification by the Liver

1. Patients should be observed for signs and symptoms of impaired liver function; these should be evaluated, investigated, reported and/or treated with appropriate nursing measures. This is of particular importance when a patient has:
   A. Malnutrition. (See Chap. 3.)
   B. Known liver disease. (See Chap. 3.)
   C. Taken into his body toxic substances that may cause chemical injury to the liver (e.g., fumes of certain organic solvents, certain medications).
   D. Jaundice.
2. When a patient has had surgery involving the biliary tract:
   A. He should be observed closely for signs and symptoms of jaundice (or increasing jaundice), and these should be reported promptly.
   B. Careful observation must be made of any bile drainage.
      (1) The tube should be draining properly at all times.
      (2) The tube should never be clamped without specific medical orders. When the tube is clamped and there is nausea and vomiting, abdominal distention or pain, the tube should be unclamped promptly, and this should be reported appropriately.

Elimination of Carbon Dioxide in the Lungs

1. Patients should be observed for signs and symptoms of the inadequate elimination of carbon dioxide; these should be evaluated, investigated, reported and/or treated with appropriate nursing measures. This is of particular importance when the patient has:
   A. Circulatory failure. (See Chap. 1.)
   B. Respiratory problems. (See Chap. 2.)
2. When a patient has difficulty in expiration (e.g., as in emphysema):
   A. Physical and emotional rest should be encouraged.
   B. The use of the abdominal muscles in expiration should be taught and encouraged.
   C. Oxygen should be administered only when ordered, and then with great caution.

8

Enzymes and Hormones

Normal body functioning depends upon the presence of
certain enzymes and hormones.

ANATOMY AND PHYSIOLOGY

Enzymes

1. Enzymes are organic catalysts produced by a living organism. The
   production of enzymes depends upon good nutrition and normal
   metabolic processes. (See Chap. 3.)
2. Enzymes play an important role in such body processes as:
   A. The digestion and absorption of food.
   B. The metabolism of carbohydrates, fats and proteins.
   C. Intracellular oxidation and reduction.
   D. Muscle contractions.
   E. Blood clotting.

Hormones

1. Hormones are chemical regulators produced by endocrine glands.
   A. Hormones that affect various digestive processes are produced by
      certain glandular cells in the gastric and duodenal mucosa.
   B. Hormones are carried by the blood to the tissues that they affect.
2. The pituitary gland lies centrally in the brain, partly within a bony
   concavity. The gland is divided into two lobes.
   A. The anterior lobe produces at least six known hormones (and
      doubtlessly many more). These hormones seem to affect nearly
      all body activities, partly because different hormones affect the
      secretions of other endocrine glands (e.g., adrenocorticotropic
      hormone, thyrotropic hormones, gonadotropic hormones).
      (1) The thyrotropic hormone stimulates the secretion of thy-
          roxine. (See No. 3.)
      (2) The adrenocorticotropic hormone stimulates the secretion of
          adrenocortical hormones. (See No. 5.)
      (3) The growth hormone (or somatropin) stimulates the devel-
          opment and enlargement of tissues.

(4) The gonadotropic hormones affect the development of sexuality. (See Chap. 19.)

B. The posterior lobe produces two hormones—vasopressin and oxytocin.

(1) Vasopressin, which is sometimes called the antidiuretic hormone, contracts smooth muscles, especially those of the arterioles, and stimulates the reabsorption of water in the kidneys.

(2) The primary action of oxytocin is to stimulate forceful contractions of the uterus. It is questionable that oxytocin affects normal labor and delivery, but oxytocin is used therapeutically to produce uterine contractions.

(3) These hormones are not released into the blood continuously. Their release is under nervous control.

3. The thyroid gland is located in front of the trachea just below the larynx. The gland lies on both sides of the trachea, but a narrow strip extends across the trachea. The chief hormone secreted is thyroxine.

A. Thyroxine contains a high percentage of iodine.

B. Thyroxine is gradually released to the bloodstream. It eventually enters the cells, affecting the metabolic rate primarily through affecting cellular oxidation.

4. The parathyroid glands are imbedded in the posterior thyroid, two in each lobe. The parathyroid hormone affects calcium and phosphorus metabolism.

A. A steady concentration of calcium in the extracellular fluid is essential to normal neuromuscular mechanisms.

B. Parathyroid hormone stimulates the release of calcium from the bones.

5. There is an adrenal gland located on the top of each kidney. The outer portion is called the cortex, and it secretes many hormones referred to as adrenocortical hormones. The medulla (the interior) secretes epinephrine and norepinephrine.

A. The adrenocortical hormones are generally divided into three groups according to their actions: the mineralocorticoids, the glucocorticoids and the androgens.

(1) The mineralocorticoids (including desoxycorticosterone and aldosterone) regulate the extracellular concentrations of sodium and potassium by their effects upon reabsorption in the kidney tubules.

(a) The body tends to reabsorb sodium and excrete potassium.

(b) The reabsorption of sodium is accompanied by the absorption of water, so blood volume is affected.

(c) There is a normal increase in the secretions of mineralocorticoids when there is physical stress and when there is a low concentration of sodium.

(2) The glucocorticoids (including hydrocortisone) affect the metabolism of protein, fat and carbohydrates primarily. They are of tremendous importance at times of physical stress (e.g., infections, severe traumas), because these hormones stimulate catabolism and the production of energy.

(3) The androgens are involved in masculinization.

B. Secretion of both the mineralocorticoids and the glucocorticoids is increased at times of stress. The stimulus for increased secretion may be direct through the sympathetic nervous system or indirect through stimulation by epinephrine.

6. The pancreas is both an exocrine and endocrine gland. The hormone it produces is insulin. Insulin is essential to the proper metabolism of glucose. (See Chap. 3.)

PATHOLOGY

Pituitary Gland

1. Signs and symptoms of abnormal hormone production by the pituitary gland may include:

    A. Abnormal growth patterns (e.g., dwarfism, acromegaly, gigantism).

    B. Signs and symptoms of problems with the other endocrine glands.

    C. Excessive urine production accompanied by polydypsia, weight loss and weakness.

2. Problems with the pituitary gland may be caused by disturbances of growth and function taking place within the gland or by increased pressure against the gland.

    A. Hyposecretion of the growth hormone before adolescence causes dwarfism.

    B. Hypersecretion of the growth hormone before adolescence causes gigantism.

    C. Hypersecretion of the growth hormone after adolescence causes acromegaly, a condition in which there is a thickening of bones transversely. This can be noted mainly in the mandible, the nose and the bones of the hands and feet.

    D. Abnormal secretion of the gonadotropins causes disturbances in the normal development of secondary sex characteristics and in normal sexual functioning.

    E. Hyposecretion of the antidiuretic factor causes a condition called diabetes insipidus, in which there is a decreased reabsorption of water by the kidneys. This results in the loss of huge quantities of water. (See Chap. 4.)

Thyroid Gland

1. Signs and symptoms of abnormal hormone production by the thyroid gland may include:
   A. Enlargement of the thyroid gland (goiter).
   B. Those signs related to hyposecretion and its resulting lowered metabolic rate.
      (1) In childhood there may be physical and mental retardation, retarded sexual development and a general slowdown in all body functions.
      (2) After adolescence there may be generalized edema of subcutaneous tissues, mental dullness, susceptibility to cold, a decrease in reproductive functions and a general slowdown in all body functions.
   C. Those signs related to hypersecretion and its resulting increased metabolic rate. These include:
      (1) Enlargement of the thyroid gland (goiter).
      (2) Excessive weight loss accompanied by excessive appetite.
      (3) Tachycardia.
      (4) Nervousness, tremors, hyperirritability.
      (5) Hot, moist skin with hypersensitivity to heat.
      (6) Dyspnea upon exertion (due to oxygen deficiency).
      (7) Exophthalmia.
2. Problems with the thyroid gland may be caused by disturbances of growth and function taking place within the gland, removal of the gland, or by problems related to the pituitary gland.
   A. A lack of iodine in the diet causes enlargement of the thyroid gland as the cells attempt to produce sufficient hormone (endemic goiter).
   B. Hyposecretion of thyroid hormone in the child is called cretinism.
   C. Hyposecretion of thyroid hormone in the adult is called myxedema.
   D. Hypersecretion of thyroid hormone may be referred to as thyrotoxicosis, toxic goiter or Graves disease. In hyperthyroidism, the increased metabolic rate requires increased oxygen and food; heat production is increased and there is excessive neuromuscular irritability. When thyrotoxicosis abruptly becomes very severe it may be called a thyroid crisis. There is extreme hyperthermia and the condition can lead to heart failure.

Parathyroid Gland

1. Signs and symptoms of abnormal hormone production by the parathyroid glands include:
   A. Those related to hyposecretion. These include:
      (1) Numbness and tingling, especially in extremities.

(2) Carpopedal spasms, muscle twitchings, tetany.

(3) Laryngeal spasms.

B. Those related to hypersecretion. These include:

(1) Anorexia, vomiting, constipation.

(2) Frequent formation of renal calculi.

(3) Frequent pathological fractures.

2. Problems with the parathyroid glands may be caused by problems of growth and function taking place within the gland, problems related to the thyroid gland or removal of the thyroid gland.

Adrenal Glands

1. Signs and symptoms of abnormal hormone production by the adrenal cortex include:

A. Those related to hyposecretion. These include:

(1) Signs and symptoms related to hypotension. (See Chap. 1.)

(2) Muscular weakness, fatigue.

(3) Gastrointestinal disturbances (e.g., anorexia, vomiting).

(4) Bronzing of the skin.

(5) Poor response to stress situations.

(6) Signs and symptoms related to fluid and electrolyte imbalance. (See Chap. 4 and 5.)

(7) Feminism in the male.

B. Those related to hypersecretion (or overdosage). These include:

(1) Hypertension with hyperirritability.

(2) Mental aberrations.

(3) Obesity, edema or abnormal fat distribution (e.g., moon face).

(4) Signs and symptoms related to fluid and electrolyte imbalance. (See Chap. 4 and 5.)

(5) Virilism in the female, perhaps precocious puberty in the male.

2. Problems with the adrenal cortex may be caused by problems with the pituitary gland, problems of growth and function taking place within the glands, inflammations or removal of the glands.

A. Hyposecretion of adrenocortical hormones may be called Addison's disease. When the symptoms of hyposecretion become very severe abruptly, this may be referred to as Addisonian crisis. Complete circulatory collapse may result.

B. Hypersecretion of adrenocortical hormones may be due to problems involving the adrenal gland, and this condition may be called Cushing's syndrome. If the problem lies with the pituitary gland, the condition is often called Cushing's disease.

3. Signs and symptoms of abnormal hormone production by the adrenal medulla include those concerned with functions related to sympathetic stimulation (e.g., constriction of arterioles, pupil dilation,

dilation of the bronchioles, decreased peristalsis, increased glyco-genesis and others).
4. Hypersecretion of the adrenal medulla may be caused by tumor growth (pheochromocytoma). The primary symptom is hyperten-sion. (See Chap. 1.)

Pancreas

1. Signs and symptoms of abnormal hormone secretion by the pancreas include:
   A. Those related to hyposecretion. These include:
      (1) Polyuria, glycosuria. (See Chap. 4.)
      (2) Excessive thirst.
      (3) Signs and symptoms associated with inadequate nutrition (especially carbohydrates, proteins). (See Chap. 3.)
      (4) Signs and symptoms associated with acid-base imbalance. (See Chap. 6.)
2. Diabetes mellitus is a condition in which there may be hyposecre-tion of insulin, or some other problem related to the proper func-tion of insulin. It is a chronic disease and the predisposition to it may be inherited. Obesity may be a predisposing factor. Diabetes mellitus can be associated with certain injuries to the pancreas (e.g., tumors, trauma, infections).
3. Hypersecretion of insulin may occur with various disorders of the pancreas (e.g., tumor growth); it causes hypoglycemia.

NURSING APPLICATIONS

Observation

1. Patients should be observed for signs and symptoms of hormonal imbalance; these should be evaluated, investigated, reported and/or treated appropriately with nursing measures. This is of particular importance when the patient:
   A. Has a diagnosed condition, or surgery, that involves or may involve any of the endocrine glands.
   B. Is receiving hormone therapy (e.g., cortisone, thyroxine, or insulin).
   C. Is obese or has a family history of diabetes mellitus.

Thyroid Gland

1. An adequate intake of food containing iodine should be encouraged.
2. When a patient has hypothyroidism:
   A. More than usual sleep and rest should be encouraged.
   B. Emotional support should be consistant.
3. When a patient has hyperthyroidism:
   A. More than usual sleep and rest should be encouraged.

B. A diet high in calories, protein and vitamins should be encouraged.

C. Stress-producing situations (physical and emotional) should be avoided as possible.

D. Emotional support should be consistent.

E. Close observations should be made for signs and symptoms of a thyroid crisis.

4. When a patient exhibits signs and symptoms of a thyroid crisis:

A. This is a medical emergency.

B. Oxygen should be administered as indicated or ordered.

C. Appropriate drugs (e.g., cardiotonics, antithyroid drugs, sedatives) should be available for prompt administration.

D. Nursing measures for the lowering of body temperature should be started promptly.

Parathyroid Gland

1. When a patient has hypoparathyroidism and shows signs and symptoms of increasing neuromuscular excitability (e.g., carpopedal spasms, muscle twitchings):

A. This is a medical emergency.

B. Equipment should be ready for prompt intravenous administration of calcium.

C. External stimuli should be limited.

2. When a patient has hyperparathyroidism:

A. Care should be taken to prevent fractures. (See Chap. 11.)

B. Fluid intake may be encouraged.

Adrenal Glands

1. When a patient has hypofunction of the adrenal cortex:

A. Orders relative to diet and fluid intake must be followed exactly.

B. Accurate measurements of fluid intake and fluid loss should be made and recorded.

C. Stress-producing situations (emotional and physical) should be avoided (e.g., infections).

D. Careful observations should be made for signs and symptoms of an Addisonian crisis.

2. When a patient shows signs and symptoms of Addisonian crisis (e.g., when adrenal glands are surgically removed):

A. This is a medical emergency.

B. Equipment for the prompt intravenous administration of appropriate fluids and drugs should be ready.

C. Absolute physical rest must be enforced.

D. The temperature should be measured and recorded frequently and appropriate actions taken for any hyperthermia. (See Chap. 9.)

E. The blood pressure and pulse should be measured and recorded frequently and appropriate action taken for hypotension. (See Chap. 1.)

3. When a patient has hyperfunction of the adrenal cortex (e.g., as in Cushing's disease) :
   A. Orders relative to diet and fluid intake must be followed exactly.
   B. Accurate measurements of fluid intake and fluid loss should be made and recorded.
   C. Emotional support should be consistent.

Pancreas

1. Periodic urine testing for glucose should be encouraged. This is of particular importance when there is a history of diabetes mellitus in the family, and/or obesity.
2. Excessive weight gain should be discouraged or corrected (preferably under medical supervision).
3. When a patient has diabetes mellitus:
   A. He should be under medical supervision.
   B. Orders relative to diet and/or medication (to lower blood sugar) should be followed exactly.
   C. Urine testing must be done accurately at the correct time and reported appropriately.
   D. Accurate measurements of fluid intake and urine output may be required.
   E. Careful observations should be made for signs and symptoms of hypoglycemia (when medications are used to lower the blood sugar) ; these should be reported and/or treated promptly. (See Chap. 3.)
   F. Careful observations should be made for signs and symptoms of impending diabetic coma; these should be reported and/or treated promptly. (See Chap. 6.)

   (Hyperinsulinism and hypoglycemia are included in Chap. 3.)

9

Temperature Regulation

A definite temperature range is required for efficient cellular functioning and proper enzymatic activity.

ANATOMY AND PHYSIOLOGY

1. The optimal temperature for normal activity of enzymes falls within the normal body temperature range of 36° C. to 38° C., with an average of 37° C.
   A. A rectal temperature usually measures slightly higher than oral, and an axillary temperature measures less than oral. (To measure body temperature accurately, the thermometer bulb must be in full contact with the mucosa or the skin.)
   B. There is a normal diurnal variation of temperature. If the waking hours are in the day, the maximum temperature is reached in the late afternoon or early evening, and the minimum is reached in the early morning.
   C. In the female, there is usually a slight rise of temperature from the time of ovulation until menstruation (or throughout pregnancy).
2. Body cells vary in their abilities to function when their temperature is below 34° C. or above 40° C. Cells of the central nervous system usually cannot function normally at a temperature above 41° C.
3. The body temperature represents a balance between heat produced in the tissues (plus a small amount which may be acquired from the external environment) and heat lost to the environment.
   A. Heat production is due to exothermic chemical reactions.
      (1) At rest, the liver produces the greatest amount of heat.
      (2) During exercise the voluntary muscles produce the greatest amount of heat. (Children often exhibit a marked rise in body temperature during exercise.)
      (3) The rate of these chemical reactions increases as the body temperature rises, thus the basal metabolic rate is elevated during fever.
   B. Heat is distributed through the body by:
      (1) Conduction through the tissues.
      (2) The circulating blood.

C. The total amount of heat in a given area in the body is influenced by the rate of blood flow.

D. Heat is lost from the body through:
  (1) Conduction.
  (2) Radiation.
  (3) Convection.
  (4) Vaporization of sweat.

E. The amount of heat lost from the body surface by radiation and conduction varies with:
  (1) The amount of body insulation (e.g., subcutaneous fat, clothing).
  (2) The amount of skin area exposed.
  (3) The external environmental temperature.
  (4) The amount of blood flow in the peripheral capillaries.

F. The amount of heat lost from the body surface by vaporization depends upon:
  (1) The production of sweat.
  (2) The amount of skin area exposed.
  (3) The amount of blood flow in the peripheral capillaries.
  (4) The humidity of the surrounding atmosphere.
  (5) The air currents.

G. When the body loses more heat than it can produce in the basal state, the arrector pili muscles contract and there are involuntary contractions of voluntary muscles.

H. In old age, loss of subcutaneous tissue and circulatory changes may affect temperature control.

4. The physiological mechanisms for temperature regulation are controlled by nerve centers in the hypothalamus.

A. Autonomic nerves regulate vasoconstriction, sweat gland activity and the contraction of the arrector pili muscles.

B. Heat regulating mechanisms are generally not fully developed at birth, so there may be marked fluctuations in body temperature occurring during the first year of life. The external temperature is a major factor in raising or lowering the body temperature of an infant.

C. Toxins of some infective agents and other chemical substances (e.g., hemoglobin) in the body may act (directly or indirectly) on the temperature-regulating centers to raise the threshold for mechanisms operating to increase heat loss.
  (1) The first reaction is a decrease in heat loss with peripheral vasoconstriction and a sensation of chilling, which may be accompanied by shivering.
  (2) The second reaction is increased heat production followed eventually by peripheral vasodilatation and an uncomfortably warm feeling.

PHYSICS

1. Evaporation is the process whereby a substance in liquid state is changed to a vapor state, which requires heat. Evaporation is a cooling process.
2. Heat can be defined as the kinetic energy of molecules.
3. Heat travels from a point of higher temperature to one of lower temperature.
   A. Conduction is the transmission of heat through any substance.
   B. Radiation is the transmission of heat through a vacuum (space).
   C. Convection is the transmission of heat by the movement of a heated liquid or gas. Because of convection, increasing air movements will increase the loss of heat from an object.
4. Friction changes mechanical energy to thermal energy.

CHEMISTRY

1. Exothermic chemical reactions are those in which there is a liberation of heat.
2. Alcohol changes from a liquid to a gas more easily than water.

PATHOLOGY

Signs and Symptoms

1. Signs and symptoms of an abnormally elevated body temperature include:
   A. An abnormally elevated body temperature measurement (e.g., over 38° C.; over 40° C. is serious).
   B. A rapid, full pulse to a weak and rapid pulse.
   C. Rapid respirations.
   D. Hyperemia of skin (may be preceded by pale skin).
   E. Profuse sweating.
   F. Hot, dry skin and mucous membranes.
   G. General uncomfortable warm feeling, maybe hypersensitive skin.
   H. Chills.
   I. Headache, general malaise, restlessness.
   J. Delirium, loss of consciousness.
   K. Convulsions (seen fairly frequently in infants and small children).
2. Signs and symptoms of an abnormally low body temperature include:
   A. An abnormally low body temperature measurement (e.g., below 36° C.; below 34° C. can be serious).
   B. A rapid full pulse to a weak and rapid pulse.
   C. Slow respirations.
   D. "Goosebumps" on skin.
   E. Pale skin, sometimes cyanosis.
   F. Shivering, shaking, chattering of teeth.

G. General uncomfortable cold feeling, numbness in extremities.

H. Loss of sensation, loss of consciousness.

Fever

1. Fever is the elevation of body temperature due to disease; fever may be intermittent, remittent or relapsing.
2. Fever may be caused by disease conditions which affect:
   A. The production of heat in the body.
   B. The loss of heat from the body.
   C. The mechanisms that regulate body temperature.

Conditions Affecting Body Temperature

1. Conditions that may cause an abnormal increase in the production of heat in the body are those related to an abnormally increased metabolic rate. These include:
   A. Thyrotoxicosis. (See Chap. 8.)
   B. Any tissue injury that results in a general inflammatory response (e.g., trauma, injuries due to physical, chemical or microbial agents).
2. Conditions that may cause an abnormal decrease in the amount of heat lost from the body include:
   A. Obesity.
   B. Dehydration, which causes a decrease in sweat production. (See Chap. 4.)
   C. Certain skin problems which prevent sweat production.
   D. Impaired general circulation. (See Chap. 1.)
3. Conditions that may affect the mechanisms regulating body temperature include:
   A. Head injury, brain surgery.
   B. Cerebrovascular accidents.
   C. Depression of the central nervous system by drugs (e.g., general anesthetics, alcohol).
   D. Emotions.
   E. Heat stroke.
4. An individual may be born with a skin that lacks sweat glands. This is rare. (Skin diseases are included in Chap. 12.)
5. Heat stroke is a condition in which there is high fever and loss of consciousness. There is no sweating. It is brought about by a high environmental temperature. The condition is more likely to occur in older people or in people who are depressed by the excessive intake of alcohol.
6. Chills are generally caused by the entrance into the bloodstream of some foreign substance (e.g., pyrogens, hemoglobin). In some infectious diseases, series of chills and fever are common (e.g., brucellosis and malaria).

A. Brucellosis is a bacterial infection caused by *Brucella* organisms. After incubation periods within some of the body cells, the organisms erupt into the bloodstream; this causes chills and fever.

B. Malaria is a protozoan infection of the blood. The parasites enter the red blood cells, and when the schizont form develops and ruptures the cells, the entrance of these foreign substances into the bloodstream causes chills and fever.

NURSING APPLICATIONS

Observation and Evaluation

1. Patients should be observed for signs and symptoms of abnormal body temperature; these should be investigated, evaluated, reported and/or treated with appropriate nursing measures. This is of particular importance when the patient:
   A. Has a condition that may affect the production of heat in the body (e.g., infection, thyrotoxicosis).
   B. Has a condition that may affect the loss of heat from the body (e.g., skin disease, obesity).
   C. Has a condition that may affect the regulation of body temperature (e.g., brain injury, heat stroke).
   D. Has a condition that may affect the distribution of heat in the body (e.g., circulatory failure).
   E. Is at extremes of age.
   F. Is exposed to extremely high environmental temperature, especially when there is also high humidity.
   G. Is or may be exposed to the introduction of foreign substances into the bloodstream (e.g., during transfusion or other intravenous therapy, malaria).
2. Oral temperatures should not be measured within 30 minutes following the intake of hot or cold food or fluids, or when there has been active gum chewing.
3. Rectal temperature measurements should be made when oral measurements are contraindicated because of questionable accuracy or discomfort (e.g., when there is mouth breathing because of nasal congestion, nasal surgery, nasal tubes, poorly fitted dentures, oral surgery).
4. Oral temperature measurements should be made when rectal measurements are contraindicated because of questionable accuracy or discomfort (e.g., diarrhea, fecal impaction, rectal or perineal surgery).
5. Body temperature should be evaluated in relation to:
   A. Usual body temperature.
   B. Time of day.

C. Environmental temperature.
D. Amount of physical exercise (especially important with children).
E. Phase of the menstrual cycle (and/or pregnancy).
F. Age of the patient.
G. Emotional status of the patient.
H. Disease condition of the patient.
I. Method of measurement (i.e., rectal, oral or skin).

Regulating Body Temperature

1. Patients should be protected from extremes of environmental temperatures; this is of particular importance when the patient:
   A. Is at extremes of age.
   B. Has impaired general circulation.
   C. Has an abnormal metabolic rate.
   D. Is fatigued, unconscious or in a weakened state.
   E. Is physically very active or inactive.
   F. Has skin disease. (See Chap. 12.)
   G. Is emaciated or obese.
2. Body temperature may be decreased by such means as:
   A. Adjusting the environmental temperature (e.g., air conditioning).
   B. Increasing the vaporization of sweat (e.g., increased air currents).
   C. Limiting physical activity or any skin friction.
   D. Applying liquids to the skin that evaporate quickly (e.g., alcohol sponges).
   E. Applying cold objects or substances to the skin (e.g., ice packs, cool baths, changing clothing or bedding).
   F. Administering antipyretic drugs as ordered and indicated.
   G. Exposing a greater amount of skin to the air.
3. Body temperature may be increased by:
   A. Adjusting the environmental temperature (e.g., increasing room temperature).
   B. Decreasing the vaporization of sweat (e.g., eliminating draughts).
   C. Increasing physical activity (active or passive) and skin friction.
   D. Applying insulating materials around the body (e.g., blankets).
   E. Applying warmed objects to the skin (e.g., warmed blankets).
   F. Encouraging and providing warm (hot) food and fluids.
4. When a patient has a markedly abnormal body temperature:
   A. This is a medical emergency.
   B. The temperature should be measured frequently (as often as every 15 minutes if indicated) and reported appropriately.
   C. Nursing measures should be instituted promptly to raise or lower the body temperature as indicated.

10

Sleep and Rest

Body cells require periods of decreased activity during which they can restore themselves.

ANATOMY AND PHYSIOLOGY

1. Required hours of sleep and rest vary with each individual.
   A. The average number of required hours of sleep in a 24-hour period include the following:
      (1) Infants, 18 to 20 hours.
      (2) Children, 10 to 14 hours.
      (3) Adults, 7 to 9 hours.
      (4) Elderly people, 5 to 7 hours.
   B. Sleep patterns are learned.
2. During sleep the metabolic rate is reduced below the basal level. Deep sleep is more restful than light sleep.
3. The higher the metabolic rate, the greater the need for increased circulation, respiration, nutrition and excretion. Muscle activity increases the metabolic rate.
4. Decreasing the demands placed upon the body during stress allows greater total body response to stress.
5. Energy is required both for responding to a stimulus and repressing response to a stimulus.
6. Factors that interfere with sleep and rest include:
   A. Physical discomfort. (See Chap. 14.)
   B. Impulses from visual, auditory or cutaneous receptors.
   C. Psychical disturbances.
7. Sleeplessness may be accompanied by restlessness, hyperactivity and muscular tension.
8. Normal fatigue is experienced after strenuous work. A period of rest or sleep normally restores one's ability to work and a general feeling of well-being.
9. The continuous contraction of muscles leads to muscle fatigue.

PATHOLOGY

1. Signs and symptoms of insufficient rest and sleep may include:
   A. Nervousness, inability to concentrate.
   B. Inappropriate fatigue.
   C Generalized loss of muscle tone, incoordination, lassitude.
   D. Dizziness.
   E. Darkened areas around eyes and puffiness of eyelids.
   F. Reddened and burning conjunctiva, ptosis of eyelids.
   G. Yawning.
   H Excessive irritability, restlessness, muscle tension.
2. Nervousness is a state of mental and, usually, bodily restlessness. It is accompanied by a feeling of uneasiness and apprehension. It tends to interfere with productive, purposeful activities of daily living. Excessive nervousness usually causes inappropriate fatigue.
3. Nervousness most often results from interference with personality organization. The cause of the interference is generally a problem which is not obvious to the individual—some mental or emotional conflict. It is common for major mental disorders to begin with nervousness.
4. Nervousness may result from:
   A. Psychological problems.
   B. Neurological problems (e.g., brain injuries, encephalitis).
   C. Endocrine problems (e.g., thyrotoxicosis).
   D. Certain nutritional deficiencies (e.g., B vitamins).
5. Pathological fatigue cannot be relieved by rest and sleep. Possible causes of pathological fatigue include:
   A. Nervousness.
   B. Neurological problems (e.g., brain injuries).
   C. Endocrine problems (e.g., Addison's disease, diabetes mellitus, thyrotoxicosis). (See Chap. 8.)
   D. Impaired circulation. (See Chap. 1.)
   E. Inadequate oxygen. (See Chap. 2.)
   F. Hypoglycemia. (See Chap. 3.)
   G. The inadequate elimination of metabolic wastes. (See Chap. 7.)

NURSING APPLICATIONS

1. Patients should be observed for signs and symptoms of inadequate sleep and rest; these should be investigated, evaluated, reported and/or be treated with appropriate nursing measures. This is of particular importance when the patient:
   A. Is at extremes of age.
   B. Is under unusual physical or emotional stress (e.g., illness, pregnancy).
   C. Is convalescing from illness or injury.

D. Has a high metabolic rate (e.g., during fever or with thyrotoxicosis).
E. Has impaired circulation.
F. Has impaired respiratory function.
G. Has impaired endocrine function (e.g., adrenal cortical problems).
H. Has malnutrition.
I. Has a mental disorder.

2. The quantity and quality of sleep and rest may be evaluated in relation to:
A. The usual sleep and/or rest patterns.
B. Age.
C. The individual's physical condition.
D. The individual's emotional and psychic status.
E. Any drugs that have been administered to provide sleep and rest.

3. When an individual is under physical or emotional stress, more than the usual rest and sleep should be encouraged and provided.

4. Sleep and rest may be encouraged by such means as:
A. Providing a non-stimulating environment (e.g., limiting light or sound).
B. Providing physical comfort. (See Chap. 14.)
C. Providing psychological comfort.
D. Providing for muscular relaxation. (See Chap. 11.)
E. Providing both physical and mental activities and varieties of each during a 24-hour period.
F. Administering sedative or hypnotic drugs as ordered and indicated.

5. Muscle fatigue may be prevented by:
A. Providing adequate support for the body parts.
B. Changing the positions of the body parts frequently.

11

Locomotion

Bones, muscles and joints provide a means of locomotion.

ANATOMY AND PHYSIOLOGY

General Considerations

1. The skeleton is composed of a definite arrangement of bones joined together by ligaments, cartilage and muscles.
   A. The skeleton provides:
      (1) A framework for the body.
      (2) Protection for soft tissues. (See Chap. 12.)
      (3) A system of levers for locomotion.
   B. Each bone has a distinctive size and shape.
   C. The bones of the skeleton are joined to one another by connective tissue structures which permit varying degrees of movement between the adjoining bones.
      (1) The amount of motion permitted at an articulation depends upon the shapes of the adjoining bones and the arrangement of ligaments, tendons and muscles surrounding the joint.
         (a) Muscle tension interferes with joint motion.
         (b) Prolonged immobilization can cause joint stiffness and limited range of motion.
      (2) A freely movable joint has the following characteristics:
         (a) The contiguous bony surfaces are covered with hyaline cartilage.
         (b) A fibrous capsule surrounds the articulation.
         (c) Synovial membrane lines the capsule and secretes the lubricating synovial fluid.
         (d) Some joints may be divided by menisci (e.g., the knee).
      (3) A bursa is a small closed sac which contains a film of fluid; it acts as a lubricating device. Bursae may be found wherever tendons rub against resistant structures, in some joint cavities and, subcutaneously, over joints that undergo acute flexion or over bones subject to considerable pressure.

137

2. Bone is a plastic tissue composed of an organic portion which gives pliability, and an inorganic portion which gives hardness and rigidity.
   A. The amount of inorganic substance increases with age; the amount of organic substance decreases.
   B. The long bones in children are largely cartilaginous and calcification is usually not complete until the 18th to 20th year. Also the epiphyses usually do not close until this time.
   C. Bone is continually being torn down and built up, and a balance between the two processes must be maintained if bone is to be normal.
   D. The production of bone as well as its growth and repair are affected by several factors. These include:
      (1) Vitamin D and, to some extent, Vitamin A.
      (2) Parathyroid hormone.
      (3) Growth factor of anterior pituitary hormones.
   E. Pressure, stress and weight bearing can alter the shape and growth of bones.
   F. When bone is not functioning for locomotion over a prolonged period of time, some decalcification of the bones occurs.
3. All the movements of the body are brought about through the actions of muscles.
   A. Muscles are formed by groups of muscle fibers held together by connective tissue.
   B. Muscles are firmly attached to bones by connective tissue.
4. Muscle tissue performs mechanical work by contracting; that is, by a shortening and thickening of its fibers.
   A. Muscle contractions occur as a result of complex oxidation-reduction reactions (involving carbohydrates) which occur in in the muscle fibers.
   B. Continuous or frequently repeated "all-out" contractions of a muscle, or continually holding a muscle in a state of contraction, may cause injury to the muscle fibers.
   C. Violent contractions may cause tearing, stretching or even rupture of muscle fibers and the blood vessels that supply the muscle.
   D. Muscle contraction is under nervous control.
      (1) Muscles are under more or less continuous nervous stimulation, and the rotating contraction of different groups of muscle fibers within the muscle results in tonus.
      (2) The myotatic (stretch) reflex is essential for maintaining skeletal muscle tone, which in turn is essential for maintaining the normal condition of muscle fibers.
         (a) The tonus of the antigravity muscles (e.g., those of the jaw) is markedly decreased during sleep or depression of the central nervous system (e.g., with general anesthesia).

(b) The integrity of the higher centers (lying in the cerebral cortex and reticular formations) is essential for the maintenance of normal muscle tonus. These in turn are influenced by proprioceptive impulses arising within the muscle itself.

(c) Tendon jerks are examples of myotatic reflexes.

(d) Muscles that hold the body erect or are involved in locomotion lose their tone very rapidly during prolonged periods of inactivity.

(3) Clonus is caused by the repeated synchronous activation of many motor units.

(4) Tetany (prolonged contraction) is caused by the continuous nervous stimulation of muscle groups.

(5) Change in position of any body part depends upon a constant series of nervous impulses, mediated by efferent nerves, which cause smooth coordinated contractions of the agonist muscles and relaxation of the antagonist muscles involved.

5. Many areas of the cerebral cortex control motor function. The major motor area concerned with voluntary movement is located just in front of the central fissure in the frontal lobe. The baby at birth has practically no voluntary control over his muscular movements.

6. Motor pathways pass directly or indirectly (through subcortical integration centers) to the medulla where up to 85 per cent of the fibers cross before entering the spinal cord.

7. The motor fibers pass down the spinal cord in several tracts and synapse with the lower motor neurons in the anterior horns of the spinal cord.

8. The individual muscles innervated by the motor nerves lie either approximately at the same level or below the level of origin of the lower motor neurons.

9. The spinal nerves that supply the upper and the lower extremities divide, recombine and divide again in complicated patterns to form two nerve plexuses.

A. The brachial plexuses are located between the neck and the axilla in each shoulder; the nerves supply all the muscles of the upper extremities.

B. The lumbosacral plexuses are located in the lower back; the nerves supply all the muscles of the lower extremities.

10. The peripheral nerves which run very superficially in the extremities include:

A. The peroneal, in the popliteal space.

B. The ulnar, along the medial upper arm and down the ulna side of the forearm.

C. The radial, around the back of the humerus and down the radial side of the forearm.

D. The sciatic, in the hip and down the back of the thigh.

11. The functions of the cerebellum are concerned with equilibrium, postural reflexes, regulation of muscle tone and coordination of voluntary movement.

12. Proprioceptors, located in the skeletal muscles, tendons and joints, are sensitive to pressure or stretch and transmit impulses to the brain by way of the posterior columns of the spinal cord.

A. These impulses provide information about movements and the position of the limbs, and are important for muscular coordination.

B. Conscious interpretation of the impulses takes place in the temporal and parietal lobes of the cerebral cortex.

13. There are reflex mechanisms governing the orientation of the head in space, the relation of the head to the trunk, and the appropriate adjustments of the limbs to the position of the head.

A. Sensory nerve endings in the inner ear, the retina and the skeletal muscles, tendons and joints receive stimuli. (See Chap. 16.)

B. Impulses are transmitted to the spinal cord, the midbrain and the cerebellum.

C. Motor nerves cause appropriate postural adjustments.

Facts About Specific Bones, Muscles and Joints Concerned with Locomotion

1. The bones of the upper extremity include those of the shoulder girdle (clavicle and scapula), the upper arm (humerus), the lower arm (radius and ulna), the wrist (8 carpal bones), and the hand (5 metacarpal bones and 14 phalanges).

2. The shoulder joint, formed by the articulation of the head of the humerus with the scapula, is of the ball and socket type.

A. The socket is shallow.

B. The ligaments surrounding the joint are relatively loose.

C. The shoulder joint allows movement of the humerus in all directions.

D. The scapula is connected to the trunk by muscles only.

3. Muscles that originate on the trunk and insert on the shoulder girdle (acting singly or in combinations) act to adduct, abduct, elevate, depress and to rotate the shoulder girdle.

(For complete abduction of the shoulder, the humerus must be outwardly rotated after the first 90° of motion.)

4. Muscles that originate on the trunk and shoulder girdle and insert on the humerus (acting singly or in combinations) act to adduct, abduct, flex, extend and rotate the humerus.

5. The elbow joint comprises three different portions: the joints between the ulna and humerus, between the radius and humerus, and between the radius and the ulna.
   A. The joint between the ulna and the humerus is a simple hinge joint.
   B. Muscles that originate on the shoulder girdle and/or the humerus and insert on the radius or ulna act to flex and to extend the forearm.
   C. Muscles that originate and insert on the ulna and radius act to supinate and to promote the forearm.
6. The wrist joint proper, formed by the articulations of several carpal bones and the distal end of the radius, is of the gliding type.
   A. Muscles of the posterior aspect of the forearm act to extend the hand.
   B. Muscles of the anterior aspect of the forearm act to flex the hand.
   C. The flexors and extensors acting in different groupings also abduct, adduct and circumduct the hand.
7. The joints between the metacarpal and the carpal bones are of the gliding type, and have limited motion, with the exception of the first metacarpal, which is a saddle joint and allows for abduction, adduction, circumduction and opposition of the thumb.
8. The joints between the metacarpal and phalangeal bones are of the condyloid type and allow flexion, extension, limited abduction and adduction and circumduction of the fingers.
   (Flexion of the fingers can best be accomplished when the wrist is in hyperextension; the flexion should allow for the natural deviation of the fingers toward the thumb side of the palm.)
9. The joints between the phalanges of each digit are of the hinge type and allow for flexion and extension.
10. The vertebral column is composed of individual vertebrae, the bodies of which are separated by fibro-cartilaginous discs, and all are bound together by numerous ligaments that pass from one bone to another.
    A. The intervetebral discs absorb shock and permit a slight degree of movement.
    B. The vertebral column articulates with the skull and with the iliac bones of the pelvic girdle.
11. At birth and until a baby is able to hold up his head, the primary curve of the vertebral column is posteriorly convex. After the baby's muscles have developed enough so that he can hold up his head and stand and walk, the secondary curves of the vertebral column appear.
    A. The cervical curve is anteriorly convex.
    B. The thoracic curve is posteriorly convex.

C. The lumbar curve is anteriorly convex.

D. The natural curves of the vertebral column give resilience and help to absorb shock.

E. The natural curves may be changed by prolonged postural changes, variations in walking, and pregnancy.

F. In walking or sitting the pelvic girdle normally provides support for the vertebral column.

12. Muscles of the back that essentially attach vertebrae to vertebrae or vertebrae to ribs act to extend the spine and assist in rotation of the spine. (These muscles are fixator muscles and are arranged primarily for the purpose of support, not for the performance of work.)

13. Muscles that originate on the pelvic girdle and insert on the ribs act to flex the spine.

14. Muscles that originate on the vertebrae or shoulder girdle and insert on the posterior skull act to extend the head.

15. Muscles that originate on the temporal bone or cervical vertebrae and insert on the clavicle or rib cage act to flex the head.

16. The bones of the lower extremity include those of the pelvic girdle (hip bones, sacrum and coccyx), the thigh (femur), the leg (tibia and fibula), the ankle (7 tarsal bones) and the foot (5 metatarsal bones and 14 phalanges).

A. The hip bone consists of three parts: the ileum, the ischium and the pubis. The hip bones articulate anteriorly at the symphysis pubis.

B. During pregnancy a hormone causes some relaxation of the ligaments of the pelvic girdle.

17. The hip joint, formed by the articulation of the head of the femur fitting into the acetabulum of the hip bone, is of the ball and socket type.

18. Muscles that originate on the vertebrae or pelvic girdle and insert on the femur (acting singly or in combinations) act to flex, extend, abduct, adduct or rotate the femur.

19. The knee joint, formed by the articulation of the distal femur and the tibia, is both condyloid and gliding.

A. The knee movements are closely related to movements of the hip joint (e.g., flexion of femur and flexion of lower leg).

B. The patella is a flat bone located in the tendon on the quadriceps femoris in front of the knee joint; it articulates with the femur. (It helps to protect the knee joint, especially in kneeling.)

C. Menisci (small crescents of fibrocartilage) lie between the tibia and the femur and help to adapt the surfaces of these bones and obviate jars.

20. Muscles that originate on the pelvic girdle or femur and insert on the tibia (acting singly or in combinations) act to extend, flex and, in certain positions, to rotate (medially and laterally) the lower leg.

21. The ankle joint, formed by the articulation of the distal ends of the tibia and fibula and one of the tarsal bones, is both hinge and condyloid in type.
    A. Muscles that originate on the tibia and fibula and insert on the medial or lateral aspects of the tarsal or metatarsal bones act either to invert or evert the foot.
    B. Muscles that originate on the anterior aspects of the tibia and fibula and insert on the tarsal bones act to dorsiflex the foot.
    C. Muscles that originate on the posterior aspects of the femur, tibia and fibula and insert on the tarsal bones act to plantar-flex the foot. (The major muscles that act to plantar-flex the foot insert in the tendon of Achilles.)
22. The tarsal and metatarsal articulations allow limited gliding motions.
23. The metatarsal and phalangeal articulations allow some flexion, extension, abduction and adduction.
24. The interphalangeal joints permit flexion and limited extension.
25. The foot has a longitudinal arch and a series of transverse arches formed by the arrangement of the tarsal and metatarsal bones and the ligaments that bind them together. (When the body is raised on the ball of one foot, the stress on the longitudinal arch is increased fourfold.)
26. The major muscle groups may be considered to include:
    A. Flexors and extensors of the toes and fingers.
    B. Flexors, extensors and rotators of the feet and hands.
    C. Flexors and extensors of the legs and thighs.
    D. Flexors, extensors, supinators and pronators of the lower arm.
    E. Flexors, extensors and rotators of the upper arm.
    F. Extensors of the vertebral column.
    G. Adductors, abductors, elevators and depressors of the shoulder girdle.
    H. Flexors and rotators of the trunk.

Posture

1. Good posture may be defined as maintaining good anatomical relationships between body parts when the body is in different positions.
    A. The alignment of the body parts should be balanced, and there should not be undue muscle tension or strain.
    B. Correct body posture exists when the muscular forces required to balance torques produced by the weights of various parts of the body are at a minimum.
2. A good lying posture in the dorsal recumbent position is the closest possible to good standing posture.
3. A good lying posture in the supine position is the closest possible to the good standing posture with the head turned to the side.

4. A good lying posture in the side-lying position is an approximation of a good sitting posture.
5. The position of function for the hand is similar to that position used in gripping a ball.
6. The position of function for the foot is that position desirable in good standing posture.
7. The spinal muscles supply the contractions necessary for erect posture. If the reflex mechanisms necessary for this posture are lost, the muscles must be controlled voluntarily. Poor posture and fatigue result.
8. Poor posture is often related to one's emotional status (e.g., depression or excessive tension), while good posture generally accompanies a sense of well-being.

PHYSICS

1. Force is that which changes or tends to change the linear motion of a body, and the motion is in the same direction as the force.
2. Work is done by a force if the force is allowed to act through a distance.
3. Torque is that force which changes or tends to change the rotary motion of a body.
4. Gravitation is the force of attraction between two objects (e.g., the earth and an object on or near the earth).
    A. The center of gravity of a body is the point where the whole weight of a body may be considered to be concentrated. (The center of gravity in the human body is located at a point approximately 0.57 of the height of the body.)
    B. Because of gravitational pull, more force is usually required to lift a heavy object than to push or pull it along a smooth surface.
5. A body is said to be unstable if a slight tipping of the object raises its center of gravity.
    A. A vertical line drawn downward from the center of gravity of a body in stable equilibrium will fall within the base of support. (Increasing the base of support will increase stability.)
    B. In general, a change in the position of the center of gravity upsets equilibrium and, for equilibrium to be regained, changes must be made in forces and/or torques acting on the object (e.g., in standing, when there is a forward shift in the center of gravity, the muscles of the back must exert more pull to maintain body balance).
6. When a body is in equilibrium,
    A. The sum of all forces acting on the body equals zero, and
    B. The sum of all torques acting at any axis must equal zero.
7. Within the elastic limit, the stress is proportional to the strain. (Hooke's Law)

A. If the elastic limit of an object is exceeded, the object is either permanently distorted or broken.

B. Types of stress that may produce characteristic injuries in the body are tension, compression, twisting and bending.

8. A lever is a simple machine comprising a rigid bar which moves about a fulcrum (or fixed axis). Keeping lever arms short decreases the torque produced by a given load.

PATHOLOGY

Signs and Symptoms

1. Signs and symptoms of problems involving bones may include:
   A. Abnormalities in contour, alignment or continuity of a part or parts.
   B. Absence of, loss of, or change of movement of a part.
   C. Crepitus.
   D. Pain (especially with movement).
   E. Ecchymosis or hematoma of injured part.
   F. Local edema.

2. Signs and symptoms of problems involving voluntary muscles may include:
   A. Muscle fatigue.
   B. Loss of function.
   C. Muscle spasms, which may be accompanied by acute cramping pain.
   D. Lameness, aching of muscles or acute pain.
   E. Muscle atrophy.

3. Signs and symptoms of problems involving the nervous control of muscle function may include:
   A. Paralysis (flaccid or spastic).
   B. Convulsions, tics, muscle spasms, tremors.
   C. Changes in muscle contractions (e.g., strength or coordination).
   D. Difficulty in postural adjustments.
   E. Hypoactive tendon reflexes (e.g., loss of knee jerk).
   F. Hyperactive tendon reflexes (e.g., ankle clonus or tonic neck reflex).
   G. Cramping pain which may accompany muscle spasms.
   H. Burning, tingling pain along peripheral nerve.
   I. Numbness of part.

4. Signs and symptoms of problems involving the movements of joints may include:
   A. Change in contour or size of joint.
   B. Limitation of motion in joints.
   C. Swelling, redness and increased skin temperature around joint.
   D. Local aching or pain which may become acute with muscle contractions.

Bones

1. Problems affecting bones may include:
   A. Congenital or acquired deformities.
   B. Fractures, with or without dislocations.
   C. Infections.
   D. Metabolic disease (e.g., osteomalacia).
   E. Abnormal growths in or on the bone (e.g., cysts, tumors).
   (Injuries to the skull, vertebrae and thorax are included in Chap. 12.)
2. Congenital bone defects may include such things as absence of bones, positional anomalies (e.g., clubbed feet) or dislocations.
3. Bone deformities may be acquired through:
   A. Abnormal bone development because of malnutrition. (See Chap. 3.)
   B. Abnormal bone development because of hormone imbalance. (See Chap. 8.)
   C. Abnormal prolonged pressure against bones, especially during growth.
   D. Infections (e.g., tuberculosis).
   E. Bone tumors.
4. Fractures are breaks in the continuity of bone which may be caused by trauma or because of pathology of the bone itself.
   A. Fractures may be complete, incomplete, simple, compound, green-stick or comminuted.
   B. Fractures occur more easily in older people.
   C. When bone is fractured there is hemorrhage and the formation of granulation tissue (called procallus). The granulation tissue becomes dense connective tissue, and then fibrocartilaginous tissue (callus) develops between the fragments of bone. Ossification and calcification follow. Bony union is accomplished when new spongy bone invading the callus (from the periosteum of the bone fragments) makes contact and unites.
   D. The rate and quality of bone healing depends upon such factors as:
      (1) The size of the bone involved.
      (2) The alignment of the fractured parts (which may be accomplished through reduction and/or traction).
      (3) The blood supply to the part.
      (4) Adequate nutrition.
      (5) Immobilization of the part.
      (6) Protection of the part from trauma.
      (7) Absence or presence of infection.
5. Osteomalacia is a disease in which the bones become soft because of inadequate calcification. The condition may be related to malnutrition, hormonal imbalance or poor blood supply.

6. Osteomyelitis is inflammation of bone due to injury by micro-organisms. The infection usually occurs because of wound contamination, which may happen with a compound fracture or with bone surgery.

Muscles

1. Problems that affect muscles may include:
   A. Inflammation due to over-exercise, overstraining of muscle fibers or chilling.
   B. Inadequate blood supply. (See Chap. 1.)
   C. Malnutrition. (See Chap. 3.)
   D. Interference with normal innervation of muscle contractions.
   E. Traumatic injuries (e.g., with fractures, dislocations, crushing injuries, surgery).
   F. Parasites (e.g., trichinosis).
   G. Congenital or acquired weakness.
   (Problems of abdominal and perineal muscles are included in Chap. 12.)
2. Myositis is an inflammation of muscle tissue which is often due to over-exercise, prolonged stretching of muscles or sudden pull. It can also result from chilling (e.g., neck and back muscles). There is muscle tenderness which may be exquisite, and often muscle spasm which can be extremely painful (e.g., gastrocnemius muscle).
3. Trichinosis is a parasitic infestation by the *Trichinella spiralis*. The parasites are ingested and may invade many body organs. When the skeletal muscles are invaded, there is acute muscle pain, especially during muscle contraction.

Nerves

1. Problems affecting the nervous control of muscles may include:
   A. Injury to the sensory and/or motor areas of the brain.
   B. Injury to the sensory and/or motor pathways in the brain and the spinal cord.
   C. Injury to the spinal nerves, various nerve plexuses or peripheral nerves.
   D. Injury to the kinesthetic receptors in the muscles themselves.
   E. Injury to the cerebellum, midbrain or vestibular apparatus.
2. Injury to nerve tissue involved in normal muscle function may be caused by:
   A. Trauma.
   B. Pressure due to accumulating fluid (e.g., inflammatory exudate, excessive cerebrospinal fluid, or blood) or abnormal growths (e.g., cysts, tumors).
   C. Inadequate blood supply. (See Chap. 1.)
   D. Inadequate oxygen. (See Chap. 2.)

E. Malnutrition (glucose in particular). (See Chap. 3.)

F. Degenerative disorders (e.g., multiple sclerosis, Parkinson's disease).

G. Infections (e.g., encephalitis, meningitis).

H. Toxic substances in the blood (e.g., waste products of metabolism). (See Chap. 7.)

3. Injury to the motor areas of the cerebral cortex, the motor pathways in the brain and spinal cord, the anterior horn cells or peripheral nerves usually causes paralysis.

A. In upper motor neuron damage (cerebral cortex or tracts), the muscles are spastic and reflexes are exaggerated.

B. In lower motor neuron damage (anterior horn or peripheral nerve), the muscles are flaccid, reflexes are limited or lost, and muscle atrophy occurs.

4. Injury to the motor area, or to the motor pathways to the cerebellum, midbrain or vestibular apparatus may also cause other abnormal motor activity. These include:

A. Involuntary movements such as convulsions, spasms, tics, tremors.

B. Muscle rigidity.

C. Muscular incoordination.

D. Difficulty with postural adjustments.

(Injury to the vestibular apparatus is included in Chap. 16.)

5. Injury to the sensory areas of the cerebral cortex, the sensory pathways in the brain and spinal cord or peripheral nerves usually causes flaccid paralysis. There is lack of sensation from the part which is affected by the nerve damage. Positional reflexes are limited or lost. Muscle atrophy follows.

6. Tabes dorsalis is a condition which may occur in chronic syphilis. The posterior columns of the spinal cord and posterior nerve roots are injured.

7. Epilepsy is a chronic disorder that involves the cerebral cortex. It is characterized by seizures which may include convulsions.

A. Grand mal attacks involve convulsions and, frequently, loss of consciousness.

B. Petit mal attacks involve momentary losses of consciousness.

C. Psychomotor attacks may involve loss of consciousness, loss of memory, violent activity and muscular incoordination.

8. Cerebral palsy is a disturbance of the motor function and is frequently associated with birth injuries. There is spastic weakness of the extremities and exaggerated reflexes.

9. Multiple sclerosis is a degenerative disorder that involves demyelination of nerves and sclerosing of areas in the brain and spinal cord. Symptoms are determined by the areas affected. Muscle weakness, incoordination and involuntary movements (e.g., tremors, spasms or jerking movements) occur frequently.

10. Parkinson's disease is a degenerative disease which causes destruction of nerve cells in the basal ganglia. There are muscle tremors of increasing severity, muscle rigidity and general difficulty with neuromuscular control.
11. Cerebrovascular accidents usually cause some degree of paralysis and/or loss of sensation.
12. Meningitis is an inflammation of the meninges and may be caused by a number of different microorganisms, including the *Neisseria meningitidis*. There may be muscle rigidity, muscle spasms and paralysis.
13. Encephalitis is an inflammation of the brain tissue and may be caused by a number of different microorganisms, including a number of viruses. There may be signs and symptoms of motor and/or sensory difficulties, depending upon the extent of the inflammation and the severity.
14. Poliomyelitis is an acute viral infection which usually affects the anterior horn cells, causing severe muscle spasms, flaccid paralysis and muscle atrophy. (Bulbar poliomyelitis is included in Chap. 2.)

Joints

1. Problems that affect the movement of joints may include:
   A. Trauma to the various tissues in and around the joint (e.g., strains, sprains, fractures).
   B. Degenerative changes (e.g., hypertrophic arthritis).
   C. Inflammatory disease of the joint (e.g., atrophic arthritis, gout).
   D. Infections (e.g., as may occur with rheumatic fever).
   E. Accumulation of fluid within the joint cavity (e.g., blood, inflammatory exudate).
2. Hypertrophic arthritis (sometimes called osteoarthritis) involves hypertrophic changes in the joint. The joint becomes enlarged, the articular cartilages become thin, and there may be calcium deposits within the joint. This condition may result from traumatic injury, excessive use of the joint, poor posture and excessive weight bearing.
3. Atrophic arthritis (sometimes called rheumatoid arthritis) is an inflammatory condition of joints in which all the tissues show inflammatory response (e.g., changes in production of synovial fluid, edema, congestion, tissue destruction, fibrosis). The entire joint may eventually become spongy and ankylosed. Muscle spasms occur frequently. The condition is often classified as a collagen disease and may be associated with general poor physical and/or emotional health, possibly endocrine imbalance.
4. Gout is a chronic inflammatory condition of the joints in which there are deposits of sodium urate crystals in the joints, frequently in the feet. There seems to be an inherited tendency in the development of this condition.

5. Bursitis is an inflammation of bursae, which may result from traumatic injury, strain or overuse of muscles and joints around which these structures are found.

NURSING APPLICATIONS

Observation and Evaluation

1. Patients should be observed for signs and symptoms of abnormal structure and function of the bones, muscles and joints necessary to normal locomotion; these should be investigated, evaluated, reported and/or be treated with appropriate nursing measures. This is of particular importance when the patient:
   A. Is at extremes of age.
   B. Has been subjected to traumatic injury (e.g., falling, auto accidents).
   C. Has a disease or injury (e.g., surgery) involving these bones, muscles or joints.
   D. Has a disease or injury (e.g., surgery) that involves the brain, spinal cord, peripheral nerves or kinesthetic receptors.
   E. Has restricted physical activity.
   F. Is pregnant.
   G. Has extensive, severe burns.
2. The structure and function of bones, muscles and joints necessary to normal locomotion should be evaluated in relation to the:
   A. Normal size and contour of body parts.
   B. Normal alignment of body parts.
   C. Normal movements of body parts.
   D. Normal voluntary control of body movements.
   E. Normal postural reflexes.
   F. Presence of any injury or disease process that may affect the bones, muscles, joints and nervous control of locomotion.

Preventing Injury

Patients should be protected from injury to bones, muscles, joints and nervous tissues involved in locomotion by such means as:
1. Providing and encouraging the closest approach possible to normal anatomical alignment while in any posture (lying, sitting, standing).
   A. When normal alignment is not possible effort should be directed toward improving the alignment (e.g., through positioning, adjustment of equipment or environmental factors such as light).
   B. Emotional support should be consistent.
   C. Any possible emotional components should be recognized and reported appropriately.
2. Teaching and encouraging the use of good body mechanics.
   A. The body should be balanced over a firm base of support in

standing, walking, squatting or rising. (Using a wide stance and keeping the body centered over the base of support increases stability of an upright posture.)

B. When carrying heavy objects, the balance of the body should be shifted from the ankle rather than from the trunk.

C. Prolonged carrying of objects on one side should be avoided.

D. The pelvis and lower extremities should provide a firm support for the vertebral column through use of low-heeled shoes, or through standing and walking postures that provide this support.

E. The least amount of muscular effort necessary to perform a given task should be used.

   (1) Movements should be made smoothly and rhythmically.

   (2) In lifting or carrying heavy objects, the arms should be held close to the body and the object should be close to the body before lifting is done.

   (3) When moving a heavy object, the parts of the body should be placed in such a way as to face in the same direction as the force to be applied.

   (4) Objects should be moved or slid along surfaces if possible, rather than lifted.

   (5) Body weight should be utilized whenever possible to push or pull objects.

   (6) When performing tasks, the sitting position should be used in preference to standing whenever possible.

   (7) Work levels should be such that muscle strain is minimized.

F. Objects that are too heavy to be moved alone should not be lifted without adequate assistance.

G. The muscles best suited to the task to be done should be utilized.

   (1) In lifting, pushing or pulling the muscles of the lower extremities should be used rather than the muscles of the trunk.

   (2) In carrying heavy objects, the muscles of the upper extremities should be used rather than the muscles of the trunk.

   (3) When reaching upward or working at low levels, the trunk should be maintained in normal alignment and adjustments made by the lower extremities (e.g., rising on toes or squatting).

3. Providing for and encouraging whatever exercise is possible (active or passive) of the major groups of muscles daily, unless this is contraindicated.

A. The freely movable body joints of the trunk and extremities should be moved through their normal and/or anatomically possible ranges of motion, at least once a day.

B. Exercise should be increased gradually within medical orders (e.g., planned arm and shoulder exercises following radical mastectomy).

C. Over-exercising should be prevented and discouraged, and any signs and symptoms of this should be reported appropriately.

D. Patients should be encouraged to assume activities of daily living as much as possible.

4. Preventing muscle fatigue by planning and providing adequate rest periods.

5. Providing adequate support for the body parts without pressure, drag or strain (e.g., head, vertebral column, shoulders, knees, hips and feet). Supporting the head is of particular importance for the infant.

6. Providing frequent changes of position (at *least* three times daily) within medical orders. Prolonged pressure against any bone should be prevented; this is of particular importance in the young and when there is bone pathology.

7. Moving patients smoothly and maintaining the normal body alignments during the moving process.

8. Handling the body parts firmly but gently, always providing adequate support for the limb and the joints.

9. Protecting patients from accidents (e.g., falling, slipping, striking hard objects).

10. Encouraging and providing good nutrition and weight reduction as indicated. (See Chap. 3.)

11. Preventing chilling of body parts (e.g., neck or shoulders).

12. Using strict aseptic technique when there is a compound fracture or internal skeletal devices.

13. Encouraging and providing as possible well-fitting and appropriate wearing apparel.

A. Clothing should not add heavy weight or pull over the shoulders.

B. Foundation garments should be well-fitting and constructed for the purpose for which they are worn (e.g., corsets or braces).

C. Shoes and hosiery should be the correct size and shape. High heels should be discouraged for regular wear; this is of particular importance for the pregnant woman or a patient who has spinal problems.

14. Using caution in the administration of intramuscular injections (e.g., site of injection, amount of injection and type of fluid injected).

15. Encouraging competent medical supervision during pregnancy, labor, delivery, the post partum period.

16. Observing for signs and symptoms of inadequate circulation and taking appropriate action. (See Chap. 1.)

17. Observing for signs and symptoms of peripheral nerve damage and taking appropriate action promptly (e.g., notifying physician, bivalving a cast if necessary).

18. Observing for signs and symptoms of local or systemic infection and

reporting these appropriately. This is of particular importance when there is a compound fracture or internal fixation devices.

19. Protecting the patient from injury to bones, muscles, joints and peripheral nerves is of particular importance when the patient:
    A. Is dependent upon others for physical care or protection. These patients include those who:
       (1) Have psychic disturbances.
       (2) Have loss of consciousness (e.g., brain injury, general anesthesia).
       (3) Have difficulty with vision, hearing, touch or equilibrium.
       (4) Are infants, children or elderly.
       (5) Are weak, fatigued or debilitated.
       (6) Are mentally incompetent.
    B. Is subject to or having convulsions (e.g., epilepsy).
    C. Is subject to loss of consciousness (e.g., hypertension, emotional disturbances or epilepsy).
    D. Has specific problems involving locomotion.

Nursing Treatments

1. When fracture of a bone has occurred or is suspected:
   A. The affected part should be left in the position assumed until medical assistance is available or,
   B. If transportation is necessary, it should be accomplished with the least possible amount of motion of the injured part.
      (1) The affected part should be splinted if possible.
          (a) A traction-type splint is preferable for simple fractures of the extremities.
          (b) A splint without traction is preferable for compound fractures.
          (c) Splinting of bones requires immobilization of the joints above and below the injury.
          (d) If the knee or elbow is injured and no traction is available, the full lengths of the articulating bones should be splinted in the position that has been assumed.
      (2) If the hip is injured, movement of it should be avoided, and the extremity affected should be allowed to remain in the position of comfort.
   C. Cold applications may be helpful.
2. Muscle relaxation may be promoted by:
   A. Massage.
   B. Positive relaxation exercises.
   C. Positioning.
   D. Extra warmth.
   E. Providing a non-stimulating environment.

F. Providing physical comfort.

G. Providing emotional comfort.

3. When a patient has simple muscle spasm (cramping):
    A. The affected muscle may be carefully placed on stretch (e.g., spasm of the gastrocnemius may be relieved by dorsal flexion of the foot).
    B. Gentle massage of the muscle may be helpful. (This should not be done if there is possibility of a circulatory problem.)
    C. Warm applications may be helpful.

4. When a patient has severe muscle spasms and/or there is spastic paralysis:
    A. The muscles affected should be put at rest in position of comfort.
    B. Deformities should be prevented by providing normal alignment and positions of function as much as possible (e.g., by use of pads, pillows, sandbags, rubber balls for hands, special splints).
    C. Heat should be applied effectively as ordered and indicated.
    D. Antispasmodic drugs should be administered promptly as ordered and indicated.

5. When a patient has flaccid paralysis, the affected part:
    A. Must be supported in good alignment at all times.
    B. Must be protected from pressure, stretching, or abnormal motion.

6. When periarticular structures (e.g., ligaments, muscles or bursae) are inflamed, torn or stretched:
    A. The involved joint should be immobilized.
    B. Warm or cold applications may be helpful, depending upon the time elapsed since the injury. Cold may be helpful immediately; warmth, later on.

7. When a patient has inflammation of a joint (e.g., in arthritis):
    A. The body parts should be maintained in an alignment as normal as possible. The hands and feet should be kept in position of function.
    B. The affected joint should be kept immobilized as ordered.
    C. Exercises involving the affected joint should be done as ordered. (These may be preceded by applications of heat and/or the administration of pain-relieving medications.)
    D. The joint should be handled gently and kept well supported.
    E. Applications of heat should be carried out effectively as ordered and indicated.
    F. Observations should be made for signs of increasing limitations of motion or deformity, and these should be reported appropriately.

8. When a patient has sustained injury to structures concerned with locomotion, medical orders relative to positioning, exercise, immobilization and/or traction should be explicit and followed exactly.

Any problems related to these factors or accidental trauma to the affected part should be reported promptly.

9. When a patient has a cast applied:
   A. The body part extending beyond the cast or partially movable within the cast should be kept in the same alignment as the body parts held immovable by the cast.
   B. The injured part should be supported in good alignment at all times.
   C. The injured extremity may be elevated as permitted by medical orders.
   D. The cast should be protected from dampness.
   E. The cast should be protected from pressure while it is drying (e.g., with pillows). The patient should be turned on the unaffected side only.
   F. The affected part should be observed closely for signs and symptoms of an inadequate blood supply. (See Chap. 1.)
   G. He should be observed closely for signs and symptoms of peripheral nerve damage. If these should occur, the physician should be notified at once and, if necessary, the cast should be bivalved promptly.

10. When a patient has traction applied and the objective is to immobilize and align a part:
    A. The injured part should be maintained in the exact alignment in which it was placed by the physician.
    B. The traction apparatus should be maintained as it had been arranged (e.g., weights and alignment of pulleys).

11. When a patient has traction applied and the objective is to stretch contracted muscles or to relieve pain:
    A. The traction may be interrupted for nursing care as permitted.
    B. Changes of position may be made as permitted.

12

Bones, Muscles and Fluid That Protect and Support

Some bones, muscles and body fluid serve to protect and support underlying soft tissues.

ANATOMY AND PHYSIOLOGY

1. The bones of the skull protect the contents of the cranium, including the brain, the meninges, the blood vessels and the cerebrospinal fluid.
2. Some of the bones of the skull (frontal, parietal, temporal and occipital) are united in suture lines that are immovable joints. The suture lines are not united at birth and there are unossified areas between the bones.
   A. The anterior fontanel lies between the two parietal and frontal bones, and normally closes within one and one-half years.
   B. The posterior fontanel lies between the two parietal and the occipital bones, and normally closes within 6 months.
3. Cerebrospinal fluid is produced constantly in the lateral ventricles. From there it circulates through the ventricles and into the subarachnoid space. The fluid circulates in this space around the brain and spinal cord. The fluid is reabsorbed into the venous system, primarily in the dural sinuses.
   A. Cerebrospinal fluid is watery, yellowish and somewhat similar to tissue fluid.
   B. In the adult there is about 125 ml. of cerebrospinal fluid.
   C. The fluid has a protective function (among others), in that it serves to cushion the brain and spinal cord.
4. The vertebral column protects the contents of the neural canal.
   A. The vertebrae are connected by anterior and posterior ligaments and intervertebral discs.
   B. The neural canal, containing the spinal cord, meninges and spinal fluid, is formed by the bodies and processes of the vertebrae.

C. Spinal nerves emerge from the neural canal through the inter-vertebral foramina, which are posterior to the bodies of the vertebrae and between the bases of successive arches.

D. The intervertebral discs have an outer layer of fibrous tissue and an inner soft elastic tissue called the nucleus pulposa. The discs act as shock absorbers.

5. The thoracic cage is composed of 12 thoracic vertebrae, which articulate with the 12 pairs of ribs, some of which articulate anteri-orly with the sternum and clavicle.

A. Within the thoracic cage lie the lungs, the heart and the great vessels.

B. Movement of the ribs by costal muscles plays an important role in breathing.

C. The diaphragm, which plays an important role in breathing, originates in part on the ribs and sternum.

6. The pelvic girdle is composed of the hip bones, the sacrum and the coccyx.

A. The hip bones articulate anteriorly at the symphysis pubis. They articulate with the sacrum posteriorly in the sacroiliac joints.

B. The true pelvis contains the bladder, rectum and (in the female) the non-pregnant uterus and vagina.

7. The muscles of the abdominal wall are flat muscles which extend from the pelvic girdle or lumbodorsal fascia to the costal cartilages; they help to support and protect the abdominal and pelvic viscera.

A. The separated rectus abdominis muscles extend from the pubes to the anterior rib cage, and are relatively weak muscles. The umbilicus lies between the separated rectus muscles and trans-mits the umbilical cord in the unborn child.

B. The inguinal canal (which transmits the spermatic cord in the male and the round ligament in the female) runs through the lower portion of the abdominal muscles above the inguinal liga-ment. It has two openings: a superficial one in the external oblique close to the body of the pubis, and a deep opening, which lies more laterally and opens into the abdominal cavity.

C. The femoral canal lies in the femoral sheath. Its base is the femoral ring, which lies behind the inguinal ligament. It trans-mits numerous lymphatic vessels.

8. The muscles of the pelvic floor support part of the weight of the abdominal viscera and pelvic viscera. These muscles include the paired levator ani and coccygeus muscles. During childbirth the muscles of the pelvic floor are markedly stretched.

9. The abdominal muscles are contracted and exert pressure against the abdominal and pelvic viscera during:

A. Forced expiration.

B. Coughing.

C. Vomiting.
D. Voluntary compression during such processes as micturition and defecation.
E. Flexion of the vertebral column.
F. Lifting legs when lying in horizontal position.

PATHOLOGY

Signs and Symptoms

1. Head injury:
   A. Abnormality in contour or alignment or contiguity of skull bones.
   B. Headache.
   C. Observable bleeding (e.g., from injured area, nose, mouth, ears).
   D. Drainage of cerebrospinal fluid (e.g., from nose, ears, wound).
   E. Signs and symptoms of brain injury (e.g., due to increased intracranial pressure). These may include:
      (1) Changes in cardiovascular function. (See Chap. 1.)
      (2) Changes in respiratory function. (See Chap. 2.)
      (3) Nausea and/or vomiting (often projectile). (See Chap. 3.)
      (4) Problems related to elimination. (See Chap. 7.)
      (5) Hyperthermia. (See Chap. 9.)
      (6) Excessive irritability, hyperactivity. (See Chap. 10.)
      (7) Changes in motor function. (See Chap. 11.)
      (8) Changes in sensory function. (See Chap. 11 and 16.)
      (9) Changes in mental functions. (See Chap. 17.)
      (10) Changes in speech. (See Chap. 18.)
2. Spinal injury:
   A. Abnormality in contour, alignment or contiguity of vertebral column.
   B. Headache, local pain at site of injury or pain along paths of sensory nerves.
   C. Loss of locomotive function involving muscles attached to trunk. (See Chap. 11.)
   D. Drainage of cerebrospinal fluid (e.g., from wound).
   E. Signs and symptoms of spinal cord injury (dependent to some extent upon the level of injury). These may include:
      (1) Changes in respiratory function. (See Chap. 2.)
      (2) Problems related to elimination. (See Chap. 7.)
      (3) Changes in motor function. (See Chap. 11.)
      (4) Changes in sensory function. (See Chap. 11 and 16.)
3. Injury to the bones of the thoracic cage:
   A. Abnormality in contour, alignment or contiguity of the bones of the thoracic cage.
   B. Sharp pain, especially with respiratory movements.

C. Changes in respiratory function. (See Chap. 2.)

D. Changes in heart action. (See Chap. 1.)

4. Injury to the bones of the pelvic girdle:
   A. Abnormality in contour, alignment or contiguity of bones of the pelvic girdle.
   B. Loss of locomotive function involving muscles attached to pelvic girdle. (See Chap. 11.)
   C. Pain, local or radiating down leg.
   D. Urine retention, constipation or abnormal drainage.
   E. Problems related to the uterus (pregnant or non-pregnant).

5. Injury to the abdominal musculature:
   A. Weakness of loss of function of the abdominal muscles.
   B. Abnormal lumps (especially in groin, scrotum or umbilicus).
   C. Pain (especially with muscle contractions).
   D. Wound separation, possibly with evisceration.

6. Injury to the muscles of the pelvic floor:
   A. Incontinence or retention of urine.
   B. Incontinence or retention of feces.
   C. Feeling of pressure or dragging sensation in pelvic area.
   D. Prolapsed uterus.
   E. Dysmenorrhea.

(Basic pathology related to bones and muscles is included in Chap. 11.)

Injuries and Disturbances of Function

1. A traumatic head injury can result in:
   A. Loss of consciousness (which may be momentary or prolonged).
   B. Bone fracture (with depression or splintering of fragments).
   C. Inflammatory response with hyperemia and edema and eventual fibrosing.
   D. Hemorrhage.
   E. Loss of cerebrospinal fluid or interference with the production and/or absorption of this fluid.

2. Hydrocephalus is a condition in which there is interference with the normal production and/or drainage of cerebrospinal fluid.

3. A traumatic injury of the vertebral column can cause injury to the spinal cord and nerve roots. Such injury may be the result of:
   A. Stress, caused by tension, compression, twisting or bending.
   B. Fractures with or without displacement.
   C. Bone pathology (with subsequent destruction and collapse).
   D. Ruptured or slipped intervertebral disc.

4. Intervertebral discs can become softened and the nucleus pulposus can become displaced. This stretches the posterior ligament. Sometimes the disc can actually herniate into the neural canal and press on nerve roots.

5. Traumatic injury to the bones of the thoracic cage (splintering, crushing or displacement of bones) can result in injury to the respiratory muscles, pleura, lungs, heart and great vessels.

6. Traumatic injury to the bones of the pelvic girdle can result in injury to the urinary tract, uterus, lower intestinal tract, spinal nerves and large blood vessels.

7. Weakness of the abdominal musculature may be congenital or acquired. A surgical wound that has not healed well is one way of acquiring weakness. When the weak (or injured) muscles are strained (e.g., with strenuous exercise, lifting, obesity, pregnancy, abdominal distention, paroxysmal coughing), a hernia may result. When there is a surgical wound, the wound may open and abdominal viscera be exposed.

   A. An abdominal hernia is the protrusion of peritoneum and intestine through a weakened area of the abdominal musculature. It may be reducible or non-reducible. If the blood supply to the protruding tissues is cut off, it is called a strangulated hernia.

      (1) An indirect inguinal hernia involves the protrusion of peritoneum and intestine into the inguinal canal and, in the male, on into the scrotum.

      (2) A direct inguinal hernia involves the protrusion of peritoneum and intestine through the posterior inguinal wall.

      (3) A femoral hernia involves the protrusion of peritoneum and intestine into the femoral canal.

      (4) An umbilical hernia involves the protrusion of peritoneum and intestine into an umbilical ring that has not closed or is weak.

   B. If an abdominal incision fails to heal properly, the wound may open, exposing the abdominal viscera. Viscera may actually come to the outside. Shock often results, and peritonitis may follow.

8. Weakness of the pelvic floor may be congenital or acquired. It is frequently acquired through childbirth when there is considerable trauma, when there are tears (not repaired or improperly repaired) or when episiotomies have failed to heal properly. Uterine displacement occurs and occasionally the uterus may actually prolapse through the vagina. Rectoceles and cystoceles are frequent results of this problem. (See Chap. 7.)

NURSING APPLICATIONS

1. Patients should be observed for signs and symptoms of problems involving bones, muscles and fluid that serve to protect and support underlying soft tissue; and these should be investigated, evaluated, reported and/or be treated with appropriate nursing measures. This is of particular importance when the patient:

A. Is at extremes of age.
B. Has sustained a traumatic accident (e.g., falling, auto accident).
C. Is pregnant or has borne children.
D. Has a disease condition or has sustained an injury that involves the head, the cerebrospinal fluid, the vertebra, the thoracic cage, the pelvic girdle, the abdominal musculature or the muscles of the pelvic floor.

(Ways of preventing injury to bones, muscles and joints is included in Chap. 11.)

2. When a patient has sustained a head injury, or this is suspected:
   A. He should be maintained absolutely quiet in a horizontal position until there are medical orders otherwise.
   B. His head should be supported and immobilized until there are medical orders.
   C. The injured area should be protected from any trauma (e.g., pressure).
   D. No object remaining in a head wound should be moved or removed.
   E. Strict aseptic technique should be used in the care of any open wound.
   F. Careful observations should be made for signs and symptoms of brain injury; these should be reported and/or treated with appropriate nursing measures.
   G. Careful observations should be made for leakage of cerebrospinal fluid, which should be reported promptly.

3. It is especially important that infants (up to the age of about one and one-half years) be protected from injury to the fontanelles.

4. When a patient has sustained traumatic injury to the vertebrae, or this is suspected:
   A. He should be kept quiet in the position he is in until medical orders are available. If it is absolutely necessary to transport him or to change his position without medical supervision:
      (1) Flexion of the spine should be avoided.
      (2) He may be placed on his back if the cervical region is involved.
      (3) He may be placed on his abdomen if the thoracic or lumbar region is involved.
   B. Medical orders relative to positioning, traction, immobilization or exercise of limbs must be followed exactly.
   C. The trunk should be well-supported and in good alignment at all times. Any quick movements should be discouraged.
   D. Careful observations should be made for signs and symptoms of injury to the spinal cord; these should be reported and/or treated with appropriate nursing measures.

E. Any appliance (e.g., brace, corset) should be properly fitted and properly applied.

5. When a patient has injury to the bones of the thoracic cage (e.g., as in traumatic accident or chest surgery), or this is suspected:

   A. He should be kept quiet in the position he is in until medical orders are available. If it is necessary to transport him or change his position, the chest wall should be well-supported and immobilized.

   B. The injured area should be protected from any trauma (e.g., pressure, movement of any object in chest wall).

   C. Close observations should be made for any signs and symptoms of respiratory problems; these should be reported and/or treated with appropriate nursing measures.

   D. Close observations should be made for any signs and symptoms of circulatory problems; these should be reported and/or treated with appropriate nursing measures.

6. When a patient has traumatic injury to the bones of the pelvic girdle, or this is suspected:

   A. He should be kept quiet and the injured part immobilized in the position of comfort until medical orders are available.

   B. The injured area should be protected from any trauma (e.g., pressure).

   C. Close observations should be made for any signs and symptoms of problems related to the elimination of urine and/or feces (e.g., retention, incontinence, abnormal drainage); these should be reported promptly.

   D. Close observations should be made for any signs and symptoms of problems related to a pregnancy (e.g., vaginal bleeding, premature labor); these should be reported promptly.

   E. Close observations should be made for any signs and symptoms of problems related to peripheral nerve injury; these should be reported promptly.

7. When a patient has a weakened area in the abdominal musculature (e.g., a congenital weakness, a poorly healed surgical wound, or a hernia):

   A. Strenuous activity involving these muscles should be discouraged (e.g., lifting, stretching, descending stairs).

   B. Increased intra-abdominal pressure should be avoided as much as possible. This includes:

      (1) Distention and constipation. (See Chap. 7.)
      (2) Urinary retention. (See Chap. 7.)
      (3) Excessive coughing. (See Chap. 15.)
      (4) Vomiting. (See Chap. 3.)

   C. The weakened area should be adequately supported (e.g., well-fitted and properly applied corsets, binders, trusses); this is of particular importance when there is sneezing, coughing, laughing or vomiting.

D. Positioning should minimize tension on affected muscles (e.g., by flexion of femurs).

E. Careful observations should be made for signs and symptoms of intestinal obstruction, which should be reported promptly.

F. Careful observations should be made for signs and symptoms of wound dehiscence or evisceration (following abdominal surgery); these should be reported promptly and treated with appropriate nursing measures.

    (1) Any exposed organ should be covered promptly with sterile saline compresses and a supportive dressing. (A supportive dressing is adequate for an open wound.)

    (2) The patient may be placed in low Fowler's position.

    (3) The patient should be kept absolutely quiet and given consistent emotional support.

8. When a patient has weakened muscles of the pelvic floor,

A. Prolonged standing (or sometimes even sitting) should be discouraged.

B. Increased abdominal pressure should be avoided as much as possible. (See No. 7, B.)

C. Any pessary should be well-fitted and properly inserted.

D. Careful observations should be made for signs and symptoms of a prolapsed uterus, which should be reported promptly.

E. Careful observations should be made for signs and symptoms of urine retention, which should be reported promptly. (See Chap. 7.)

F. Careful observations should be made for signs and symptoms of constipation, which should be reported. (See Chap. 7.)

13

Skin and Mucous
Membrane

Unbroken healthy skin and mucous membranes serve as
first lines of defense against harmful agents.

ANATOMY AND PHYSIOLOGY

The Integument

1. The skin is the largest organ of the body. It envelopes the entire
   surface of the body. Its epithelium is continuous with the epi-
   thelium of the external orifices of the digestive, respiratory and
   genitourinary tracts.
2. The healthy intact skin:
   A. Prevents water loss.
   B. Is very important in temperature regulation.
   C. Is impermeable to most microorganisms.
   D. Is resistant to many potentially injurious chemical compounds.
   E. Is resistant to considerable trauma.
   F. Is resistant to considerable cold, heat and some radiation (e.g.,
      ultraviolet rays)
   G. Supplies information about the external environment.
3. The skin is composed of two layers.
   A. The epidermis is the outer layer.
      (1) It is avascular, nourished by tissue fluid only.
      (2) The cells of the outermost stratum contain considerable
          keratin; they are dead and constantly being shed, to be
          replaced by cells moving up from the lower strata.
      (3) The epidermis varies in thickness from about 0.10 mm. on
          most parts of the body to about 1.0 mm. on the soles of
          the feet.
      (4) Rubbing and pressure cause increased thickening of the
          epidermis.

B. The dermis (or corium) lies beneath the epidermis.
   (1) It is composed of connective tissue which contains:
      (a) Elastic fibers.
      (b) Blood and lymph vessels.
      (c) Nerves for pain, touch or pressure, heat and cold.
      (d) Sebaceous glands and sweat glands.
   (2) The thickness varies but is probably about 1.0 mm. to 3.0 mm. (on soles of feet).
   (3) It is connected to loose connective tissue (or hypodermis), which in many places is subcutaneous fatty tissue. The hypodermis is connected with underlying deep fascia, aponeuroses or periosteum.

4. The skin may be dry, moist, rough or smooth, depending upon the nature and amount of keratinized epidermis and the amount and nature of the secretions of the cutaneous glands.
  A. Sebum is an oily secretion produced by the sebaceous glands.
    (1) It keeps the skin soft and supple.
    (2) It prevents the passage of water through the skin.
    (3) There is decreased production when circulation is impaired (e.g., in old age).
    (4) There may be increased production in some of the glands when the secondary sex characteristics are being developed (e.g., glands of face, apocrine glands in axilla and around external genitalia.)
  B. Sweat glands are distributed over the entire body. They produce sweat continuously and normally increase production when there is an increased need to lose body heat. (Sweat is included in Chap. 4.)
  C. Ceruminous glands are modified sweat glands in the external auditory canal. They secrete cerumen (wax), which softens and protects.
  D. Rubbing and pressure normally causes great thickening of the epidermis. Infants and small children have soft and delicate epidermis.

5. The brown pigment, melanin, is produced in the lower epidermis as fine granules within the cells. Individuals vary markedly in the amount of this pigment, which is produced normally or can be produced in response to ultraviolet rays.

6. Individual skins vary in their resistance to injury. Factors which affect this resistance include:
  A. The general health of the cells.
  B. The amount of subcutaneous tissue.
    (1) Very much or very little subcutaneous tissue tends to decrease resistance.
    (2) There is loss of adipose tissue in old age.

(3) When there is lack or loss of tissue over the boney prominences, pressure over these prominences shuts off the blood supply very quickly.

   C. The amount of melanin (in relation to ultraviolet rays).

   D. Maintenance of a pH that is neutral or very slightly acidic.

7. Normal cutaneous vascular response to injury may include:

   A. The white reaction (vasoconstriction).

   B. The red reaction (vasodilatation).

   C. The wheal or hive (localized edema).

   D. The blister (serous fluid collection between layers of epidermis).

8. The temperature of the skin depends largely upon the amount and rate of blood flow through its vessels.

9. Normal physiologic response to externally applied heat or cold depends upon:

   A. Normal sensory perception.

   B. Normal vasomotor activity.

10. Prolonged coldness causes a decrease in sensation and can lead to tissue injury.

11. Prolonged heat can result in adaptation of the sensory receptors for heat and can cause tissue injury.

12. Itching is an unpleasant cutaneous sensation which provokes scratching.

   A. The sensation can occur in the epidermis, the epithelial layer of transistional epithelium (e.g., in pharynx) and mucocutaneous junctions (e.g., anus, female perineum, auditory canal, nares).

   B. The sensation may be stimulated chemically (e.g., by histamine-like substances), mechanically (e.g., tickling, crawling insects), thermally and electrically.

   C. The sensation may continue long after stimulation has ceased.

   D. The nerve endings are made more sensitive by increased heat (e.g., increased blood flow, friction, external heat).

   E. The sensation can occur through stimulation by the higher centers (i.e., neurogenically).

   F. The scratch reflex involves basically:

      (1) Sensory receptors and sensory pathways in the spinal cord.

      (2) Subcortical centers in the midbrain and thalamus.

      (3) Motor pathways in the spinal cord and peripheral motor nerves.

   G. It is difficult to voluntarily refrain from scratching. Distraction of attention can be helpful sometimes.

13. The nails are horny plates which develop continuously from cells in the epidermis.

14. Hairs are horny threads which develop from epidermis. Each hair arises from a hair follicle which begins in the hypodermis. One or more sebaceous glands are connected with each hair.

Mucous Membranes

1. The respiratory, gastrointestinal and genitourinary tracts are lined with mucous membranes.
2. Healthy, intact mucous membranes:
   A. Prevent water loss.
   B. Are impermeable to many microorganisms.
   C. Are resistant to many injurious chemical compounds (e.g., digestive juices).
   D. Have some resistance to trauma.
   E. Have varying absorptive power.
   F. Contain goblet cells which secrete mucus.
3. Mucus serves to:
   A. Keep the membrane moist.
   B. Act as a lubricant.
   C. Act as a protectant against some chemical and microbial agents.
4. Irritation of mucous membrane generally causes an increase in mucus production; but may cause a reduction.
5. The mucous membrane of the mouth is similar in structure to the skin. It is very sensitive. It is attached to underlying structures by a loose submucosa, except where food is crushed and rubbed (e.g., the hard palate). Some glands in the mucosa and submucosa produce saliva, which contains mucus, water, ptyalin, salts and some proteins.
6. The epithelial lining of the vagina is lubricated by mucus from the cervix, and this is normally made acid by fermentative action (bacteria and glycogen).

PHYSICS

1. Friction is that force which opposes motion between two contacting surfaces.
   A. Friction is caused by surface irregularities.
   B. Friction may be decreased by decreasing the irregularities (e.g., by smoothing surfaces or separating the surfaces with lubricants).
2. Friction produces heat.

CHEMISTRY

1. Surface tension of water may be decreased by soaps and detergents.
   A. Soaps are metallic salts of fatty acids. Some are highly alkaline.
   B. Synthetic detergents can be more efficient than soap in lowering surface tensions.
2. Lowering of surface tension aids in the emulsification of fats.
3. Some of the chemical compounds in body fluids (e.g., proteolytic enzymes) are extremely irritating to the skin.

4. Some of the body fluids can be decomposed by microorganisms to produce irritating chemical compounds (e.g., ammonia from urine, certain protein breakdown products from apocrine sweat glands).

PATHOLOGY

Signs and Symptoms

Signs and symptoms of problems that affect the skin and/or mucous membranes may include:
1. Abnormal pigmentation.
2. Abnormal texture or turgor.
3. Abnormal skin temperature.
4. Lesions.
5. Pruritis.
6. Tenderness, soreness, pain.
7. Edema.
8. Bleeding.
9. Desquamation.
10. Alopecia.
11. Abnormal nails.

Conditions Affecting Skin and Mucous Membrane

1. Problems that affect (or may affect) skin and/or mucous membrane include:
   A. Inadequate blood supply, including hypoxia. (See Chap. 1 and 2.)
   B. Malnutrition. (See Chap. 3.)
   C. Fluid and electrolyte imbalance. (See Chap. 4 and 5.)
   D. Inadequate elimination. (See Chap. 7.)
   E. Hormonal imbalance. (See Chap. 8.)
   F. Hyperthermia. (See Chap. 9.)
   G. Injuries that may result from trauma, excessive heat or cold, dryness, excessive moisture, chemicals, microorganisms, parasites, insect bites, radiation.
   H. Specific disease conditions that may involve metabolic problems, allergic response, specific infections, abnormal growths, neurogenic factors.
2. Disorders of the skin and mucous membranes may be caused by such factors as:
   A. Inflammatory response to irritants.
      (1) Dermatitis is inflammation of the skin caused by sensitivity to external or internal irritants.
         (a) The inflammatory response may involve erythema, edema, blisters, oozing of exudates, crusting, desquamation, thickening, fissuring and hyperpigmentation.

(b) Predisposing causes appear to include such factors as general physical health, susceptibility to allergic reactions, nervous tension, health of skin and nutritional status.

(c) Immediate causes involve specific irritants (e.g., certain chemical compounds, microorganisms, dusts, radiation).

(2) Eczema is a dermatitis which seems to be related more to predisposing factors than to immediate causes.

(3) Contact dermatitis is caused by actual contact with irritants in the environment.

(4) Exfoliative dermatitis is frequently caused by drugs and involves massive desquamation.

(5) Neurodermatitis, sometimes called atopic eczema, is due to neurogenic factors in some individuals.

(6) Urticaria is associated with allergic response, and involves hives and sometimes generalized edema. Itching is severe.

B. Inflammatory responses to unknown causes.

(1) Psoriasis is a condition in which there are patches of dry and scaly eruptions. These are generally accompanied by remissions and exacerbations.

(2) Pemphigus is a condition characterized by large bullae in skin and mucous membrane. There is crusting and scarring.

(3) Mycosis fungoides is a fatal skin disease characterized by tumors and tissue destruction.

(4) Scleroderma is a collagen disease (possibly related to hypersensitivity), in which the skin becomes pale, firm and attached to underlying tissues. It is usually fatal.

C. Various skin manifestations may occur with some communicable diseases (e.g., a macular rash with measles, vesicles with chicken pox, macules, papules, vesicles, pustules with small pox, erythema with scarlet fever and rheumatic fever, rosy maculo-papular rash with typhoid fever).

Pigmentation

Abnormal pigmentation of the skin and mucous membranes may be the result of:

1. An increase in yellow pigment. This may occur with high intake of carotene in the diet or with jaundice. (See Chap. 7.)

2. An increase in melanin or melanoids. This may occur locally with exposure to ultraviolet rays, scratching or chafing, some cancers, some vitamin deficiencies, sometimes with pregnancy, and in Addison's disease.

3. An increase in oxyhemoglobin (hyperemia or erythema). This occurs when there is an increased blood flow and peripheral vasodilation. It may occur with inflammatory response, with high body tempera-

ture, as a response to a high skin temperature, or as an early response to a low skin temperature.

4. A decrease in hemoglobin (pallor). This occurs when there is decreased blood flow and vasoconstriction. It occurs as an immediate response to injury and as a response to cold. It can be noted in scar tissue because of the poor blood supply.
5. An increase in reduced hemoglobin cyanosis or mottling. This occurs when there is venous stasis.
6. A decrease in pigmentation (or visible pigmentation). This occurs with edema and maceration. It may occur when there is excessive desquamation.
7. The presence of abnormal pigments. This may occur as a result of the intake of certain chemical substances that may be deposited in the skin and/or mucous membranes.

Lesions

Lesions of the skin and mucous membranes include:
1. Macule—a flat, usually small, discolored spot.
2. Papule—an elevated, usually small, discolored eruption.
3. Exanthem or rash—rosy areas of erythema or areas of macules and papules (may be extensive).
4. Vesicle—a blister containing serous exudate.
5. Pustule—an elevated skin lesion which contains purulent exudate.
6. Bulla—a large blister which may contain serous or purulent exudate.
7. Crusts—dried exudate.
8. Scales—flakes of dead epidermis.
9. Nodule—a small, usually firm swelling.
10. Wheal or hive—swollen, hot raised area, which may vary in size from tiny to very large. It may be white and then redden. There is generally hyperemia around it. It is characterized by itching.
11. Wart (verrucae)—an elevated brownish swelling, which may appear in crops.
12. Mole—flat or raised plaque or nodule which has excessive pigment (e.g., yellow, brown, greenish black). It can vary in size from tiny to very large.
13. Comedo (blackhead)—discolored plugs of dried sebum found in sebaceous glands.
14. Corns, calluses—hypertrophied thickened horny epidermis.
15. Chancre—a small sore, may be a hard plaque or an ulceration located at site of inoculation of causative microorganisms of syphilis or chancroid.
16. Gumma—a sticky ulceration which may occur anywhere in the body (third stage syphilis).
17. Excoriation—a break or abrasion.

18. Ulcer—erosion, necrosis of tissue.
19. Cicatrix (scar)—fibrous replacement of injured tissue.

Pruritus

Pruritus may be associated with such things as:
1. Crawling insects, parasites and their bites (e.g., scabies, pediculi, mites, fleas).
2. Urticaria.
3. Some types of dermatitis.
4. Emotional or psychological disturbances.
5. Dryness.
6. Some skin infections.

Infections

1. Those infections caused by fungi include:
   A. Epidermophytosis (athlete's foot) characterized by superficial vesicles and scaling; occurs frequently between the toes, but may occur in other areas of body.
   B. Tinea (ringworm) of scalp, nails, hands, trunk—characterized by scabs, vesicular or pustular lesions, distorted or lost nails.
   C. Actinomycoses—may involve the skin, causing discolored lumps with open sores.
   D. Thrush (moniliasis)—may involve the vagina or the mouth of newborn, characterized by erythema and white patches.
2. Those infections caused by bacteria include:
   A. Acne vulgaris—involves secondary infections of sebaceous glands, frequently associated with secondary sex characteristics.
   B. Erysipelas—caused by a strain of streptococcus and characterized by areas of erythema and edema.
   C. Furuncles and carbuncles (boils)—localized infections usually caused by staphylococci or streptococci, originating in a hair follicle and associated glands. If the infective material gets outside the protective wall it can cause cellulitis.
   D. Impetigo contagiosa—caused by a streptococcus, characterized by pustules and crusting.
   E. Syphilis—caused by a spirochete. In the first stage there is a hard chancre at the point of inoculation; in the second stage there is a rash; in the third stage there may be gummas involving the skin or mucous membranes.
   F. Chancroid—involves a soft chancre; caused by a bacillus.
   G. Leprosy—caused by a bacillus. It may involve a nodular skin lesion which often ulcerates; the skin affected may become thick and leathery.
3. Those infections caused by viruses:
   A. Warts.

    B. Herpes simplex (cold sore or canker sore)—characterized by a group of small blisters which rupture, crust and heal slowly.

    C. Herpes zoster (shingles)—characterized by a chain of blisters which follow the path of sensory nerve trunks from the spine around to the front, associated with great pain and itching.

Pressure

Unusual or prolonged pressure.
1. Corns and calluses occur frequently on the feet due to such factors as poorly fitting shoes or fallen metatarsal arches.

Growths

Abnormal growths (e.g., neoplasms) :
1. Leukoplakia are raised flat shiny lesions of the mucous membrane (especially of mouth), which may become cancerous.
2. Pigmented moles are often precancerous, especially those which are very dark.
3. Senile keratosis precedes cutaneous epithelioma, and may appear as small reddish or brownish scaling spots, usually on or about the face.
4. Any nodule may be potentially cancerous (e.g., sarcomas, fibrosarcomas).

Venous Stasis

Venous stasis (or impaired circulation) :
1. Stasis dermatitis is a condition, usually of the lower extremities, characterized by redness, edema, itching and dryness.
2. Varicose ulcers may result from the death of skin due to inadequate circulation.

Burns

1. Burns may be caused by certain chemical compounds (e.g., strong acids and bases), radiation, electricity and excessive heat. They are generally classified as:
    A. First degree—when there is erythema.
    B. Second degree—when there is blister formation, but regeneration of epithelium is possible.
    C. Third degree—when all the layers of the skin are destroyed and regeneration cannot occur.

Wound Healing

1. Healing may occur by:
    A. Recuperation of the injured cells.
    B. Regeneration, which involves reproduction and organization.
        (1) Regeneration depends upon such factors as:
            (a) The type of cell involved.

(b) The severity of the injury (e.g., approximation of wound edges).

(c) The presence of infection.

(d) The blood supply.

(e) The nutritional status.

(f) The age of the individual (healing is more rapid in the young).

(2) Nerve tissue, muscle tissue and elastic tissue have practically no ability to regenerate, although squamous cells are easily regenerated.

C. Fibrous tissue substitution, which involves the formation of granulation tissue and fibrosis:

(1) Granulation tissue is composed of connective tissue, blood vessels and lymphatics. It is soft, grayish red and bleeds easily.

(2) As collagen fibers and hyaline substance increase in amount, contraction occurs and the blood vessels are closed off, and the scar becomes nearly avascular.

(3) Scarring is helpful by establishing continuity, reinforcing the area, and walling off infective agents.

(4) Scarring can result in contractures when it occurs around joints. Stretching of the fibrous tissue helps the fibers to become longer.

2. Wounds may heal by first or second intention.

A. Healing by first intention involves:

(1) The formation of a blood clot which closes the wound, protects underlying tissues from injury and provides a framework for new growth.

(2) The growth of epithelial tissue across the wound.

(3) The development of granulation tissue and subsequent fibrous tissue substitution; generally the wound is covered and granulation tissue formed by the seventh or eighth day after injury.

B. Healing by second intention involves the extensive development of granulation tissue, because epithelial tissue cannot cover the wound. This may occur with a particularly large wound or because of wound infection. Healing requires a much longer time and scarring is extensive.

NURSING APPLICATIONS

Observation and Evaluation

1. Patients should be observed for signs and symptoms of problems involving the skin and mucous membranes; these should be investi-

gated, evaluated, reported and/or treated with appropriate nursing measures. This is of particular importance when the patient:
A. Is at extremes of age.
B. Is known to have a sensitive or delicate skin.
C. Has impaired circulation. (See Chap. 1.)
D. Is subject to having irritating substances on the skin or mucous membranes (e.g., sweat, urine, feces, gastrointestinal secretions, various exudates).
E. Depends upon others for physical care or protection (e.g., infants and young children, weak or debilitated, mentally incompetent, unconscious, immobilized or bed-ridden).
F. Has appliances or equipment in contact with skin or mucous membrane (e.g., traction, casts, braces, trusses, tubes).
G. Is receiving treatments in which skin or mucous membranes are involved (e.g., radiation therapy, heat treatments, irrigations, ice packs).
H. Has an injury or disease condition that affects the skin or mucous membrane.
2. The condition of the skin or mucous membranes should be evaluated in relation to such factors as:
A. The age of the patient.
B. His general physical condition (e.g., circulation, nutrition, body temperature).
C. His emotional status.
D. The normal pigmentation of the individual.
E. Any injury that has occurred and the normal process of healing.
F. Any diagnosed disease condition that involves (or may involve) these structures.

The Integument

1. The skin should be protected from injury due to:
A. Trauma.
   (1) Friction should be avoided by:
      (a) Providing and encouraging the use of properly-fitted and applied shoes, clothing, supportive appliances, and dressings.
      (b) Moving the patient carefully, avoiding sliding.
      (c) Using powders on skin surfaces, especially if surfaces are in contact with each other.
   (2) Special precautions should be taken when sharp objects are used on or around the body (e.g., pins, razor blades, scissors).
   (3) Appliances with sharp edges should be carefully padded as necessary (e.g., casts).

(4) Skin care should be done gently, with appropriate materials and force.

(5) Adhered materials, exudates or secretions should be removed carefully, gently and by appropriate methods (e.g., with soaking, use of special solvents).

(6) Scratching should be discouraged and prevented as possible.

    (a) The cause of itching should be sought and removed whenever possible (e.g., an insect, irritating fabrics, irritating secretions).

    (b) Itching that cannot be controlled by nursing measures should be reported promptly.

    (c) Excessive warmth should be avoided (e.g., by removal of warm clothing or covers, or by limiting exercise).

    (d) Cool compresses or soaks may be helpful unless contra-indicated.

    (e) Cooling lotions may be helpful unless contraindicated.

    (f) Rest and sleep should be promoted as possible. (See Chap. 10.)

    (g) Prescribed medications for the relief of itching should be administered or applied promptly, as ordered and indicated.

    (h) Mittens, restraints or special coverings for the affected skin may be helpful.

(7) Caution should be used in hair removal. "Plucking" should be generally discouraged, and never done around the nose.

B. An inadequate blood supply.

(1) Prolonged pressure against any body part should be prevented (e.g., by positioning, appropriate support). This is of particular importance for the bony prominences.

(2) Exercise (active or passive) should be provided and encouraged within medical orders.

(3) Massage, especially of skin over pressure points, should be performed effectively and as frequently as necessary.

C. Drying.

(1) Emollients or protectives should be applied as needed.

(2) Excessive washing, or the use of drying soaps or other drying agents, (e.g., rubbing alcohol) should be discouraged and avoided. If frequent cleansing is necessary,

    (a) The skin should be observed carefully for signs of dryness.

    (b) Appropriate cleaning and nondrying agents should be used carefully.

    (c) The skin should be carefully dried.

    (d) Emollients and/or protectives should be applied.

(3) The humidity should be increased as possible.

(4) Good circulation to the affected part should be provided as possible (e.g., by positioning, massage).

D. Excessive moisture.

(1) The skin should be cleaned and dried carefully as necessary.

(2) Clothing and bedding that is wet should be changed promptly.

(3) Wet dressings and pads should be changed as ordered and indicated.

(4) Drying agents (e.g., powders, antiperspirants, alcohol) or protectives should be applied unless contraindicated.

(5) When the skin has to be wet for prolonged periods (e.g., frequent or continuous wet compresses or soaks) provision should be made for occasional drying. If the skin shows signs of maceration, this should be reported promptly.

E. Heat or cold.

(1) The temperature of water (or solutions) used for treatments or baths should be measured or tested, and the heat should not exceed that which is safe, comfortable and therapeutically effective.

(2) Heating appliances should be checked frequently and carefully controlled (e.g., heating pads, electric lights).

(3) When local applications of heat or cold are used, the skin should be observed frequently for abnormal circulatory changes (e.g., excessive or prolonged redness, whiteness or cyanosis).

(4) When a patient complains of discomfort that is related to hot or cold applications, the skin should be observed carefully. The treatment should be discontinued if indicated, and this should be reported appropriately.

(5) Special precautions should be used in the application of heat or cold when the patient:

(a) Has impaired circulation. (See Chap. 1.)

(b) Has impaired sensory function. (See Chap. 16.)

(c) Has impaired locomotor function. (See Chap. 11.)

(d) Has little subcutaneous tissue, or has edema of the area.

(e) Is receiving continuous applications.

(6) Burns should be prevented by appropriate measures of accident prevention.

F. Radiation.

(1) Excessive exposure to the sun's rays should be prevented and discouraged.

(2) When treatments involving radiation (e.g., ultraviolet or infrared rays) are used, the time and frequency of the treatment must be followed exactly, and the skin should be observed carefully for excessive redness.

G. Chemicals.

    (1) Medications should not be applied to the skin without medical orders. Caution should be used in the application of any potentially harmful cosmetic preparations (e.g., hair removers, antiperspirants).

    (2) Strongly alkaline soaps should not be used on the skin.

    (3) Patients should be protected from contact with any known allergens (e.g., drugs, foods, fabrics).

    (4) Irritating secretions, excretions or exudates should be removed from the skin promptly.

    (5) Special precautions should be taken to prevent harmful substances or drugs from being in contact with the skin (e.g., infiltration of irritating drugs that are supposed to be administered intravenously).

    (6) The skin should be protected against known irritants (e.g., poison ivy, poison oak).

H. Insect bites.

    (1) Appropriate means should be used to protect patients from flying insects (e.g., screens, netting).

    (2) Clothing and bedding should be maintained clean and free from insects.

    (3) The hair should be kept clean and free from insects.

I. Microorganisms.

    (1) The skin should be protected from all types of injury as possible. (See A through H.)

    (2) The skin should be kept clean and free from materials that contain (or are suspected to contain) microorganisms.

    (3) The skin should be observed for signs of injury, lesions and infection, which should be reported promptly.

2. When a patient has sustained injury to the skin (e.g., cuts, abrasions, burns, infections):

A. The injured area must be protected from injury due to trauma, excessive moisture, heat, radiation, chemicals, insects or microorganisms.

B. Tensions around any wound should be avoided.

C. The injured area should be observed closely for signs and symptoms of the following, which should be reported promptly:

    (1) Abnormal wound healing.

    (2) Infection (or additional or secondary infection).

    (3) Contractures (in case of burns).

D. Contractures should be prevented by:

    (1) Changes of position, within medical orders.

    (2) Exercise.

E. Good nutrition should be encouraged (e.g., a diet high in protein, vitamins and minerals).

3. When a patient has skin lesions (e.g., pustules, vesicles, desquamation) :
   A. The lesions should be protected from injury.
   B. The lesions should not be cleaned or any preparation applied until medical orders are available.
   C. Orders relative to cleansing, application of medications, baths and so forth should be followed exactly.
   D. Any dietary orders should be followed exactly (e.g., limitation of sweets, fats or possible allergens).
   E. Careful observations should be made for any allergic connections, and these should be reported appropriately.
   F. Careful observations should be made for emotional components, and these should be reported.
   G. Emotional support should be consistent.

The Mucous Membranes

1. The mucous membranes should be protected from injury due to:
   A. Trauma.
      (1) Friction should be avoided by:
         (a) Providing and encouraging the use of properly fitted appliances (e.g., dentures in the mouth, pessary in vagina).
         (b) The use of appropriate lubricants when performing treatments involving the gastrointestinal tract, the respiratory tract, the urinary tract or the female reproductive tract.
      (2) Sharp objects should be kept away from the mouth (e.g., pins).
      (3) Equipment used in treatments involving mucous membranes should be absolutely smooth, padded if necessary, and soft as possible.
      (4) No tube or equipment should ever be forced into a body opening. It is essential to insert and direct equipment in the proper direction and the proper distance for the desired therapeutic effectiveness.
      (5) Foods high in roughage should be discouraged (e.g., bran).
   B. Dryness.
      (1) Adequate humidity should be provided (e.g., by use of vaporizers).
      (2) The mucous membranes of the oral cavity should be kept well-moistened; this is particularly important when there is mouth breathing.
      (3) Emollients or protectives should be used as necessary, unless contraindicated.

    (4) The use of drying soaps or other drying agents should be avoided, or carefully rinsed off after use.

C. Excessive moisture.

    (1) The perineal area should be kept free from secretions, urine, feces or menstrual flow.

D. Heat.

    (1) The temperature of water or solutions used for treatments (e.g., irrigations or instillations) should be measured or tested, and the heat should not exceed that which is safe and therapeutically effective.

    (2) When local applications of heat are used, careful observations should be made for signs of excessive redness in the affected mucous membranes.

    (3) The intake of excessively hot food or fluids should be discouraged.

E. Chemicals.

    (1) No medications should be used on mucous membranes without specific medical orders.

    (2) The intake of spicy or chemically irritating foods or fluids should be discouraged.

F. Microorganisms.

    (1) Mucous membranes should be protected from all types of injury. (See A through E.)

    (2) Mucous membranes should be kept clean (e.g., good oral hygiene) and free from possibly infective exudates, or excretions.

    (3) Prolonged or excessive use of irrigations (e.g., antiseptic gargles or douching) should be discouraged.

    (4) Careful observations should be made for signs of injury, lesions or infection, and these should be reported promptly.

2. When a patient has sustained injury to mucous membranes, or has lesions:

A. The affected area must be protected from injury due to trauma, dryness, heat, chemicals or microorganisms.

B. Dietary orders must be followed exactly (e.g., roughage, hot and spicy foods).

C. The affected area should be observed carefully for signs of:

    (1) Abnormal healing.

    (2) Infection (or additional or secondary infection).

14

The Inflammatory Response and Immunity

The body is able to produce cellular elements and specific chemical substances that protect the body against injurious agents.

ANATOMY AND PHYSIOLOGY

1. The body's primary defense mechanisms are those related to natural resistance (or innate immunity). These include:
   A. Healthy, intact skin and mucous membranes.
   B. The inflammatory response to injury.
   C. The presence in the plasma of some nonspecific antibodies (slight effect only).
2. The body's secondary defense mechanisms involve those related to the development of specific antibodies (acquired immunity).
3. The body's ability to resist injury varies among species, races and individuals.
4. Individuals at extremes of age have less resistance than those in the middle years.
5. The two basic purposes of the inflammatory reaction are:
   A. Destruction, neutralization or limitation of the effects of injurious agents.
   B. Assistance with tissue repair. (See Chap. 13.)
6. The body's inflammatory reaction to local injury involves two major responses:
   A. Those related to changes in blood vessels.
      (1) After momentary vasoconstriction, there is vasodilatation with hyperemia (redness, heat, congestion).
      (2) There is increasing capillary permeability, and fluid leaks out of the capillaries into the injured tissue (swelling).

B. Those related to the mobile inflammatory cells.
  (1) White blood cells migrate to the injured area; they phago-
      cytize and digest foreign bodies and cellular debris.
  (2) The bone marrow is stimulated to produce more white blood
      cells, particularly polymorphonuclear leukocytes.
7. The mobile inflammatory cells include:
  A. Those found in the circulating blood. These include:
    (1) Polymorphonuclear leukocytes.
      (a) Neutrophils (60 to 80%). These digest material and
          liberate enzymes that dissolve themselves and other
          materials.
      (b) Eosinophils (2 to 4%). These seem to be associated in
          some way with hypersensitivity reactions.
      (c) Basophils. The precise functions of these cells are un-
          known.
    (2) Lymphocytes (20 to 30%). The precise functions of
        lymphocytes is unknown. They may be related to antibody
        production. They may be stem cells from which other in-
        flammatory cells are formed.
    (3) Monocytes (2 to 4%). These seem to be associated with the
        production of antibodies, and may be precursors of macro-
        phages.
  B. Those found in the tissues.
    (1) Plasma cells produce antibodies.
    (2) Macrophages are phagocytic, produce antibodies and can
        develop into fibroblasts.
8. There are normally 5,000 to 9,000 mature leukocytes per cu. mm. of
   blood.
  A. All the leukocytes (except lymphocytes) are developed in
     myeloid tissue in the bone marrow. Under normal conditions,
     neutrophils can be produced in as great a quantity as required.
  B. Lymphocytes are formed in lymphoid tissue, and may be found
     there as well as in the circulating blood.
9. Lymphoid tissue, which forms the lymph nodes, is present in small
   amounts in the bone marrow and the spleen. It is scattered in the
   mucous membranes of the alimentary canal, respiratory passages
   and in many other tissues of the body.
  A. Lymph nodes are small bodies located along the courses of
     lymphatic vessels. The major groups of lymph nodes that may
     be palpated easily (and become noticeably tender) when en-
     larged include:
    (1) Those of the head (e.g., occipital, around ears).
    (2) Those of the neck (e.g., submaxillary and cervical).
    (3) Those in the axilla.
    (4) Those in the groin (inguinal nodes).

B. There is a circular band of lymphoid tissue that guards the respiratory and digestive tracts. The anterior part of the ring is formed by the lingual tonsil; the posterior, by the pharyngeal tonsil (adenoids). The palatine tonsils lie on either side of the pharynx between the glossopharyngeal and pharyngopalatine arches.

C. Lymphoid tissue has the function of producing lymphocytes, and of filtering out and destroying foreign bodies, including microorganisms.

10. The fixed inflammatory cells (or fixed macrophages) are often referred to as the reticuloendothelial system.

A. The reticuloendothelial system is composed of:

(1) Kupffer cells in the liver.

(2) Sinusoidal cells in the spleen, lymph nodes and bone marrow.

(3) Histiocytes in the tissues (which in inflammation can become motile macrophages).

B. These cells are able to ingest many kinds of foreign matter.

11. Antibody (excluding those small amounts of nonspecific antibodies found in the plasma) is a specific protein substance, produced in some of the body cells in response to the introduction of a specific antigen.

A. Antibody is produced from portions of gamma globulin; each antibody has a specific chemical structure.

B. Any foreign material introduced into the body may act as an antigen (e.g., ingested, inhaled, injected, in contact with skin).

C. Antibody reacts with antigen in some specific way that prevents the harmful effects of the antigen and facilitates the work of the phagocytic cells.

D. Some antibodies disappear rather quickly, although others remain in the body tissues or circulating blood for years.

E. Once the body has made a specific antibody, it can usually produce that antibody again rather quickly if it is needed.

F. Antibodies pass from the mother to the baby through the placenta and, to some extent, through the mother's milk.

G. Hypersensitivity represents an unfavorable antigen-antibody reaction, which produces undesirable physiological responses. Histamine (or histamine-like substances) are formed in the tissues, and these compounds seem to be related to the various hypersensitivity reactions.

PATHOLOGY

Signs and Symptoms

1. Signs and symptoms of the body's inflammatory response to injury may include:

    A. Local signs and symptoms.
        (1) The cardinal signs and symptoms of inflammation include:
            (a) Pain.
            (b) Swelling.
            (c) Redness.
            (d) Heat.
            (e) Loss of function (probably due primarily to the original tissue injury).
        (2) Swelling and tenderness of lymph nodes.
        (3) Red, inflamed lymphatic vessels (seen as red lines in skin).
        (4) Presence of exudates (in body fluids, in drainage from body cavities, or from an open lesion or wound).
        (5) Lesions of the skin or mucous membranes. (See Chap. 13.)
        (6) Wound healing.
    B. Systemic signs and symptoms.
        (1) Fever (with associated signs and symptoms). (See Chap. 9.)
        (2) Tachycardia.
        (3) Leukocytosis.
    C. Systemic signs and symptoms that are frequently associated with inflammatory processes.
        (1) Lassitude.
        (2) Malaise.
        (3) Anorexia, nausea, vomiting.
        (4) Diarrhea.
        (5) Skin lesions.
2. Signs and symptoms of leukemia may include:
    A. In chronic leukemia:
        (1) Pallor.
        (2) Increasing fatigue.
        (3) Purpura.
    B. In acute leukemia:
        (1) Fever.
        (2) Malaise, prostration.
        (3) Infections of the skin and mucous membranes.
        (4) Purpura.
3. Signs and symptoms of hypersensitivity reactions may include:
    A. Persistent sneezing.
    B. Excessive lacrimal secretion (tearing).
    C. Excessive watery nasal discharge.
    D. Wheezing, dyspnea.
    E. Skin lesions (e.g., rashes, urticaria).
    F. Nausea and vomiting.
    G. Diarrhea.
    H. Those related to anaphylactic shock. (See Chap. 1.)

The Inflammatory Reaction

1. The causative agents of inflammatory reactions are injurious chemical substances. The sources of these chemical substances may be:
    A. External (e.g., insect bites, toxins produced by microorganisms outside the body and ingested, toxins produced by pathogenic microorganisms inside the body, certain drugs).
    B. Internal (e.g., digestive juices in the submucosa or on serous membrane, cellular injuries that result in the release of intracellular substances, the breakdown products of cellular debris, and chemical substances formed in faulty metabolic processes).
    C. Both internal and external (as demonstrated by the antigen-antibody reactions that occur with infections and in hypersensitivity).
2. When microorganisms capable of causing disease gain entrance into the superficial skin or mucous membrane, there is normally a localizing process (e.g., pimples, furuncle, abscesses are formed).
    A. Polymorphonuclear leukocytes, fibrin and edema fluid containing nonspecific antibodies surround the microorganisms. Lymphocytes surround these, then macrophages, which cause some granulation.
    B. Phagocytosis and proteolytic action can cause the formation of pus (an inflammatory exudate containing dead or dying leukocytes, tissue debris, products of proteolytic digestion, and the microorganisms, which may be dead or alive).
    C. This inflammatory exudate may be absorbed by the body, drained from a body opening (naturally or through surgical intervention), or forced from a body opening, as in coughing.
3. When the localizing process fails, the microorganisms:
    A. May cause a spreading cellulitis (which occurs most frequently in loose tissues such as the subcutaneous tissue).
    B. May travel and be drained with tissue fluid into the lymphatic vessels, where they may cause an inflammation (lymphangitis).
    C. May reach the lymph nodes, where they may:
        (1) Be destroyed by the action of the mobile and fixed inflammatory cells.
        (2) Cause a local inflammation (lymphadenitis, cervical adenitis, tonsillitis).
4. When microorganisms capable of producing disease enter the circulating blood, either directly or indirectly through lymph drainage:
    A. The fixed inflammatory cells of the liver, bone marrow and spleen attempt to destroy the microorganisms, and may be successful.
    B. The liver, spleen and bone marrow may become the sites of inflammation.

C. A state of septicemia exists and all the tissues of the body are subject to infection.

(When microorganisms reach the lymphatic vessels that drain the face, they can reach the venous sinuses of the brain and may cause a meningitis, and possibly a venous sinus thrombosis.)

Conditions Affecting Defense Mechanisms

1. The production of specific antibodies, if possible and rapid enough, facilitates the actions of the inflammatory cells against specific microorganisms or their toxins.
   A. The rapidity of antibody production depends largely upon whether or not the body has produced the specific antibodies before, and the type of microorganism involved.
      (1) The body would have produced the antibodies before if the person has had certain specific diseases (e.g., typhoid fever, measles), or has been vaccinated successfully.
      (2) Some antibodies that the body produces against certain microorganisms cannot be "recalled" by the body quickly when these particular pathogens cause an infection (e.g., viruses of the common cold).
   B. Antibody production is slower and not as effective in the aged and in the very young.
   C. Antibody production is decreased when there is generally poor physical health, whatever the cause.
2. If both primary and secondary defense mechanisms fail to destroy or neutralize injurious agents:
   A. The inflammatory process may become chronic.
   B. The injurious agents may cause increasing tissue destruction and, eventually, death.
3. Problems that interfere with primary defense mechanisms include those concerned with:
   A. Inadequate circulation. (See Chap. 1.)
   B. Severe malnutrition. (See Chap. 3.)
   C. Injury to the skin and mucous membranes. (See Chap. 13.)
   D. An excessive amount of adrenocortical hormone in the blood (e.g., in adrenal disease or with therapeutic administration).
   E. Toxemia, which may be due to:
      (1) Poisons.
      (2) The inadequate elimination of toxic substances produced in the body. (See Chap. 7.)
   F. The inadequate production of hydrochloric acid by gastric glands (e.g., as occurs in some gastric disorders).
   G. The inadequate production or function of inflammatory cells (e.g., as with leukemia, Hodgkin's disease, liver disease, agranulocytosis).

4. The fixed inflammatory cells of the reticuloendothelial system (in the liver, spleen, bone marrow, lymph nodes and body tissue themselves) may be injured by:
   A. Trauma.
   B. Injurious agents such as toxic drugs, radiation and toxic substances produced in the body (e.g., by the body or by microorganisms).
   C. Neoplasms.
5. Hodgkin's disease is a condition in which the lymph nodes becomes enlarged and are unable to function properly. The condition may be acute or chronic, but sooner or later, it causes death, which is generally due to uncontrolled infections.
6. Agranulocytosis involves leukopenia, in which there is a marked decrease in granulocytes. This condition is caused by injury to the bone marrow by such things as radiation, certain drugs and poisons. Ulcerations of the mucous membranes of the respiratory and digestive tracts are early manifestations of this problem.
7. Leukemia is a relatively rare, progressively malignant, and (at present) fatal condition, in which there is progressive proliferation of bone marrow or lymphoid tissue that produces white blood cells. There is a great excess of white blood cells in the circulating blood.
   A. The four major types of leukemia are:
      (1) Lymphocytic (lymphatic or lymphogenous).
      (2) Myelocytic (granulocytic or myelogenous).
      (3) Plasmocytic.
      (4) Monocytic.
   B. Each type has an acute and chronic form. The chronic form usually begins after the age of 40; the acute form may occur at any age, but is seen most often in childhood.
   C. When the bone marrow is affected (myelocytic leukemia), the condition is complicated by anemia and thrombocytopenic purpura. (See Chap. 1.)
   D. In lymphocytic leukemia, lymphoid tissue all over the body becomes tremendously enlarged, and often presses on vital structures.
   E. In chronic leukemia, the white blood cell count may go up to several hundred thousand per cubic millimeter of blood, and there are many immature forms that cannot function properly.
   F. In acute leukemia, the white blood cell count is lower than in the chronic form, but there are many immature cells also.
   G. Some disease conditions of lymphoid tissue (e.g., Hodgkin's disease and some neoplasms) appear to develop into a lymphatic leukemia.
   H. Death may occur because of uncontrolled infections, hemorrhages, or the pressure of enlarged nodes upon vital structures.

8. Hypersensitivity (or allergic response) represents an inflammatory condition caused by antigen-antibody reactions.
   A. A hypersensitive state exists only when the body has produced antibodies in response to a specific antigen, and these are present in the body in sufficient quantity to cause reactions when the allergen is present.
   B. The severity of an allergic response depends upon:
      (1) The degree of sensitivity of the individual (the amount of antibodies).
      (2) The amount of the antigen present.
   C. Hypersensitivity reactions include:
      (1) Local reactions involving primarily skin or mucous membrane (e.g., hyperemia, edema, hemorrhages, necrosis, hives).
      (2) Systemic reactions, which may include generalized edema, extensive skin lesions, swollen lymph nodes, inflammation of joints, malaise, fever, bronchiolar constriction, purpura.
      (3) Anaphylactic shock, in which there is vascular collapse or asphyxia, due to edema or contractions of smooth muscles of the respiratory tract.

PHYSICS

1. Gravitation is the force of attraction between two objects.
2. The law of gravitation states that any two objects in the universe are attracted to each other with a force that is proportional to the product of their masses, and inversely proportional to the square of the distance between them.

NURSING APPLICATIONS

Observation and Evaluation

1. Patients should be observed for signs and symptoms of their inflammatory reactions (favorable or unfavorable); these should be investigated, evaluated, reported, and/or treated with appropriate nursing measures. This is of particular importance when the patient:
   A. Is at extremes of age.
   B. Has impaired circulation. (See Chap. 1.)
   C. Has malnutrition. (See Chap. 3.)
   D. Has injured skin or mucous membranes. (See Chap. 13.)
   E. Is fatigued, weak or debilitated.
   F. Has a toxic condition (e.g., uremia).
   G. Has a liver disease.
   H. Has a known infection.
   I. Has a history of hypersensitivity.
   J. Has problems which involve the white blood cells and/or the reticuloendothelial system.

    K. Is receiving medications or preparations which are frequently associated with hypersensitivity reactions (e.g., sera, desensitizing drugs).

2. An individual's inflammatory response should be evaluated in relation to such factors as the:

    A. Normal inflammatory response.

    B. Normal immune reaction.

    C. Diagnosed disease condition.

Nursing Measures

1. When a patient has a superficial infection (e.g., a pimple, furuncle, canker sore):

    A. The affected area should be protected from any trauma (e.g., squeezing). (This is of particular importance when the infection is on the face.)

    B. Warm, moist applications may be helpful.

    C. The affected area should be observed for signs of increasing infection, and these should be reported appropriately.

    D. The affected area should be observed for signs and symptoms of healing, and these should be reported appropriately.

2. When a patient has drainage of exudate from an inflamed or infected area (e.g., an infected ear), the positioning of the patient should promote drainage.

3. When a patient has problems involving impaired body defense mechanisms:

    A. Special precautions must be used to protect him from any injury.

      (1) Special precautions should be used to protect him from any traumatic injury.

      (2) Special precautions should be used to protect the skin and mucous membranes from injury. (See Chap. 13.)

      (3) Special precautions should be used to protect the patient from infections. (See Chap. 20.)

    B. More than usual rest and sleep should be provided and encouraged. (See Chap. 10.)

    C. Foods high in protein, vitamins and minerals should be encouraged and provided (within medical orders).

4. Patients should be discouraged from taking unprescribed medications.

5. It is important that any known sensitivities to various chemical substances (e.g., in foods or drugs) should be ascertained and patients should be protected from contact with these substances.

6. When pharmaceutical preparations likely to cause hypersensitive reactions are administered (e.g., desensitizing drugs, antitoxins):

    A. The patient should be observed for signs and symptoms of local or systemic reaction for at least 15 minutes after the injection.

B. Epinephrine and equipment for its administration should be ready for immediate administration.
7. When a patient develops signs and symptoms of a hypersensitive reaction:
   A. This should be reported promptly.
   B. Any possibly causative agent (e.g., a drug or blood transfusion) should be discontinued (transfusions may be either slowed or stopped as indicated by the severity of symptoms) until medical orders are available.

15

Physical Discomforts

Sensations of physical discomfort indicate injury or threat of injury to the body.

ANATOMY AND PHYSIOLOGY

1. The simplest and most widely distributed sensation is that of pain.
   A. Several kinds of stimuli are adequate to elicit pain (e.g., electrical, mechanical, chemical and thermal).
      (1) Pressure against pain fibers causes pain.
      (2) Metabolic wastes of cellular activity can cause tissue injury.
   B. Some regions of the body give rise primarily, or almost exclusively, to the sensation of pain (e.g., the teeth, tympanic membrane or cornea). When an area is supplied primarily by pain fibers, localization of pain is difficult.
   C. Muscles and tendons possess exquisite pain sensitivity.
      (1) Exercising ischemic muscles usually causes severe cramping pain.
      (2) Muscles are very sensitive to pinching or squeezing.
   D. Pain fibers adapt very slowly, if at all.
   E. Tolerance for pain increases with age.
2. The three kinds of pain that are generally recognized and designated are:
   A. Superficial or cutaneous.
   B. Deep (from muscles, tendons, joints and fascia).
   C. Visceral.
3. The viscera are relatively insensitive to many stimuli, but pain may result from:
   A. Tension or stretch of smooth muscle fibers.
   B. Chemical irritation, especially when the organ is ischemic (e.g., in myocardial infarction or strangulated hernia).
4. Irritation of the viscera may be manifested by:
   A. Referred pain.
      (1) Pain is felt in the body surface although originating in the viscera.

190

(2) Pain is felt in dermatomes associated (because of their nerve supplies) with posterior roots through which the afferent impulses from the viscera reach the spinal cord (e.g., heart pain may be felt in upper shoulders and possibly as radiating down the arms).

B. Poorly localized pain.

C. Excessive sensitivity to pain and pressure over and around the affected organ (e.g., discomfort above and around an inflamed appendix).

D. Autonomic reflexes such as sweating or vasomotor changes.

E. Somatic reflexes (e.g., muscular rigidity over the affected area).

5. A painful stimulus (visceral) is received by a visceral receptor and impulses are transmitted to the brain by the following routes:

A. To the spinal cord and to the thalamus by way of the spino-thalamic tract.

B. Directly to the thalamus by way of a cranial nerve.

6. A painful stimulus (cutaneous or deep) is received by a somatic receptor, carried to the spinal cord by a spinal nerve, across the gray commissure, and to the spino-thalamic tract to the thalamus.

7. The thalamus gives rise to a crude, uncritical form of consciousness, and diffuse and unlocalized pain may be perceived at this level.

8. Sensory fibers for pain pass from the thalamus to the somesthetic area of the cerebral cortex, where more discriminative perception of pain may be made.

9. If the axon of a specific nerve fiber or its dorsal root is irritated, the pain is perceived as coming from the terminal end.

10. Brain tissue itself has no pain receptors.

11. Sense perception centers for pain can become hypersensitive after repeated stimulation. This results in an increased sensitivity to pain.

12. An individual's emotional attitude toward pain affects his sensitivity to pain. Attitudes are learned.

13. The pain that an individual experiences depends upon his perception of the pain and his personal reaction to the pain perceived.

14. Some of the factors that affect an individual's personal reaction to pain are:

A. His state of consciousness.

B. The integrity of his cerebral functions.

C. His past experience with pain.

D. The total amount of pain experienced.

E. His understanding about the origin and significance of the pain.

F. Training.

G. The amount of fatigue he has.

H. The amount of attention paid to the pain.

I. His emotional status (e.g., anxious, fearful, composed).

15. Unpleasant organic sensations may cause:
    A. Insomnia.
    B. Restlessness and bad dreams.
    C. Increased irritability to external stimuli.
    D. Increasing emotional tension.

PATHOLOGY

Signs and Symptoms

1. Signs and symptoms of physical discomfort may include:
   A. Crying, moaning, yelling.
   B. Unusual quietness, withdrawal.
   C. Generalized or local muscle rigidity, writhing.
   D. Pained facial expressions (e.g., grimaces).
   E. Unusual postures (e.g., knees drawn up to abdomen).
   F. Pulse and blood pressure changes (may be increased or decreased).
   G. Respiratory changes (e.g., increased, decreased, irregular).
   H. Changes in skin color and temperature (may be red and hot, or pale and cold).
   I. Anorexia, nausea, vomiting.
   J. Excessive perspiration.
   K. Rubbing, scratching.
   L. Restlessness, insomnia.
   M. Behavioral changes (e.g., excitement, irritability, depression).
2. Pain can excite automatic defense reactions through stimulation of the sympathetic division of the autonomic nervous system.
   A. "Fight or flight" reactions can occur with cutaneous pain.
   B. There may be failure of defense reactions (e.g., fall in blood pressure, weakness, nausea) with severe deep or visceral pain.
3. The threshold for pain may be lowered (hyperalgesia) when there is trauma or inflammation of an area (e.g., the sunburned skin is more sensitive to painful stimuli than the normal skin).
4. Visceral pain occurs when the viscera are inflamed, or when there is traction or tension that affects the tissues.
5. Central pain is that which does not originate in the periphery, but results from injury involving the nerve trunks, pain tracts or areas of the brain concerned with the perception of pain.
6. Causalgia is burning pain experienced as coming from the periphery, but the pain is actually caused by injury to peripheral nerve trunks. (This sometimes occurs when there has been amputation of a limb.)
7. Significant information about experienced pain includes:
   A. The type of pain (e.g., aching, burning, griping, cramping, constrictive, dull, sharp, stabbing, stinging).
   B. The location of the pain and any spreading or localization of it.

C. The time of occurrence.
D. The constancy of the pain.
   (1) Pain is rarely constant for long periods of time.
   (2) Pain indicates that tissue damage is occurring, and when the damage has reached a certain point, even the pain receptors are damaged.
E. Any recurrence of the pain.
F. The severity of the pain.
8. Factors that can be helpful in estimating the severity of the pain experienced by a patient include:
   A. The age, cultural background, emotionality, objectivity.
   B. His facial expression.
   C. His postural attitude.
   D. The amount of muscular rigidity.
   E. The degree and type of physical activity (e.g., hyperactivity, depression).
   F. Vital signs (which may be increased or decreased).
   G. His emotional status (e.g., fearful, angry, withdrawn, crying).
   H. His distractability from the pain.

Conditions Causing Discomfort

1. Hunger (differentiated from appetite) is an uncomfortable visceral sensation indicating the body's need for food. Contractions of an empty stomach can become extremely painful. Hypoglycemia causes the sensation of hunger. (See Chap. 3.)
2. Thirst is an uncomfortable sensation felt in the mouth and pharynx. Thirst is experienced when there is an increase in the salt concentration of the body fluids, when there is abnormal fluid loss, and when there is dryness of the oral and pharyngeal mucous membranes. (See Chap. 4.)
3. Nausea is an unpleasant visceral sensation, which usually precedes vomiting but may occur without it. When nausea is caused by gastric irritation, the sensation can usually be relieved by vomiting. (See Chap. 3.)
4. Coughing, although a protective mechanism, can become exhausting and self-perpetuating (in terms of continual irritation of the trachea and bronchi). Paroxysmal coughing can cause strain of the diaphragm, thoracic muscles and abdominal muscles.
5. Dizziness is a feeling of giddiness or light-headedness, which is generally momentary and may result in syncope. It may occur when there is hypotension, hypoglycemia and a decrease in the blood level of carbon dioxide (e.g., in emotional hyperventilation), or in anoxia of the brain.
6. Vertigo involves false sense perception (movement of self or environment), related to disturbance of equilibrium.

A. Vertigo is usually associated with lack of muscle coordination, nystagmus, and is frequently accompanied by nausea and vomiting.

B. Possible causes of vertigo include:
   (1) Problems involving the labyrinths (aural vertigo). (See Chap. 16.)
   (2) Problems involving the eighth cranial nerve.
   (3) Problems involving the brain stem, cerebellum or forebrain.
   (4) Some psychological disturbances.

7. Headache may be caused by painful stimuli within the cranium or outside the cranium.

A. Causes of headache occurring within the cranial cavity include:
   (1) Traction on certain veins, arteries, cranial or cervical nerves.
   (2) Displacement of brain tissue (e.g., following loss of cerebro-spinal fluid).
   (3) Abnormal dilatation of certain arterial vessels.
   (4) Inflammations around certain areas that are sensitive to pain (e.g., the venous sinuses).

B. Causes of headache occurring outside the cranium include:
   (1) Sustained contractions of muscles of the head and neck (tension headache).
   (2) Systemic effects of fever, septicemia.
   (3) Nasal and paranasal congestion.
   (4) Eye problems.

C. Headache caused by problems with the cranial cavity is often made more severe by contractions of muscles of the head and neck.

D. Migraine headache tends to occur in families. It appears to be associated with increasing emotional tension, which results in the abnormal dilatation of certain arterial vessels within the cranial cavity. The headache tends to be associated with photophobia, irritability, nausea, and often is accompanied by abdominal distension, cold extremities and sweating. Usually there are sustained contractions of neck and head muscles and this increases the pain experienced. The headache may last for minutes, hours or days.

NURSING APPLICATIONS

Observation and Evaluation

1. Patients should be observed for signs and symptoms of physical discomforts; these should be investigated, evaluated, reported and/or treated with appropriate nursing measures. This is of particular importance when the patient:
   A. Is at extremes of age.

    B. Is not responsible (e.g., psychic disturbances).

    C. Has loss of consciousness.

    D. Has problems with verbal communication (e.g., because of psychic, emotional or speech problems).

    E. Has an emotional attitude about physical pain that tends to minimize the discomfort experienced.

    F. Is likely to have discomfort (e.g., due to his physical or emotional condition; any diagnostic or therapeutic procedures).

    G. May develop a complication related to his physical condition.

2. Patients should be encouraged to report and discuss their physical discomforts.

3. Precise and complete information about physical discomforts should be sought persistently and reported appropriately.

4. A patient's physical discomfort should be evaluated in relation to:

    A. The diagnosis of the patient and discomforts commonly associated with his physical problems, or with possible complications of his condition.

    B. Any diagnostic or therapeutic procedures and discomforts that may be associated with these.

    C. The severity and duration of the discomfort.

    D. His general physical condition.

    E. His emotional status.

    F. His age.

    G. Any disturbing environmental factors (e.g., noise, visitors, bright lights, disagreeable odors).

5. Physical discomforts that should be reported promptly include:

    A. Any sudden new pain or tenderness.

    B. Any severe pain.

    C. Discomfort that cannot be alleviated by nursing measures.

    D. Discomfort associated with skeletal fixation devices, newly applied casts or constrictive bandages (e.g., tingling, numbness, burning).

Alleviating Discomfort

1. Nursing measures that may be helpful in alleviating pain include:

    A. Alleviation of pressures within body organs:

        (1) Decreasing the size of meals may be helpful.

        (2) Providing good elimination from the gastrointestinal tract and the urinary bladder may be helpful. (See Chap. 7.)

    B. Alleviation of pressure against body parts:

        (1) Changes of position may be helpful.

        (2) Soft support for the affected part may ease discomfort.

        (3) Constricting bandages or binders may be loosened (unless contraindicated).

        (4) Affected body parts should be handled very gently.

(5) Lightweight coverings or no covers over the affected part may be helpful.

(6) Flexion of thighs may be helpful when there is abdominal discomfort.

C. Alleviation of joint and muscle strain:
   (1) Good body alignment should be provided.
   (2) Frequent position changes may be helpful.
   (3) Adequate support for body parts should be provided.

D. Provision for rest of painful part:
   (1) Immobilization of the affected part may be helpful.
   (2) Good support of the affected part should be provided and the part should not be jarred.

E. Provision for relaxation of tense, contracted muscles:
   (1) Massage may be helpful.
   (2) Warmth may be helpful.
   (3) Active or passive exercise may be helpful (unless contra-indicated.
   (4) Position changes and good support may be helpful.

F. Alleviation of congestion within a part:
   (1) Elevation of the affected part may be helpful (unless contra-indicated).
   (2) Active or passive exercise may be helpful (unless contra-indicated).

G. Elimination of annoying, irritating, disturbing factors in the immediate environment:
   (1) Bright lights should be avoided if possible.
   (2) Noise should be minimized.
   (3) Disturbing visitors should be discouraged.
   (4) Privacy from other people (e.g., patients) may be helpful.

H. Provision for emotional support.

I. Administration of pain-relieving drugs (e.g., narcotics or drugs that have specific action related to cause of pain) or sedatives as ordered and indicated.
   (1) New pain, not yet evaluated by a physician, should not be masked by drugs.
   (2) Drugs should be administered in time to prevent severe pain or nervous tension.

2. When a patient experiences hunger, food and/or high carbohydrate fluids should be provided (unless contraindicated).

3. When a patient experiences thirst and oral intake of fluids is limited:
   A. Frequent oral hygiene should be done.
   B. The mouth should be rinsed frequently.
   C. Gargling may be helpful.
   D. Sucking ice chips may be helpful (if allowed).
   E. Gum chewing may be helpful (if allowed).

    F. Mouth breathing should be discouraged as possible.

    G. The intake of any fluid that is allowed should be spaced to provide the greatest comfort.

4. When a patient experiences nausea:

    A. The nausea and any vomiting may be discouraged. (See Chap. 3.)

    B. Vomiting may be encouraged by:

       (1) Tickling the uvula or posterior pharynx (causing gagging).

       (2) Encouraging sips of fluid, possibly carbonated beverages (within medical orders).

5. When a patient experiences intestinal cramping related to diarrhea, nursing measures for preventing diarrhea should be utilized. (See Chap. 3.)

6. When a patient has persistent coughing:

    A. Sips of fluid may be helpful (warm or cold may be tried).

    B. Steam inhalation may be helpful.

    C. Cough medications should be provided and administered as ordered or indicated (e.g., cough drops, lozenges, cough syrups).

7. When a patient experiences dizziness or vertigo:

    A. He should be placed in a horizontal position or seated, as necessary.

    B. All body motion should be discouraged, especially that of the head.

    C. When changes of position are necessary, they should be made slowly and preferably be controlled by the patient.

    D. Closing the eyes may be helpful.

    E. Medications for motion sickness should be administered as ordered and indicated.

8. When a patient experiences a headache:

    A. A quiet environment should be provided.

    B. Physical rest should be encouraged and provided as possible.

    C. Emotional comfort should be provided as possible.

    D. Bright lights (or any light) should be avoided as possible.

    E. Coughing or straining should be avoided (especially important when there is hypertensive headache or migraine headache).

    F. Gentle massage of neck and shoulder muscles may be helpful.

    G. Exercise of neck and shoulder muscles may be helpful (in case of tension headache).

    H. Drainage of any congested sinuses should be promoted (e.g., by positioning, steam inhalation).

9. When a patient is insensitive to painful stimuli (e.g., comatose, central nervous system damage):

    A. He should be observed very closely for signs and symptoms of injury.

    B. Special precautions should be used to protect him from injury (e.g., careful positioning and changes of position, provision for adequate elimination, prevention of skin irritation).

16

The Sensory Processes (Excluding Pain)

Vision, hearing, smell, taste, touch and discernment of temperature provide the body with information about the external environment.

Vision

1. The eye, the organ of vision, is a spherical body lying within a bony orbit.
2. The wall of the eyeball consists of three concentric layers.
   A. The external layer consists of:
      (1) The sclera, a white fibrous covering of the sides and posterior part.
      (2) The cornea, a transparent tissue of the anterior region.
   B. The middle layer consists of:
      (1) The choroid, containing many blood vessels.
      (2) The ciliary body.
      (3) The iris, a muscular diaphragm that has a circular aperture called the pupil.
   C. The innermost coat, the retina, lines the posterior part and sides of the eyeball and contains the receptors for the optic nerve.
3. The cavity of the eye contains:
   A. The aqueous humor, a watery fluid filling the space between the cornea and the lens.
   B. The vitreous body, a gelatinous substance filling the cavity posterior to the lens.
   C. The crystalline lens, a transparent, biconvex circular structure which lies behind the center of the pupil.
4. The exposed part of the eyeball is covered by delicate epithelial tissue, the conjunctiva, which is reflected onto the inner surfaces of the eyelids.

    A. The eyelids are covered with skin on the outer surface. Eye lashes are attached to the free edges.

    B. The meibomian glands, or tarsal glands, are located on the inner surfaces of the eyelids. There are approximately 30 of them on each lid. They are modified sebaceous glands.

5. The conjunctival surfaces are kept moist and clean by a film of tears, a slightly hypertonic, clear, watery fluid secreted by the lacrimal glands.

    A. Tears are delivered through several fine ducts into the conjunctival fornix.

    B. Continuous reflex movements of the eyelids keep the exposed cornea moist with tears.

    C. Tears drain through the lacrimal duct to the nose. (This process is dependent upon blinking and gravity.)

    D. Tear secretion is induced reflexly by stimulation of the cornea or conjunctiva. (This reflex may be annulled either by interference with the sensory nerves from the cornea or conjunctiva, or with the motor nerves supplying the lacrimal gland.)

    E. Fluids having a salt concentration greater than 1.5 per cent, or less than 0.16 per cent, are irritating to the eyes of most people.

6. The cornea is supplied by a rich plexus of pain fibers that have a low threshold, but it has very few blood vessels.

7. The eyeball has a relatively large blood supply in the choroid, in the internal surface of the eyeball and in the conjunctiva.

8. The intraocular fluids are produced continually and drain through tiny channels into some of the veins of the eye.

    A. The normal intraocular pressure of fluids in the eye chambers is 20 to 25 mm. of mercury.

    B. The intraocular pressure reflects very closely changes in the choroidal capillary and venous blood pressures (e.g., a sudden rise in the arterial blood pressure causes a corresponding change in the intraocular pressure).

9. The optic nerve, formed by many nerve fibers from the retina, leaves the eyeball at a point called the optic disc.

10. The optic nerves pass backwards to the optic chiasm, where some fibers cross to the opposite side. From here the two optic tracts pass backwards through the midbrain and, eventually, to the visual cortex in the occipital lobe of the cerebrum.

    A. Areas in the midbrain contain centers that serve to correlate eye movements and movements of the eyelids and the body, which protects the eye from injury.

    B. Sensations of light are perceived in the visual cortex.

    C. Interference with any part of the optic nerves, chiasm or tracts, by such means as pressure, causes visual defects.

D. "Conscious vision" probably is a function of large portions of the cerebral cortex.

11. Blinking, a voluntary or reflex act, is accomplished by movements of the eyelids.
    A. Movement of the eyelids helps to protect the eye from the entrance of foreign particles.
    B. Closure of the eyes is accomplished by the contraction of muscles around the eye, which are under the control of branches of the facial nerve.
    C. Opening of the eyes is accomplished by the contraction of muscles of the eyelid under the control of the oculomotor nerve.
    D. Stimulation of the cornea or conjunctiva normally causes blinking.

12. Light rays enter the eye through the pupil, and the refraction of them, primarily through the cornea and crystalline lens, normally causes them to focus on the retina.
    A. The iris serves as an opaque screen which adjusts the amount of light allowed to enter the eye.
       (1) Parasympathetic stimulation of circular muscles in the iris causes constriction of the pupil.
       (2) Sympathetic stimulation of radial muscles in the iris causes dilation of the pupil.
       (3) In bright illumination the pupil is constricted; in dim illumination, dilated.
       (4) Constriction of the pupil helps to prevent blurred images.
    B. The adjustment of the eye, by which it focuses the image of both near and far objects on the retina, is called accommodation.
       (1) Accommodation is accomplished by changes in the convexity of the anterior surface of the crystalline lens.
       (2) Convergence of the eyes and constriction of the pupils occur when there is accommodation for near objects.
       (3) The accommodation reaction originates in the visual cortex.
       (4) Generally, the ability to accommodate is fairly poor in a child up to the age of 2 to 3 years.
       (5) Generally, the ability to accommodate decreases after the age of 45.

13. The retina is stimulated most effectively by light, but crude visual sensations can be evoked by mechanical forms of stimulation (e.g., pressure).

14. Concentrated sources of light situated near an object being observed causes glare.
    A. When there is glare, visual acuity is decreased and eye strain occurs.
    B. Squinting helps to reduce glare.

15. How much illumination is desirable for ideal vision depends largely upon such factors as the amount of visual acuity demanded for the job, and the contrast between light and dark in what is being observed. (A general over-all illumination of a room with an increased illumination on the working surface produces a minimum of eyestrain and glare.)

16. The extrinsic eye muscles move the eyeball in its orbit.
   A. The eye muscle movements are under the control of cranial nerves. (Voluntary movements are controlled by the motor cortex.)
   B. At birth the eyes are not associated with each other, but act as two independent sense organs. By about the third month the child begins, by trial and error process, to move his eyeballs in such a way as to gain a common visual direction and, in this way, his eyes can become associated.
   C. Eye and head movements are closely associated with the vestibular apparatus.
      (1) Nystagmus involves abnormal eye movements, caused by the stimulation of motor nerves through the vestibular nuclei.
      (2) Visual disturbances are often associated with vertigo and nausea.

17. Binocular vision is important for depth perception and for the largest possible visual field.

Hearing

1. The ear is the receptor of sound, and also contains end organs for the sense of balance.
   A. The outer ear is composed of the pinna and the auditory canal.
      (1) The pinna contains elastic cartilage and is covered with skin.
      (2) The auditory canal is an S-shaped passage approximately one and one-quarter inches long. It ends blindly at the flexible tympanic membrane.
         (a) The ear canal in the child is relatively straight.
         (b) The canal is lined with skin that contains cerumen-secreting glands.
   B. The middle ear is a tiny chamber situated in the temporal bone; it contains three articulating miniature bones (ossicles).
      (1) The malleus articulates with the tympanic membrane, the incus is in the center and the stapes articulates with the oval window in the posterior wall.
      (2) The middle ear is filled with air, maintained at atmospheric pressure by means of an air passageway through the eustachian tube.

(3) The middle ear is lined with mucous membrane, which is continuous with that of the eustachian tube, the nasopharynx and the mastoid antrum.

(4) The posterior wall of the middle ear has an opening into the mastoid antrum.

    (a) The mastoid process is the posterior portion of the temporal bone.

    (b) The mastoid contains a deep grove for the lateral sinus of the brain.

    (c) The mastoid antrum is separated from the brain by only a thin plate of bone.

    (d) The mastoid cells are spaces containing air, located in a section of the mastoid process. There is also air in the antrum, which communicates with the tympanic cavity.

    (e) A branch of the facial nerve lies very close to the middle ear.

C. The internal ear, called the labyrinth, consists of two parts.

(1) The osseous labyrinth is a series of cavities within the temporal bone; the membranous labyrinth is a series of communicating sacs and ducts that lie within the osseous labyrinth.

(2) The osseous labyrinth consists of the vestibule, the semicircular canals and the cochlea. Each contains perilymph, a clear fluid.

    (a) The vestibule is the central portion, and its lateral wall contains the oval window.

    (b) There are three bony semicircular canals which open into the vestibule. They are unequal in length, and lie in different directions.

    (c) The cochlea is a conical structure, with spirals that form a canal.

(3) The membranous labyrinth consists of the utricle and the saccule within the vestibule; the semicircular ducts within the semicircular canals; and the cochlear duct within the cochlea. All contain a fluid, endolymph.

    (a) Hair cells in the utricle, saccule and semicircular ducts act as rotary and gravity receptors. Nervous impulses are carried to the brain by way of the vestibular nerve, which becomes the acoustic nerve.

    (b) Specialized cells in the cochlear ducts (organ of Corti) act as receptors for sound. Nervous impulses are carried to the brain by way of the cochlear nerve, which becomes the acoustic nerve.

2. Normally, the tympanic membrane is forced into vibrations by

sound waves, and the vibratory motions are transmitted through the ossicles to the fluid in the inner ear. In old age, movement of the ossicles may be lessened.

3. Continued stimulation of the auditory nerves gives rise to general fatigue and nervous irritability.

4. The cochlear division of the acoustic nerve (auditory nerve) leaves the cochlea, and passes to the midbrain (where there are centers for auditory reflexes); it then passes to the temporal lobes of the cerebral cortex for conscious perception.

5. Hearing is generally the last sense to be lost when there is loss of consciousness.

6. Labyrinthine stimulation is the primary factor in the nausea and vomiting of motion sickness, and that associated with vertigo. Impulses from the vestibular organs appear to pass to the vomiting center.
   (Equilibrium is included in Chap. 11, and vertigo is included in Chap. 15.)

7. The fluid in the semicircular canals, when heated or cooled quickly, gives rise to sensations of position change which may cause vertigo.

Superficial Touch and Pressure

1. Objects brought into contact with the skin produce the sensation of touch or pressure through the stimulation of end organs located in the skin and subcutaneous tissues.

2. Nerve fibers that carry impulses of touch and pressure from the periphery to the brain pass either:
   A. Up the cord in the posterior columns (gracilis and cunneatus tracts) and cross in the medulla, or
   B. Up the anterolateral spinothalamic tracts, crossing at different levels of the cord.

3. Sensations of pressure and touch are perceived in the somatic sensory area of the cerebral cortex, primarily in the postcentral gyrus.

Heat and Cold

1. The receptors for heat and cold are located in the skin and mucous membranes. Mucous membrane has fewer sensory nerve endings than the skin.

2. Sensory impulses for heat and cold travel through peripheral nerves to the spinal cord, up the spinal cord by way of the lateral spinothalamic tracts, through the medulla to the thalamus, and, finally, to the cerebral cortex, where the sensation is perceived.

Taste and Smell

1. The olfactory end organs, located in the olfactory area of the nasal mucosa, are sensitive to chemical stimulation.

2. Nerve impulses are carried by way of the olfactory nerves to the temporal lobes of the cerebral cortex, where smell is perceived.
3. The taste buds, embedded in the tongue, are sensitive to chemical substances in solution.
4. Nerve impulses are carried by way of the facial and glossopharyngeal nerves to the postcentral gyrus, where taste is perceived.
5. The number of functioning taste buds decreases with age.
6. Smell is more acute than the sense of taste.

PHYSICS

1. Light is a form of electromagnetic radiation (gamma rays, x-rays, ultraviolet rays, visible light rays and infrared rays).
2. Illumination varies with three factors:
   A. The power of the source of light.
   B. The distance from the source of light.
   C. The angle of incidence at which the light strikes a surface and is reflected.
3. Refraction is the bending of a ray of light when it passes from one medium to a medium of a different density.
4. A converging lens causes, through refraction, the convergence of parallel light rays on the opposite side of the lens at a point called the principal focus.
5. Sound originates in vibrations, and the waves, which are set up in some medium (solid, liquid or gas), travel outward from the source of sound.
6. Pitch indicates the brain's interpretation of the frequency of sound waves.
7. The intensity of sound is heard as loudness.
8. Pressure is the force exerted on a unit area.
9. Pressure exerted on a confined liquid is transmitted undiminished to all parts of that liquid.
10. Heat is a form of energy, and temperature is the measure of the intensity of heat.

PATHOLOGY

Vision

1. Signs and symptoms of problems concerned with vision may include:
   A. Visual disturbances. These include:
      (1) Partial or complete loss of vision in one or both eyes.
      (2) Blurring of vision, loss of visual acuity.
      (3) Diplopia (double vision).
      (4) Spots before the eyes (often floating spots).
      (5) Visual hallucinations.
      (6) Sudden flashes of light.

B. Abnormal positions or movements of eyeballs (e.g., squint, nystagmus).

C. Abnormal pupil sizes (e.g., irregularities, constriction or dilatation of one or both pupils that is inappropriate to lighting).

D. Photophobia.

E. Difficulties in postural adjustments and other body movements (e.g., handling of objects).

F. Pain (e.g., generalized headache, frontal or occipital headaches or pain in or behind the eyes).

G. Frowning, squinting, muscular twitchings in eyelids or around the eyes.

H. Excessive blinking, redness, burning of conjunctiva.

I. Lesions of eyelid or eyeball.

J. Edema, itching of eyelids.

K. Abnormal drainage from the eye (e.g., excessive tearing, purulent exudate).

L. Bleeding in eye, or bleeding from around the eyeball.

M. Vertigo, nausea and vomiting.

2. Eyestrain, leading to fatigue, occurs when the ciliary muscles become tired due to prolonged contraction (e.g., when used for performing fine work for long periods of time).

3. Malnutrition may be a cause of eye damage:

A. An inadequate dietary intake of Vitamin A can result in abnormal cellular changes in the conjunctiva and cornea, as well as impaired night vision.

B. An inadequate dietary intake of B vitamins can result in retinal damage.

4. Myopia is nearsightedness (i.e., light rays are focused in front of the retina). Objects must be at close range to be seen clearly. The problem may be due to increased refraction by the cornea or lens, or to the length of the eyeball.

5. Hyperopia is farsightedness (i.e., light rays are focused in back of the retina). Objects must be at a far range to be seen clearly. The problem may be due to decreased refraction by the cornea or lens, or to the shortness of the eyeball.

6. Presbyopia is a condition in which vision is blurred due to a hardening of the lens, so that accommodation cannot occur normally.

7. Astigmatism is a condition in which all vision is blurred to some extent, because of abnormal curvatures of the lens.

8. Photophobia is an unusual intolerance to light. It often occurs with inflammations of the eyes or eyelids. It may occur with some communicable diseases (e.g., measles), and with some brain injuries. Referred pain may be involved.

9. A sty (or hordeolum) is an infection of the sebaceous glands

and/or hair follicles of the eyelid. The condition is often associated with eyestrain or poor physical health.

10. A chalazion is a small hard cyst of a meibomian gland of the eyelid. The cyst can irritate the eyeball.

11. Inflammation of the conjunctiva and eyelids may be caused by:
    A. Trauma (e.g., foreign particles).
    B. Heat.
    C. Hypersensitivity reaction. (See Chap. 14.)
    D. Microorganisms.

12. Conjunctivitis neonatorum is an infection of the conjunctiva of a newborn baby; it may be caused by a number of microorganisms, most particularly the Gonococcus. The baby's eyes contact these pathogens during birth.

13. Acute conjunctivitis involves excessive catarrhal exudate, discomfort and photophobia. The inflammation is often caused by microorganisms, but may be associated with other irritants.

14. Blepharitis is an inflammation of the eyelids, usually caused by microorganisms. The hair follicles and meibomian glands are the structures affected primarily. There may be edema and redness of the lid, exudate production, and small ulcerations along the eyelid.

15. Ulcerations of the cornea may occur as a result of trauma or infections.

16. Keratitis is an inflammation of the cornea, which may be the result of traumatic injury, certain systemic infections (e.g., syphilis), some hypersensitive reactions or invasion of microorganisms. When the inflammation is severe, blindness results.

17. Uveitis is an inflammation of the iris (iritis), choroid (choroiditis) and ciliary body. These inflammations may occur in association with certain systemic diseases, some local infections or certain toxic reactions. The condition may contribute to the development of glaucoma.

18. Glaucoma, a major cause of blindness, is a condition in which there is increased intraocular pressure due to faulty drainage of aqueous humor. There may be an inherited tendency for this condition, or it may occur as a consequence of a problem within the eyeball, such as abnormal growths or an inflammatory process. Glaucoma may be acute (requiring immediate treatment), or chronic (requiring continued medical supervision). The increased ocular pressure is damaging to all the structures of the eyeball.

19. A cataract is an opacity (or cloudiness) of the lens, caused by chemical changes within it. The condition may be inherited, acquired early in fetal development, a degenerative process occurring with the aging process, or caused by some kind of injury to the lens.

20. When the retina becomes separated from the choroid, or when the layers of the retina becomes separated, the condition is called "detached retina." The separation may occur as a result of head injury, tumor growth, inflammation of the choroid, hemorrhage, and even sudden physical exertion by an individual who is in poor general health. It may occur in one or both eyes, and causes various visual disturbances, possibly complete loss of vision.
21. Sympathetic ophthalmia is the involvement of the heathy eye with an inflammatory process of the injured eye.
22. Degenerative problems of the eye occur frequently in the retina, and, more specifically, in the tiny blood vessels of the retina. Retinal hemorrhages are often associated with diabetes mellitus and with hypertension.
23. Vision may be affected by injuries or disease conditions that affect the optic nerves, the optic tract, the midbrain or the occipital lobe of the cerebral cortex (e.g., cerebrovascular accidents, tumors, increased intracranial pressure).
24. Retrolental fibroplasia is a condition in which there is a proliferation of some of the retinal cells, an increase in blood vessels, edema and possible retinal separation. It occurs in premature infants, and seems to be related to the prolonged administration of high concentrations of oxygen after birth.
25. Strabismus (squint) is a condition in which both eyes cannot be used at the same time to see an object. The line of vision of only one eye is directed at the object to be seen. A baby may be born with this condition, or it may develop as a result of some other condition. Muscles that move the eyeball inward or outward may be overactive or underactive. The squinting eye may move in the same direction as the good eye, but not on the same line of vision. In monocular squint one eye is used constantly for vision; in alternating squint, either eye may be used for vision and the other eye becomes the squinting eye. Sometimes squint is caused by refractory problems.

Hearing

1. Signs and symptoms of problems concerned with hearing may include:
   A. Auditory disturbances:
      (1) Absence of hearing.
      (2) Loss of hearing (pitch or intensity).
      (3) Tinnitus (buzzing, roaring, ringing, pounding sounds in ears).
      (4) Auditory hallucinations.
   B. Signs and symptoms of deafness, such as:
      (1) Faulty speech (especially in childhood).
      (2) Inattentiveness, unresponsiveness.

(3) Strained or intense facial expressions.
(4) Tendency toward withdrawal.
C. Pain in or around the ear, may vary from dull ache to excruciatingly sharp pain.
D. Feeling of fullness in the ears.
E. Drainage from the auditory canals (e.g., blood, exudates).
F. Lesions of the auditory canal, redness, swelling, itching.
2. Signs and symptoms of facial paralysis may include:
A. Inability to close eye on affected side.
B. Inability to use facial expressions on affected side (e.g., smiles, frowns).
C. The mouth drawn over to the unaffected side.
3. Signs and symptoms of inflammation of the mastoid cells may include:
A. Swelling of the mastoid region.
B. Tenderness in the mastoid region, which may become severe pain.
4. The auditory canal may be injured by:
A. Trauma (e.g., foreign bodies inserted into the canal).
B. Allergic manifestations (e.g., eczema).
C. Microorganisms (e.g., fungus infections, furuncles).
5. The tympanic membrane may be ruptured by:
A. Severe trauma to the side of the head.
B. The pushing of foreign objects through it (e.g., hairpins, match-sticks).
C. Pressure exerted against the membrane by accumulating exudate in the middle ear.
D. Pressure exerted again the membrane by fluids injected into the auditory canal (e.g., accidentally during irrigation).
E. Excessive pressure of air against the membrane when the eustachian tubes are closed or plugged.
6. Otitis media, inflammation of the middle ear, may be acute, chronic, purulent, catarrhal. The inflammation may be caused by:
A. Abnormal pressures in the middle ear (e.g., with high altitude flying, or when eustachian tubes become plugged because of infection).
B. Microorganisms (e.g., may enter the middle ear through the eustachian tubes or through a ruptured ear drum).
7. Inflammatory processes of the middle ear can result in permanent damage to the structures of the middle ear, including the ear drum.
8. A purulent otitis media usually involves the mastoid cells, causing abscess formation. If exudate cannot drain out through the middle ear, the pressure produced in the mastoid process causes great pain. Infection in the mastoid cells can spread to the meninges, the lateral venous sinuses, or the brain itself.

9. Otosclerosis is a condition in which the bony capsule of the labyrinth becomes spongy, and the stapes becomes ankylosed in the
   oval window. The other ossicles may also become ankylosed. There
   seems to be an inherited tendency in the development of this
   condition.
10. Deafness may be due to:
    A. Some disturbances in the transmission of sound from the external
       environment to the cochlea (conduction deafness).
    B. Some problem of the nerve tissue involved with hearing (e.g.,
       auditory nerves, cerebral pathways, auditory centers in the
       temporal lobes of cerebral cortex). Problems may be caused by
       infections, tumors, head injuries, psychogenic disturbances,
       some drugs. This may be referred to as perception deafness.
    C. A combination of both (progressive deafness).
11. Some loss of hearing is common with the aging process.
12. Signs and symptoms of problems involving the sense of balance
    may include:
    A. Vertigo.
    B. Nausea and vomiting.
13. Labyrinthitis is an inflammation of the inner ear which is usually
    caused by an infection in the middle ear. Vertigo is severe.
14. Menière's syndrome involves changes in the endolymph channels
    of the cochlea, and changes in the organ of Corti. There are attacks
    of severe vertigo and tinnitus. There may be degeneration of the
    acoustic nerve.

Touch, Pressure, Heat, Cold

1. Signs and symptoms of abnormalities in the perception of pressure
   and touch may include:
   A. Anesthesia (absence of these sensations).
   B. Hyperesthesia (increased intensity of these sensations).
   C. Paresthesia (abnormal sensations).
   D. Difficulty with locomotor activities.
2. Any injury or disease condition that affects the sensory receptors,
   the peripheral nerves, the posterior nerve roots, the posterior
   columns of the spinal cord, the sensory pathways in the brain, or
   somesthetic areas in the cerebral cortex affects the perception of
   touch, pressure, heat and cold.
3. Interference with the normal functioning of the sensory receptors
   may be caused by:
   A. Problems of the skin and mucous membrane. (See Chap. 13.)
   B. Inadequate circulation. (See Chap. 1.)
4. Interference with the normal functioning of the peripheral nerves
   may result from traumatic injury, pressure, inadequate circulation.
   (See Chap. 11.)

5. Injury to the posterior nerve roots may be caused by:
   A. Injuries related to the vertebral column. (See Chap. 12.)
   B. Pathological lesions resulting from syphilis.
   C. Pressures exerted by abnormal growths.
6. Interference with normal functioning of the sensory pathways in the spinal cord and brain, or the somesthetic areas of the cerebral cortex, may result from:
   A. Degenerative diseases (e.g., multiple sclerosis).
   B. Pernicious anemia.
   C. Traumatic injuries.
   D. Increased intracranial pressure.
   E. Neoplasms.
   F. Inadequate circulation, oxygen, glucose. (See Chap. 1, 2, and 3.)

Taste and Smell

1. Lesions of the temporal lobe of the cerebrum may result in:
   A. Impairment in taste and/or smell.
   B. Olfactory or gustatory hallucinations.
2. Smell may be impaired because of inflammation of the nasal mucosa (e.g., infections, hypersensitivity reaction).
3. Inflammatory conditions of the tongue may impair taste.
4. Sometimes strong or unpleasant tastes or odors can cause nausea.

NURSING APPLICATIONS

Vision

1. Patients should be observed for signs and symptoms of problems concerned with vision; these should be investigated, evaluated, reported and/or treated with appropriate nursing measures. This is of particular importance when the patient:
   A. Is at extremes of age.
   B. Has loss of consciousness.
   C. Has an injury (including surgery) or a disease condition that involves or may involve:
      (1) The structures of the eyeball.
      (2) The eyelid.
      (3) The extrinsic eye muscles.
      (4) Nerve tissue concerned with vision.
2. The condition of a patient's eyes or vision should be evaluated in relation to:
   A. Normal vision, eye movements, pupil size, tearing, blinking, color.
   B. The individual's normal vision (e.g., as corrected by lenses).
   C. His diagnosed condition.
3. Patients should be protected from eye injury; this is of particular importance when the patient:

    A. Is at extremes of age.

    B. Is irresponsible (e.g., children, patients with psychic problems).

    C. Has loss of consciousness.

    D. Has a problem involving one or both eyes already.

4. Patients should be protected from eye injury by:

    A. Encouraging and providing appropriate lighting.

       (1) Adequate lighting for the type of work being done by the eyes should always be provided.

       (2) When pupils are dilated, bright lighting should be avoided.

       (3) Glare or sudden bright lights in the eyes should be avoided (e.g., by placement of light, looking away, use of good sun glasses).

    B. Encouraging and providing frequent rest for the eyes, which is of particular importance when fine work is being performed.

    C. Protecting the eyes from irritating chemical substances (e.g., soaps, creams, sprays, fumes).

    D. Protecting the eyes from trauma.

       (1) Eyes should not be rubbed.

       (2) Great caution should be used with the manipulation of equipment near the eyes; this is of great importance when the patient is irresponsible or lacks control.

       (3) Only very soft materials (e.g., cotton) should be used in eye treatments.

       (4) When eye irrigations are done, no force should be used.

       (5) Appropriate means of accident prevention should be encouraged at all times; this is of particular importance with children.

    E. Protecting the eyes from heat (e.g., steam or overly-hot compresses).

    F. Maintaining cleanliness (or sterile technique if indicated) in all eye care.

    G. Encouraging and providing good nutrition. (See Chap. 3.)

    H. Encouraging and providing (as possible) prompt medical attention for any eye discomforts or abnormalities in structure or function.

    I. Encouraging frequent ophthalmologic examinations; this is of particular importance if the patient is over 45 years of age, wears glasses, or has a known eye problem.

    J. Discouraging eye irrigations or the use of any eye drops or ointments, unless done under medical supervision.

    K. Providing proper emergency treatment for eye injuries.

       (1) When irritating chemical substances get into the eyes, the eyes should be irrigated immediately with large amounts of water (or physiological saline solution if available).

(2) When there is a foreign body on the conjunctiva,
  (a) The eye should never be rubbed.
  (b) Strict cleanliness of the hands or any equipment must be observed.
  (c) The lower lid and then upper lid should be checked for the object.
  (d) The eyeball or lid can be gently lavaged with physiological saline solution (or water if necessary).
  (e) If medical help is not immediately available and a foreign body is not embedded or on the cornea, a soft object (e.g., cotton swab) may be used to gently remove the object.
(3) When a foreign object is embedded, is on the cornea or cannot be removed by simple lavage, the lid should be closed, the eye covered lightly with a bandage or patch, and the patient seen by a physician promptly.
(4) When a patient exhibits signs of a possible detachment of the retina (e.g., sudden loss of part or all of vision following a head injury or a sudden physical exertion):
  (a) He should be placed in a horizontal position immediately (possibly a slight Trendelenberg).
  (b) He should be kept absolutely quiet with no head movement.
  (c) His eyes should be lightly covered (to avoid eye movements).
  L. Performing appropriate prophylaxis in care of newborn's eyes.
5. When a patient has facial paralysis involving the orbicularis muscle, has corneal anesthesia, or is unconscious, the eyes should be protected from injury by:
  A. Covering them with a light dressing or with an eye patch.
  B. Moistening and cleaning the conjunctiva with physiological saline solution frequently.
6. When a patient has traumatic injury (including surgery) or a disease condition that involves the internal structures of the eyeball (e.g., glaucoma, uveitis, detached retina):
  A. Medical orders relative to these factors must be followed exactly:
    (1) The use of protective covering over the affected eye.
    (2) The lighting allowed (usually a darkened room or dark glasses are desirable).
    (3) The type and extent of physical activity permitted.
    (4) Positioning.
  B. A pleasant but non-stimulating environment should be provided.
  C. Stability of the head should be promoted (e.g., no jerking move-

ments, no jarring, careful changes of position, use of sandbags).

D. Emotional support should be consistent.

E. Sneezing, coughing, vomiting, laughing strenuously, straining should be prevented as possible. (Coughing is included in Chap. 15, vomiting in Chap. 3, and constipation in Chap. 7.)

F. He should be observed closely for any signs and symptoms of increasing intraorbital pressure (e.g., headache, local pain) or abnormal drainage from the eye, and these should be reported promptly.

7. When a patient has an inflammatory process that involves the eyelid, conjunctiva or cornea:

A. The affected part should be protected from further injury.

(1) The affected part should never be rubbed.

(2) Treatments should be performed with sterile technique.

(3) Lighting should be as dim as necessary to prevent discomfort.

(4) The eyes should not be used for fine work and should not be used beyond the point of comfort.

B. Very special precautions should be used to prevent the spread of any infection from one eye to the other.

8. When a premature infant is receiving prolonged oxygen therapy, the concentration of oxygen should not exceed 40 per cent (unless an increased concentration is specifically ordered).

9. When a patient is partially or totally blind:

A. He should be given adequate information about his environment to provide for his physical and psychological comfort.

B. He should be assisted with the activities of daily living only as necessary.

C. His immediate environment should be arranged in such a way as to allow him to meet his own needs safely and satisfactorily.

D. Emotional support should be consistent.

E. Special precautions should be taken to prevent accidents.

F. He should be encouraged in specialized training (e.g., vocational, braille).

10. When an eye has been removed:

A. The condition of the eye socket should be observed carefully, and any abnormalities reported promptly (e.g., irritation or exudate).

B. The eye socket should be kept clean and dry.

C. Any artificial eye should be removed carefully and gently and cleaned daily.

D. Special precautions should be taken to protect the unaffected eye from any injury.

Hearing

1. Patients should be observed for signs and symptoms of problems concerned with hearing; these should be investigated, evaluated, reported or treated with appropriate nursing measures. This is of particular importance when the patient:
   A. Is at extremes of age.
   B. Has an injury (including surgery) or a disease condition that involves or may involve:
      (1) The structures of the ear (external, middle or inner).
      (2) The pharynx or eustachian tubes.
      (3) Nerve tissue concerned with hearing.
2. A patient's hearing should be evaluated in relation to:
   A. Normal hearing ability.
   B. The patient's usual hearing.
   C. Any diagnosed condition.
3. Patients should be protected from ear injury by:
   A. Discouraging and preventing the insertion of small objects into the auditory canals (especially important with children).
   B. Never using any hard or sharp object to clean wax from the auditory canals.
   C. Discouraging the use of any medications in the ear, unless done under medical supervision.
   D. Discouraging forceful or persistent nose blowing.
   E. Encouraging gentle nose blowing with both nostrils open (if cleaning of nose in this way is deemed necessary).
   F. Using great caution in performing any treatments involving the ear, which is of particular importance when the patient is a child or lacks control.
   G. Providing for cleanliness or sterile technique in care of ears (as indicated by the patient's problem).
   H. Promoting any drainage from the auditory canal (e.g., by positioning or not plugging the canal).
   I. Encouraging prompt otologic examination when there is any noticeable change in one's hearing (pitch or intensity).
   J. Encouraging and providing (as possible) prompt medical attention when the patient has:
      (1) Impacted cerumen in the auditory canal.
      (2) A foreign object in the ear.
      (3) Acute or chronic infection of the nose, sinuses, pharynx or eustachian tubes.
      (4) Any signs and symptoms of problems involving the ear (e.g., pain, drainage, swelling, tinnitus, lesions).
4. When a patient has traumatic injury (including surgery) or a

disease condition that involves the middle or inner ear (e.g., otitis media, fenestration):

A. Medical orders relative to these factors must be followed exactly:
  (1) The use of protective bandaging over the affected ear (e.g., pressure, changing, reinforcing).
  (2) Positioning.
  (3) The extent and type of physical activity permitted.
  (4) The diet (usually liquid or soft).
B. Loud or unpleasant noises should be avoided.
C. Stability of the head should be promoted; this is particularly important when the inner ear is affected (e.g., no jarring of bed, no quick or jerky movements, careful changes of position at patient's own rate).
D. Emotional support should be consistent.
E. Sneezing, coughing, blowing the nose should be discouraged and prevented (as possible).
F. The patient should be observed closely for signs and symptoms of:
  (1) Facial nerve damage.
  (2) Injury to the mastoid cells.

5. When a patient has a problem that involves the sense of balance (e.g., labyrinthitis, Menière's syndrome):
A. Stability of the head should be promoted.
B. Appropriate means of accident prevention should be utilized.
C. The patient should be maintained in a horizontal position while vertigo exists; keeping the eyes closed may be helpful.
D. The patient should be encouraged to move only at his own rate.
E. Emotional support should be consistent.

6. No cold drops or solutions should be introduced into a patient's ear.

7. Patients should be protected from continuous noise or loud noises.

8. When a patient is comatose, verbal communications should be continued as if the patient is able to hear, which he may be.

9. When a patient is partially or totally deaf:
A. He should be helped with communications as possible.
  (1) Learning lip reading should be encouraged.
  (2) Any lip reading ability should be facilitated by the position of the speaker, lighting of the face and careful speech.
  (3) The use of hearing aids should be encouraged if they may be helpful.
  (4) Speech training may be encouraged, especially when there is only partial deafness.
  (5) Note writing can be used as necessary.
B. Emotional support should be consistent.
C. Appropriate methods of accident prevention should be utilized.

Touch and Pressure

1. Patients should be observed for problems involving perception of superficial touch and pressure; these should be investigated, evaluated, reported or treated with appropriate nursing measures. This is of particular importance when the patient:
   A. Is at extremes of age.
   B. Has injury or a disease condition that involves or may involve:
      (1) Peripheral nerves.
      (2) The spinal cord or brain.
   C. Has peripheral vascular problems.
2. When a patient is unable to perceive superficial pressure and/or touch normally:
   A. He may require varying amounts of assistance with some of his locomotor activities (e.g., walking, handling of objects).
   B. Special precautions should be taken to prevent accidents (e.g., falling, dropping potentially harmful objects).

Heat and Cold

1. Patients should be observed for signs and symptoms of problems involving the perception of heat and cold; these should be investigated, evaluated, reported and/or treated with appropriate nursing measures. This is of particular importance when the patient:
   A. Has injury of the skin or mucous membranes.
   B. Has injury or a disease condition that involves or may involve:
      (1) The peripheral nerves.
      (2) The spinal cord or brain.
   C. Is having hot or cold applications.
2. When a patient has decreased sensitivity for heat or cold:
   A. Special precautions should be taken to prevent accidents such as burns (e.g., when lighting cigarette).
   B. Temperatures of hot solutions used for treatments should be within safe limits and measured accurately.
   C. Heating equipment should not be used on a person who is in shock or who is unconscious.

Taste and Smell

1. Patients should be observed for signs and symptoms of problems involving perception of taste and smell; these should be investigated, evaluated, reported and/or treated with appropriate nursing measures. This is of particular importance when the patient:
   A. Has inflammations involving the tongue or nasal mucosa.
   B. Has or may have brain injury.
2. When the senses of taste and/or smell are diminished:
   A. Foods with strong tastes may be encouraged (within orders).

    B. Flavoring of food may be increased (e.g., salting, sweetness, herbs).

3. Odors that are annoying or unpleasant to a patient should be avoided or eliminated from the patient's environment as effectively as possible (e.g., perfumes, tobacco fumes, body wastes).

4. When a bitter-tasting drug is administered orally:

    A. Solids should not be allowed to dissolve any more than necessary.

    B. Liquids should miss the tongue as much as possible (e.g., with use of drinking tube).

    C. Unpleasant aftertastes may be eliminated with additional fluid intake or a sweet tasting substance (within orders).

17

Cognition, Memory and Association of Ideas

Normal functioning of the cerebral cortex is essential to the mental faculties of cognition, memory and association of ideas.

ANATOMY AND PHYSIOLOGY

1. The cortical gray matter is the chief organ of the psychic life of man.
2. The mental capacity of an individual seems to be a function of the cerebral cortex as a whole. The quantity of cortex may be more important than any specific locations.
3. Intelligence depends upon a knowledge of the external world received through sensory processes. Stimuli are received, perceived and stored as memories in the cerebral cortex.
4. Perceiving is a function of the cerebral cortex. It is a process of organizing present sensory data, and interpreting it on the basis of past experience.
5. Perception implies the dynamic organization of external and internal stimuli into a meaningful whole; this organization is one of the determinants of behavior.
6. Learning implies changes in behavior based on changes in the central nervous system.
7. The association areas of the cerebral cortex (located in all lobes) are those areas in which complex sensory, motor and behavior patterns are integrated. Extensive association areas seem to be located in the temporal lobes.
8. The prefrontal lobes of the cerebral cortex are probably important in highly associative abstract thought and may also be associated with emotional feelings.
9. Gradual development of the mental faculties occurs during the normal growth and development of individuals.

PATHOLOGY

1. Signs and symptoms of the impairment of mental faculties may include:
   A. Faulty sensory perceptions.
   B. Mental confusion, disorientation.
   C. Inability to reason.
   D. Inability to learn (e.g., locomotor activities, speech, abstract concepts).
   E. Loss of memory (recent or remote).
   F. Changes in usual behavior patterns (e.g., lack of restraint or judgement, inattentiveness, unusual aggressiveness or withdrawal).
2. Injury to the nerve cells, projection fibers or association fibers of the cerebral cortex may be caused by:
   A. Traumatic injury of the head (e.g., birth injuries, accidents).
   B. Increased intracranial pressure (e.g., due to bleeding, edema, tumors).
   C. Inadequate blood supply. (See Chap. 1.)
   D. Inadequate oxygen supply. (See Chap. 2.)
   E. Inadequate glucose. (See Chap. 3.)
   F. Hyperthermia. (See Chap. 9.)
   G. Toxemias (e.g., resulting from accumulation of certain metabolites, or caused by bacterial toxins or certain drugs).
   H. Abnormal growths.
   I. Degenerative problems (e.g., due to such conditions as arteriosclerotic changes or multiple sclerosis).
3. Mental retardation may be associated with such conditions as hypothyroidism (Chap. 8), microcephaly or mongolism.
4. Mongolism appears to be caused by problems in embryologic development. The condition can often be recognized at birth by some typical physical defects, such as the structure of the head and face, lack of muscle tone, and a protruding tongue. Both physical and mental development are slow, and rarely does the intellectual level progress beyond the age of 7 years.
5. The impairment of mental faculties may be associated with psychogenic disturbances, such as psychoneuroses, and psychoses.
6. Unconsciousness involves the loss of awareness. There are degrees of unconsciousness:
   A. There may be only mental confusion, disorientation and hyper-irritability to external stimuli.
   B. There may be drowsiness with very slow responses to stimuli, incoherent speech.
   C. There may be stupor, with only reflexive muscle responses to painful stimuli.

D. Deep coma involves total lack of response to stimuli. The sense of hearing is the last sense to be lost.

NURSING APPLICATIONS

1. Patients should be observed for signs and symptoms of impairment of their mental faculties; these should be investigated, evaluated, reported and/or treated with appropriate nursing measures. This is of particular importance when the patient:
   A. Is at extremes of age.
   B. Has an injury or disease condition that involves or may involve the cerebral cortex (e.g., head injury, cerebrovascular accident, toxic states, some virus infections).
   C. Has impaired general circulation.
   D. Has respiratory problems.
   E. Has malnutrition (especially available glucose).
   F. Has hyperthermia.
   G. Has emotional or psychic disorders.
   H. Is receiving or has received drugs that effect the central nervous system (e.g., ethyl alcohol, general anesthetics).
2. When a patient has impaired mental faculties:
   A. He should be protected from causing harm to himself or others (e.g., close observation, control of environment and activities).
   B. He should be helped as much as necessary or possible in meeting his basic physiological needs.
   C. Emotional support should be consistent.
3. When a child shows signs of slow mental development:
   A. Prompt medical supervision should be encouraged and provided as possible.
   B. Specialized education should be encouraged as possible.

18

Speech

Speech provides a means of communication.

ANATOMY AND PHYSIOLOGY

1. The larynx produces vocal sounds, but the actual articulation of words is accomplished by the shape given to the mouth and throat and the movement and positions of the lips and tongue.
   A. Vocal sounds are produced by the vibration of the vocal folds in the larynx, caused by the controlled passage of air through the larynx.
   B. Changes in the position and tension of the vocal folds (causing changes in pitch of voice) are brought about largely by intrinsic muscles that move some of the cartilages of the larynx.
2. The function of speech involves both sensory and motor elements in the use and understanding of symbols for the expression of ideas.
   A. The function of speech includes, on the sensory side, the abilities to understand both the written and the spoken word.
   B. The function of speech includes, on the motor side, the abilities both to speak and to write words.
3. The function of speech is thought to involve the cerebral cortex as a whole.
   A. The motor speech area (Broca's area) is located in the motor area of the frontal lobe of the cerebral hemisphere which is not dominant (i.e., in the left hemisphere in a right-handed person). It controls the complex coordinated movements of many respiratory, laryngeal, lingual, pharyngeal and labial muscles involved in verbal expression.
   B. The sensory areas of speech are considered to be largely in the occipital and temporal lobes.
4. Speech is learned.
   A. A child hears sound and copies them. He connects these sounds with objects in the external world and stores them as memories. Auditory speech is eventually associated with visual symbols of speech (the written word). Then, by association of both auditory and visual experiences he learns to write.

221

B. Understanding the spoken word starts early in life, generally in a few months.
C. The formulation of intelligible words by a child usually begins at the ages of 9 to 18 months.
D. Writing and understanding the written word can be learned generally after the fourth or fifth year, sometimes earlier.

PATHOLOGY

1. Signs and symptoms of problems related to speech may include:
   A. Inability to use voice.
   B. Hoarseness.
   C. Production of unclear, slurred, garbled words or meaningless noises.
   D. Inappropriate or unusual kinds of speech.
   E. Confused speech.
   F. Inability to express self in written and/or spoken word (motor aphasia).
   G. Inability to understand the written and/or spoken word (sensory aphasia).
2. The larynx may be injured by trauma, inflammatory processes (e.g., infections, hypersensitivity reactions, overuse of vocal cords) and tumors.
3. The muscles involved with verbal expression may be paralyzed, due to some kind of injury to the motor speech area or to the motor nerves (e.g., trauma, infections, bleeding, increased pressure).
4. Deafness prevents the learning of speech through normal means.
5. See Chap. 17, Pathology, 2 for possible causes of injury to the nerve cells, projection fibers, association fibers of the cerebral cortex.

NURSING APPLICATIONS

1. Patients should be observed for signs and symptoms of problems related to verbal communications; these should be investigated, evaluated, reported and/or treated with appropriate nursing measures. This is of particular importance when the patient:
   A. Is at extremes of age (and there is a possibility of deafness).
   B. Has possible or known brain damage.
   C. Has a condition that affects the anatomical structures concerned with the production of sound and the formation of words.
2. When a patient is hoarse:
   A. He should be discouraged from using his voice.
   B. Steam inhalations may be helpful.
   C. He should be encouraged to seek medical supervision promptly when hoarseness persists.

3. When a patient is unable to use speech effectively for communication (e.g., following a tracheotomy, with deafness, brain damage):
   A. It is necessary to use writing or to develop another means of communication.
   B. He should be encouraged in seeking and using specialized training for learning speech or another form of communication (e.g., learning to speak with air in esophagus, learning hand language).
   C. Emotional support should be consistent.
   D. He should be observed closely for indications of his needs, which may be communicated in other ways.

19

Reproduction

Human sexuality provides for reproduction of the human species.

ANATOMY AND PHYSIOLOGY

Female

1. The female organs of reproduction include:
   A. The external genitalia (the structures of the vulva), which include:
      (1) Mons pubis.
      (2) Labia majora and labia minora.
      (3) The clitoris.
      (4) The vestibule, which has four openings.
          (a) The urinary meatus.
          (b) The vaginal orifice.
          (c) Ducts of the Bartholin glands, located on either side of the vagina; they produce a mucoid secretion during sexual excitement.
          (d) Ducts of Skene's glands, which lie on either side of the urethra.
   B. The internal organs.
      (1) The ovaries are two nodular bodies located on either side of the uterus and attached to the back of the broad ligament of the uterus.
          (a) At birth each ovary contains thousands of germ cells (the primordial ova).
          (b) The ovaries function in the development and expulsion of the ova and in the secretion of estrogen and progesterone.
      (2) The two uterine tubes (fallopian tubes) extend from either side of the uterus outward toward each ovary.
          (a) The tubes are composed of smooth muscle; they are lined with mucous membrane that is continuous with that in the uterus, and are covered with peritoneum.

224

(b) The outer ends of the uterine tubes are fimbriated and open to the abdominal cavity. One fimbria of each tube is attached to the ovary on that side.

(c) The uterine tubes provide a means for the ova to reach the uterine cavity, and a means for the spermatozoa to reach an ova. Fertilization generally occurs in a tube.

(3) The uterus is a hollow and thick-walled muscular organ which lies (in the non-pregnant state) between the bladder and the rectum.

(a) The smooth muscle fibers of the uterine wall are arranged in all directions, allowing the uterus to expand and to compress downwards (during contractions) in all directions. During pregnancy there is considerable hypertrophy of the muscle fibers.

(b) Blood vessels, nerves and lymphatics lie between the muscle layers.

(c) There is a large blood supply to the uterus, and this supply increases during pregnancy.

(d) Sympathetic nerves cause muscle contractions and vaso-constriction; parasympathetic nerves inhibit contractions and allow vasodilation.

(e) Mild contractions of the uterus occur fairly frequently and without sensation, but strong contractions cause cramping discomfort, which can become severe. Dilation of the cervical canal causes contractions felt as cramping discomfort.

(f) The cervix is the lower constricted cylindrical portion of the uterus which projects into the vagina. It becomes effaced and dilates during labor.

(g) The uterus is lined with mucous membrane, which is called endometrium.

(h) The cervical mucosa contains glands which secrete a clear viscid mucus.

(i) The uterus is suspended and freely movable. It is supported by three sets of ligaments (broad, round and uterosacral) and the pelvic floor. The lower anterior wall of the uterus is connected to the bladder by a layer of connective tissue.

(j) The position of the uterus is normally slightly anti-flexed, but its position is influenced by the position of the individual, the size of the bladder and the rectum.

(4) Through hormonal effects, the endometrium of the uterus is periodically prepared for the implantation of a fertilized ovum. When a fertilized ovum implants in the endometrium, the uterus normally retains it, provides for its nourishment,

enlarges as the products of conception grow, and expels the baby and placenta at term.

(5) The vagina is a dilatable muscular tube (about 3 to 5 in. long in the adult), which extends from the vestibule to the uterus.

   (a) The vaginal walls are arranged in thick folds and are lined with mucous membrane.

   (b) The vagina ends in a blind vault into which the cervix projects. The recesses around the cervix are called fornices.

   (c) The vagina is kept slightly moist by secretions from the cervical glands.

   (d) The hymen is a thin fold of mucous membrane which lies across the vaginal orifice. It is sometimes imperforate, sometimes partly torn, and sometimes absent.

2. The secondary sex characteristics appear at puberty. These include:
   A. Development of the female body form with enlargement of breasts.
   B. Growth of axillary and pubic hair.
   C. Ovulation and menstruation.
   D. Emotional changes related to sexual awareness, sexual drive.

3. At puberty, gonadotropins produced in the anterior pituitary gland exert effects upon the ovaries, which brings about sexual maturity.
   A. The follicle-stimulating hormone (FSH) causes the periodic development of the graafian follicles (and ova), and the production of estrogen by the follicles.
   B. The interstitial cell-stimulating hormone (luteinizing hormone or ICSH) is responsible for the development of the corpus luteum in the ruptured follicle and the subsequent production of progesterone.
   C. The leuteotrophic hormone (prolactin) initiates and maintains the production of progesterone by the corpus luteum. It is responsible for lactation following delivery of a baby.

4. Ovulation involves the periodic development of a graafian follicle and the ovum it contains, and the release of that ovum into the fimbriated end of the uterine tube. Following ovulation, a yellow body (the corpus luteum) developes in the ruptured follicle.

5. Estrogen is the primary female sex hormone, it is responsible for the development and maintenance of female sexuality. It causes the periodic development of the endometrium in preparation for the implantation of a fertilized ovum.

6. Progesterone, produced by the corpus luteum, increases the growth of the endometrium and glandular activity (the secretion of mucin, which is high in glycogen content).

7. If the mature ovum is not fertilized within about 36 hours of its release from the ovary, the production of estrogen and progesterone

gradually decreases, and this hormonal change brings about the breakdown of the proliferated endometrium. The blood, mucus and epithelial cells from the endometrium escape from the uterine cavity through the vagina (menstruation).

8. The periodic preparation of the uterus for implantation of a fertilized ovum is called the menstrual cycle.
   A. The menstrual cycles begin at puberty (normally between the ages of 10 and 16 years, with the average being 12 years). Climate, race and general physical health may affect the onset of menstruation.
   B. Menstrual cycles continue from puberty until menopause (except during pregnancy).
   C. The menstrual cycle averages 28 days, but it may vary with different individuals and, to some extent, from month to month. Ovulation generally occurs about midway through the cycle, but may, in some individuals, occur at other times during the cycle.
   D. The onset of menstruation indicates the end of a menstrual cycle.
      (1) The amount of flow differs between individuals, sometimes from month to month, and usually decreases in amount as menopause approaches.
      (2) The average menstrual flow may vary normally from about 2 oz. to 8 oz. and last from 4 to 6 days.
      (3) A few days prior to menstruation and at the onset of menstruation, there may be some pelvic discomfort (feeling of pressure, fullness, a mild backache). There may be varying degrees of breast tenderness, and varying degrees of emotional instability (e.g., a mild depression). There may be a slight degree of water retention, which can be noted in some ankle edema and feeling of abdominal fullness; there may be some tendency toward constipation.
   E. The menstrual cycles may be temporarily interrupted (or delayed) by such factors as changes in environment (e.g., moving to an area in a different climate), marked changes in daily activities (e.g., a new job) and strong emotional upsets.

9. Normally, there may be a slight amount of mucoid vaginal discharge. This discharge may increase in amount (or appear) just before menarche and just before a menstrual period begins. Occasionally, in some individuals there may be a very slight brownish discharge at the time of ovulation.

10. Menopause indicates the cessation of ovarian activity and the end of the female reproductive period.
    A. Menopause may occur as early as age 40 or as late as the middle 50's. The average age is 45 years.
    B. Menstrual periods become scanty, then miss, and then cease altogether.

C. Hormonal changes are probably responsible for some of the vasomotor symptoms (e.g., hot flashes), which may be associated with menopause.

D. Following menopause there are gradual atrophic changes in the reproductive organs, including their lining (e.g., the vaginal mucosa).

E. Menopause is often accompanied by psychic changes, associated with a woman's personal reactions to the aging process and the cessation of her reproductive capacity.

Male

1. The male reproductive organs include: the gonads, which form the sex cells; a series of tubes, which carry the sex cells to the exterior; and accessory structures, which produce secretions in which the sex cells are transported and can survive outside the body.

2. The testes are two glandular structures which form the male sex cells (spermatozoa) and secrete the male sex hormone, testosterone.

   A. The testes are in the abdominal cavity in early fetal life, but normally they descend along the inguinal canal into the scrotum before birth.

   (1) The testes are suspended in the scrotum by the two spermatic cords. These cords extend from the abdominal inguinal ring to the back part of each testis. The cords are composed of arteries, veins, lymphatics, nerves and the excretory ducts of the testes (the ductus deferens).

   (2) Mammalian spermatozoa cannot adjust to the high environmental temperature inside the body.

   (3) Each testis consists of many lobules. Each lobule consists of minute convoluted tubules (the seminiferous tubules).

   (a) Specialized cells within the seminiferous tubules are transformed into spermatozoa (the male sex cells).

   (b) The tubules are supported by loose connective tissue, which contains groups of "interstitial cells."

   (4) The tunica vaginalis is the serous covering of the testes. It is derived from the peritoneum when the testes descend from the abdominal cavity.

   (5) The cremaster is a thin layer of muscle located in the inguinal canal, and extends in loops around the spermatic cord as far as the testes. When the cremaster muscles contract, the testes are drawn upward toward the subcutaneous inguinal ring.

3. The seminiferous tubules merge into progressively larger convoluted ducts that become one long tortuous channel—the epididymis—which lies on the side of the testis.

4. The vas (or ductus) deferens is a continuation of the canal of the epididymis. It passes in the spermatic cord up through the inguinal canal and the abdominal inguinal ring, and then it enters the pelvic

cavity, where it crosses in front of the ureter, and then downward toward the seminal vesicles.

5. The seminal vesicles are two membranous pouches located between the fundus of the bladder and the rectum. They secrete a fluid which is added to the spermatozoa. The lower part of each seminal vesicle joins each ductus deferens to form the two ejaculatory ducts.

6. The ejaculatory ducts run downward between the lobes of the prostate gland and open into the prostatic portion of the urethra. The urethra then continues to the outside (acting as a passageway for both semen and urine).

7. The prostate gland consists of glandular and smooth muscle tissue. The glandular tissue produces a secretion which is part of the semen. The gland is located just below the bladder (around the urethra) and in front of the rectum.

8. The bulbourethral glands (Cowper's glands) are tiny bodies located behind the membranous portion of the urethra. Their excretory ducts open into the cavernous urethra. They secrete a viscid fluid which becomes part of the semen.

9. The penis contains the greatest part of the urethra. It is composed of three cylindrical sections of cavernous tissue (tissue that contains spaces) bound together by fibrous tissue and a strong outer capsule.
   A. The medial cavernous body (the corpus cavernosum urethrae) contains the urethra.
   B. The penis is covered with skin; at the end of the penis the skin leaves the surface and becomes folded on itself to form the prepuce (or foreskin).
   C. The covering of the glans penis is continuous with the urethral mucous membrane and the internal layer of the prepuce.
   D. The glans penis is the anterior end of the corpus cavernosum urethrae, expanded into a cone shape.
   E. Under cerebral or spinal stimuli, the arterial blood supply to the blood sinuses of the cavernous tissue is increased. The increased blood causes compression of the veins, preventing venous return. The engorgement of the cavernous tissues with blood is responsible for the erection of the penis.

10. The erect penis and the contractions of smooth muscle along the male reproductive tract provide for the introduction of semen into the female reproductive tract.

11. Semen is composed of spermatozoa and fluid produced in the seminal vesicles, the prostate gland and the Cowper's glands.

12. At puberty (approximately 12 years of age), hormones bring about the secondary sex characteristics. These include:
    A. The male body form.
    B. Growth of facial and body hair.
    C. Voice change.
    D. Sexual maturity.

13. The anterior lobe of the pituitary gland produces:
   A. Follicle-stimulating hormone (FSH), which stimulates the formation of spermatozoa in the seminiferous tubules.
   B. Interstitial cell stimulating hormone (ICSH), which stimulates the interstitial cells in the testes to secrete testosterone, the male sex hormone.
14. The adrenal cortex secretes androgens that contribute to male sex characteristics.

PATHOLOGY

Female

1. Signs and symptoms of problems related to the female reproductive organs or reproductive functions may include:
   A. Absence of secondary sex characteristics.
   B. Menstrual abnormalities.
      (1) Amenorrhea (except as related to pregnancy).
      (2) Prolonged or marked dysmenorrhea.
      (3) Menorrhagia (prolonged, profuse menstruation).
   C. Gross vaginal bleeding, clots, pieces of tissue.
   D. Abnormal vaginal discharge (e.g., purulent, bloody, profuse leukorrhea, watery discharge, irritating discharge).
   E. Abdominal or pelvic pain, tenderness.
   F. Cramping sensation in pelvis, dragging sensation in pelvis.
   G. Inflammatory changes in external genitalia, vagina.
   H. Lesions of external genitalia.
   I. Urine or feces draining from vagina.
   J. Changes in contour of abdominal wall (not associated with pregnancy).
   K. Scanty lochia following childbirth.
   L. Masculinization.
   M. Infertility, habitual abortions.
   N. Painful or difficult coitus.
   O. Signs and symptoms of ectopic pregnancy, which may include:
      (1) Amenorrhea (generally no more than two months).
      (2) Sudden sharp pain in lower abdomen.
      (3) Shock. (See Chap. 1.)
   P. Signs and symptoms of menstrual problems, which may include:
      (1) Nausea and vomiting at oneset of menstruation.
      (2) Severe cramping, which may precede onset of menses and extend through first day or so of menstrual period (or may just be associated with the beginning of the period).
      (3) Marked dependent edema or abdominal "bloating" prior to menstruation.

(4) Marked psychic or emotional upsets prior to or during menstruation (e.g., depression).

(5) Abdominal pain at time of menstruation.

Q. Signs and symptoms of abortion (miscarriage or premature labor), which may include:

(1) Vaginal bleeding.

(2) Uterine cramping.

(3) Loss of products of conception.

R. Signs and symptoms of menopausal problems, which may include:

(1) Frequent or extensive vasomotor disturbances (e.g., hot flashes).

(2) Marked psychic or emotional disturbances (e.g., anxiety or depression).

2. The normal development of secondary sex characteristics in the female may be delayed or prevented by such factors as:

A. Hypothyroidism. (See Chap. 8.)

B. Decreased production of gonadotropins. (See Chap. 8.)

C. Severe malnutrition.

D. Debilitating illnesses.

E. Excessive fatigue.

F. Excessive production of androgens in adrenal cortex (e.g., with congenital adrenal hyperplasia).

G. Congenital abnormalities (e.g., absence of ovaries, uterus).

H. Ovarian problems (in which production of estrogen is decreased).

3. Dysmenorrhea may be associated with:

A. Intrapelvic pressure due to constipation, congestion of blood in the pelvic vessels, tumor growths.

B. Hormonal problems (gonadotropins, ovarian hormones).

C. Hypersensitivity of uterus to painful stimuli.

D. Psychic or emotional problems related to sexuality or menstruation.

E. Strictures of cervical canal.

4. Amenorrhea, other than that associated with pregnancy, may be associated with:

A. Those factors listed in No. 2.

B. Imperforate hymen.

C. Strong emotional upsets.

5. Infertility of the female may be caused by such factors as:

A. Mucosal secretions of the wrong pH.

B. Displaced uterus.

C. Abnormalities in the reproductive organs (congenital or acquired).

D. Ovarian problems (in production of ova or hormones).

6. Uterine displacement (antiflexion, retroversion, prolapse) may be caused by such factors as:

     A. Congenitally weak ligaments, strain of pregnancy on ligaments.
     B. Adhesions following surgery, infections.
     C. Injury of muscles of pelvic floor (e.g., with childbirth).
     D. Tumor growth.

7. Menorrhagia may be associated with:
     A. A bleeding tendency. (See Chap. 1.)
     B. Endocrine disturbances (gonadotropins, ovarian hormones).
     C. Tumors of the reproductive tract.
     D. Pelvic inflammatory disease.

8. Metrorrhagia may be associated with:
     A. A bleeding tendency. (See Chap. 1.)
     B. Uterine tumors.
     C. Pelvic inflammatory disease.

9. Vaginitis may be caused by many types of microorganisms (bacteria, fungi, protozoa).
     A. Infections are more likely to occur when there is trauma to the tissues, a poor blood supply, atrophic changes in the membrane, or malnutrition.
     B. Infections usually cause local discomfort (e.g., itching, burning) and exudate production. The exudate usually varies with the causative organisms (e.g., purulent, watery, white, yellow, sanguinous) and may be important in diagnosis.
     C. Trichomoniasis is an inflammation of the vagina caused by a protozoa (*Trichomonas vaginalis*); which may invade the cervix. Itching and burning are usually severe.
     D. Moniliasis is caused by a fungus (*Monilia albicans*).

10. Fistulas (resulting from such factors as radiation injury, trauma, infections) may occur between the bladder and vagina, a ureter and the vagina, or the rectum and vagina.

11. Cervical problems may be caused by:
     A. Infections.
     B. Trauma, as with childbirth.
     C. Erosions of unknown cause.
     D. Tumor growths. Malignancies of the cervix usually spread very rapidly throughout the surrounding tissues and the entire pelvis.

12. Problems of the body of the uterus may include:
     A. Infections (e.g., following poor technique in childbirth, retained placenta, poor drainage of lochia following childbirth).
     B. Tumor growths.
         (1) Fibroids are benign fibroid tumors within the uterus. They may be a cause of sterility. They are often a cause of vaginal bleeding.
        (2) Hydatidiform mole is a benign neoplasm in the uterus caused by degeneration of placental growth. There is enlargement of the uterus and uterine bleeding.

(3) Tumors may press on a ureter and be a cause of urinary disturbance. (See Chap. 7.)

13. Ectopic pregnancies occur outside the uterine cavity. They may occur in a fallopian tube, in the uterine horn, in the cervix or in the abdominal cavity. They occur most frequently in a fallopian tube. The tubal wall usually ruptures by the third month. Severe pain and shock result.

14. Problems of the fallopian tubes may be caused by:
    A. Infections.
    B. Strictures, which may be congenital or due to inflammation.

15. Ovarian problems may include:
    A. The formation of cysts, which may become quite large. Sometimes endometrial cysts occur on the ovary. They fill with blood during the menstrual cycle and then rupture into the abdominal cavity.
    B. Tumor growths (malignant or benign). Some benign tumor growths cause changes in sexuality, such as masculinity or increased femininity.
    C. Infection.

16. Endometriosis is a condition in which pieces of endometrial tissue occur in the pelvic cavity. The tissue responds to hormonal changes, causing menstrual bleeding into the pelvic or abdominal cavity each month. This condition causes abdominal or pelvic discomfort, and adhesions of the structures in these cavities usually result.

17. Pelvic inflammatory disease may involve the fallopian tubes, ovaries and other structures of the pelvis (e.g., peritoneum, blood vessels, connective tissue).
    A. The original infection may result from:
       (1) A systemic infection such as tuberculosis.
       (2) Peritonitis (e.g., resulting from a ruptured appendix).
       (3) Microorganisms that gain entrance through the vagina (e.g., gonococcus, streptococcus, staphylococcus.)
    B. The inflammatory process usually localizes in abscesses. Adhesions form.
    C. There may be foul-smelling and possibly purulent vaginal discharge.
    D. There is usually chronic abdominal discomfort, sometimes acute pain and, generally, systemic effects such as malaise, fever, nausea and vomiting.
    E. Pelvic inflammatory disease is a cause of menstrual problems, sterility and ectopic pregnancies.

18. An abortion is the termination of a pregnancy before the fetus has reached the stage of viability.
    A. An abortion is threatened when, in early pregnancy, there is vaginal spotting and possibly some mild uterine cramping.

B. An incomplete or partial abortion is one in which only part of the product of conception is passed. Bleeding (which may be profuse) persists until remaining tissues are lost or surgically removed.

C. A complete abortion is one in which, accompanied by bleeding and usually some cramping, the products of conception are lost. The cramping and bleeding then subside.

D. Abortion may occur because of:
   (1) Some defect in the product of conception.
   (2) A result of severe acute infection or heart disease.
   (3) Abnormalities of the female reproductive tract (e.g., an infantile uterus).
   (4) Severe trauma.

Male

1. Signs and symptoms of problems related to the male reproductive organs or reproductive functions may include:
   A. Urgency, frequency, burning related to urination.
   B. Abnormal discharge from the urethra (e.g., purulent, bloody).
   C. Lesions of the external genitalia or groin.
   D. Enlargement, swelling, tenderness, pain, heat of scrotum or in groin.
   E. Inability to retract or reduce the foreskin.
   F. Absence of testes in the scrotal sac.
   G. Lack of development of the secondary sex characteristics (e.g., small genitalia, sparse pubic and axillary hair, lack of libido).
   H. Feminization (e.g., fatty deposits in mammary and trochanteric regions).
   I. Impotency.
   J. Involuntary childlessness.

2. The development of secondary sex characteristics may be delayed or prevented by:
   A. Decreased production of gonadatropins in pituitary. (See Chap. 8).
   B. Problems of the testes, in which there is a lack of testosterone.
   C. Problems of the adrenal cortex, in which there is a lack of androgens.

3. Sterility of the male may be caused by:
   A. Abnormalities in the reproductive organs (congenital or acquired).
   B. Problems of the testes that affect the production and/or maturation of spermatozoa, or the production of testosterone (e.g., exposure to radiation, alcoholism, cryptorchidism).
   C. Excessive fatigue, debilitating illnesses, malnutrition.

4. Cryptorchidism is a condition in which one or both testes have failed to descend into the scrotum.
   A. This condition is found most frequently when there has been a premature birth.
   B. Failure of descent may occur from:
      (1) Anatomical defects.
      (2) Hormonal deficiency.
   C. The warmth of the abdominal cavity interferes with the development of spermatozoa within the seminiferous tubules. Eventually the testes atrophy.
5. Phimosis is a condition in which the foreskin cannot be retracted behind the glans penis. It may be a congenital problem or acquired because of an inflammatory process (frequently balantitis infection of the glans penis). Paraphimosis is a condition in which the foreskin cannot be reduced after retraction; this can cause stricture of the urethra. It is usually caused by an inflammatory edema resulting from infection or trauma.
6. Problems of the penis may include:
   A. Tumor growths.
   B. Skin problems. (See Chap. 13.)
   C. Trauma.
7. Urethritis, inflammation of the urethra, is generally caused by invasion of the urethra by microorganisms that have gained entrance from the outside. There is usually urgency, frequency and burning related to urination. There is frequently a discharge. Infections can continue along the reproductive tract, thus affecting the glands, the vas deferens, the epididymis and the testes.
8. The prostate gland is a frequent site of tumors, benign or malignant. Prostatic problems usually cause some degree of urinary obstruction. (See Chap. 7.)
9. A variocele involves the enlargement of the veins of the spermatic cord. There is discomfort in the groin.
10. A spermatocele is a cystic tumor of the epididymis and contains sperm.
11. Orchitis is an inflammation of the testes; it may be caused by trauma and by various infections (e.g., tuberculosis, gonorrhea, syphilis, mumps).
12. Mumps, a communicable viral disease which causes inflammation of the salivary glands, frequently causes orchitis.
13. A hydrocele is a collection of serous fluid in the testes.
14. A testis or a spermatic artery may become twisted by sudden contraction of the cremaster muscle. This causes sudden pain, tenderness and swelling. When an artery is involved, the circulation is impaired, which can result in tissue damage.

Venereal Diseases

Venereal diseases are those infections usually spread by sexual activities (e.g., kissing and sexual intercourse). These include syphilis, gonorrhea, chancroid, lymphogranuloma venereum and granuloma inguinale.

1. Syphilis is a constitutional disease caused by a spirochete. The causative organism enters the body at the contact site, usually the genitalia, sometimes the lips. The primary local lesion is the chancre. (See Chap. 13.) The infection then becomes general. In the secondary stage, there is generally a mild rash, which may be erythematous, papular or even ulcerative. There may be alopecia and patches of erosive lesions in the mouth or around the genitalia. In the third stage, which has periods of latency and relapses, the spirochetes may invade practically every part of the body. This includes bones, skin, heart, blood vessels, eyes, ears and central nervous system.

2. Gonorrhea in adults is an acute infection of the urogenital system. It is caused by a bacteria, the gonococcus. The organisms nearly always gain entrance into the body through the genital tract. The infection is characterized by an acute inflammation of the vagina in the female and the urethra in the male. There is profuse purulent exudate. Unless promptly and adequately treated the infection spreads throughout the entire reproductive tract.

3. Chancroid is a local genital sore caused by a streptobacillus. There may be some involvement of neighboring lymph nodes. There are usually no complications.

4. Lymphogranuloma venereum is an infectious disease of the genitals, characterized by a small sore followed by marked inflammation and ulceration of the inguinal and pelvic lymph nodes. The causative organism is rickettsia-like.

5. Granuloma inguinale is an infection caused by a specific bacillus. There is chronic spreading ulceration of the skin and mucous membranes of the genitalia.

NURSING APPLICATIONS

Female

1. Female patients should be observed for signs and symptoms of problems related to the reproductive organs or reproductive functions; these should be investigated, evaluated, reported and/or treated with appropriate nursing measures. This is of particular importance when the patient:
   A. Is a newborn.
   B. Is at the age of puberty.
   C. Is pregnant (known or suspected).

D. Is about the age of menopause, going through menopause or past menopause.
E. May have been exposed to a venereal disease.
2. A female patient should be encouraged to seek medical attention when:
A. Secondary sex characteristics fail to appear within the expected age limit.
B. Secondary sex characteristics appear precociously.
C. There is a tendency toward masculinization.
D. Marriage is imminent.
E. There are problems related to menstruation (e.g., severe dysmenorrhea, profuse or scanty menstrual flow, marked water retention).
F. There are problems related to achieving satisfactory sexual relations.
G. There is involuntary childlessness.
H. There is suspected pregnancy.
I. There are problems related to menopause.
J. There is any abnormal vaginal discharge.
3. Menstrual periods should be evaluated in relation to:
A. The age of the individual.
B. The average menstrual cycle, and that which is usual for the individual.
C. The average amount of menstrual flow, and that which is usual for the individual.
D. Temporary minor discomforts that are commonly associated with the menstrual period.
E. The possibility of pregnancy.
4. Female patients should be protected from injuries involving the reproductive organs by:
A. Maintaining cleanliness of the external genitalia (e.g., adequate bathing, proper cleansing following defecation).
B. Maintaining cleanliness (and sterility if indicated) when objects are inserted into the vagina (e.g., vaginal tampons, equipment used for douches).
C. Preventing trauma to the vaginal mucosa (e.g., in administration of douches, insertion of tampons).
D. Encouraging annual medical examinations with pelvic examinations (especially important after the age of forty).
E. Encouraging obstetrical check-ups following childbirth.
F. Encouraging and providing as possible appropriate medical care when there is pregnancy, threatened or incomplete abortion, or a possibility (or diagnosis) of venereal disease.
G. Using special precautions when radiation is being employed (e.g., as with certain diagnostic or therapeutic procedures).

H. Discouraging sexual activities that may lead to exposure to venereal disease.
5. Appropriate sex education should be encouraged and provided prior to puberty.
6. When a patient has dysmenorrhea:
   A. Lying in the horizontal position may be helpful.
   B. Vigorous exercise should generally be discouraged.
   C. Warmth applied to the lower abdomen may be helpful.
   D. Pelvic exercises or positions that favor venous return or changes the position of the uterus may be helpful (e.g., the knee-chest position).
   E. Constipation should be prevented as possible. (See Chap. 7.)
7. When a patient has a possible rupture of a fallopian tube due to an ectopic pregnancy:
   A. This is a medical emergency.
   B. Nursing measures for the treatment of shock should be started promptly. (See Chap. 1.)
8. When there is threatened abortion or incomplete abortion:
   A. The patient should be kept quiet in the horizontal position.
   B. The patient should be discouraged from bearing down (increasing intra-abdominal pressure).
   C. Any vaginal discharge or bleeding should be observed closely and reported appropriately. Profuse bleeding represents a medical emergency.
   D. Any tissue should be saved for medical inspection.

Male

1. Male patients should be observed for signs and symptoms of problems related to the reproductive organs or reproductive functions; these should be investigated, evaluated, reported and/or treated with appropriate nursing measures. This is of particular importance when the patient:
   A. Is a newborn or in early years.
   B. Is at the age of puberty.
   C. Is elderly.
   D. May have been exposed to a venereal disease.
2. A male patient should be encouraged to seek medical attention when:
   A. The testes have not descended into the scrotal sac.
   B. Secondary sex characteristics fail to appear within the expected age limit.
   C. Secondary sex characteristics appear precociously.
   D. There is a tendency toward femininity.
   E. He has or has been exposed to mumps.
   F. There is involuntary childlessness.

G. There is impotency.

H. There is any abnormal urethral discharge.

3. Male patients should be protected from injuries involving the reproductive organs by:

A. Maintaining cleanliness of the external genitalia (e.g., adequate cleansing of the glans penis).

B. Avoiding catheterization whenever possible. (See Chap. 7.)

C. Encouraging annual medical check-ups with rectal examinations (especially important after the age of forty).

D. Using special precautions when radiation is being employed (e.g., as with certain diagnostic or therapeutic procedures).

E. Discouraging sexual activities that may lead to exposure to venereal disease.

4. When a patient has a problem that involves the scrotum, the testes or a spermatic cord, the scrotum should be kept well-supported (e.g., with pillows, use of a suspensory).

5. When a patient has a problem involving the foreskin and/or the glans penis (e.g., circumcision), the area should be kept clean, dry and protected from trauma.

20

Microbial Injury

Some disease conditions in man are caused by microorganisms.

MICROBIOLOGY

Microorganisms

1. There are many varieties of microorganisms; most are harmless, but a few are pathogenic.
2. Microorganisms cause all the diseases that can be spread from person to person (i.e., communicable diseases).
3. Infections are caused by disease-producing microorganisms.
    A. True pathogens are virulent organisms that possess invasive ability.
    B. Some microorganisms are not truly pathogenic, but when given the opportunity, they are able to cause disease.
4. The protozoa are microscopic animals; some varieties can cause disease in man.
5. Important microscopic plants that cause disease in man include the yeasts, molds and bacteria.
    A. The basic morphological forms of simple bacteria are cocci, bacilli and spirilli.
    B. The higher bacteria include the moldlike bacteria (e.g., mycobacteria).
    C. Bacteria are capable of an extremely rapid rate of reproduction. Cell division may take place as rapidly as every 20 minutes.
6. Important ultramicroscopic forms of life that cause disease in man include the rickettsia and viruses.
7. Some bacteria give rise to resistant forms known as spores.
8. Some bacterial and protozoan forms possess flagella and can move in fluid, but other microorganisms are not able to move themselves.

Control of Microorganisms

1. Most pathogenic microorganisms are mesophilic.
    A. Microorganisms are not readily killed by low temperatures, but may be prevented from active growth by low temperatures.

Freezing of water does not necessarily destroy the microbial content.

B. Most pathogenic microorganisms can be killed at a temperature above 60° C. (140° F.), but mature spores may survive many hours of boiling temperature.

C. All living organisms can be killed by exposure to moist heat at a temperature of 121° C. (250° F.) for 15 minutes.

2. All microorganisms need moisture for growth. (Drying inhibits microbial growth, but it is an unreliable way of killing microorganisms.)

3. All pathogenic microorganisms require organic food. Cleanliness—freedom from dirt and organic materials such as body discharges and foods—discourages the growth of microorganisms.

4. Direct ultraviolet rays will kill many types of pathogenic microorganisms if there is ample exposure.

5. Chemicals that interfere with the life processes of microorganisms kill them or inhibit their growth and reproduction.

6. Sterilization is a process through which all microorganisms are destroyed. Sterilization may be accomplished by incineration, autoclaving, prolonged boiling and dry heat.

7. Disinfection is a process in which the most susceptible pathogenic, nonsporing forms of microorganisms are destroyed.

A. Disinfection may be accomplished by boiling or chemicals.

B. Raw milk can be disinfected by pasteurization.

C. Water can be disinfected by proper chlorination.

8. Bacteriostasis is a process in which the growth and reproduction of microorganisms are prevented. Bacteriostasis may be accomplished by cold, drying and chemicals.

9. The effectiveness of various methods of disinfection and sterilization depends upon:

A. The concentration of the chemical or the intensity of the physical agent used.

B. The time allowed for the process.

C. The nature of the material being treated. (The presence of organic material on objects interferes with disinfection and sterilization.)

D. The type of organisms to be destroyed.

E. The numbers of microorganisms present.

Sources of Disease-Producing Microorganisms

1. The major source of infection for communicable diseases is some person or animal who is discharging living pathogenic organisms. Carriers are persons who do not actually have clinical manifestations of an infection, but may be sources of pathogenic organisms.

2. Some bacteria normally present on or in the body may become opportunists and cause an infection.
   A. Microorganisms are always present on the outer surfaces of the body, and in cavities and tubes that have direct connection with outside of the body.
      (1) Persistently present on the skin are streptococci, staphylococci and some diphtheroids.
      (2) The mouth and throat receive many types of microorganisms (e.g., lactobacilli).
      (3) The nasal passages are constantly contaminated by inhaled air, but do not normally favor the growth of any organisms.
      (4) The external genitalia have normal flora, and usually (especially in the female) some fecal organisms.
      (5) The vagina normally has many organisms present, including lactobacilli.
   B. Microorganisms do not regularly colonize in the stomach, bladder, uterus, trachea or lungs, so these organs are free from bacterial growth.
   C. The lower small intestines and large intestines have a luxuriant growth of a number of species, including the *Escherichia coli*, Clostridia species, *Streptococcus fecalis* and many anaerobic non-spore-forming bacilli (e.g., Bacteroides species). Fecal material is composed largely of dead and living microorganisms.
   D. The remaining tissues of the body, including the blood, are normally free from microorganisms.
   E. When normal flora are destroyed, pathogenic organisms may be able to grow and reproduce to a greater extent than usual.

Transfer of Microorganisms

1. Organisms may be transferred from the source to a new host directly by:
   A. Contact with an infected part of the body or discharges which are infected.
   B. Contaminated objects (fomites).
2. Organisms may be transferred from the source to a new host indirectly by:
   A. Air (particles of dust, droplets of moisture, droplet nuclei).
      (1) Coughing, sneezing, violent talking or laughing cause the expulsion of droplets of respiratory secretions into the air.
      (2) Effective air change by good ventilation decreases the number of droplet nuclei.
   B. Sewage.
   C. Milk (provides an excellent medium for microbial growth).
   D. Food.
   E. Water.

F. Vectors (including ticks, mites, lice, fleas, mosquitoes and flies).
3. Each communicable disease is transferred in one or more rather definite ways, determined by:
   A. The way in which the pathogen leaves the source.
   B. The portal of entry of each type of pathogen.
   C. The ability of the pathogen to survive outside the host.

Some Specific Pathogenic Bacteria

1. *Salmonella typhosa* causes typhoid fever.
   A. The organisms may be found in urine, feces and blood. Organisms may be found in the gallbladder, leaving the body through the feces, months and years after the acute disease is over.
   B. The organisms may be transferred directly by fecal material, urine or blood, and indirectly by contaminated food and water. Flies may be responsible for indirect transmission.
   C. The portal of entry is the mouth.
   D. The organisms can live in ice for as long as 3 months and in moist feces as long as 2 months.
2. Other species of Salmonella cause salmonellosis (including paratyphoid fever and food poisoning).
   A. The organisms may be found in feces and vomitus of infected human beings or animals.
   B. The organisms may be transferred directly by fecal material or vomitus, and indirectly by contaminated food and water. Flies may be responsible for indirect transmission.
   C. The portal of entry is the mouth.
   D. The organisms can live outside of the host for weeks and possibly months.
3. Species of the genus Shigella cause bacillary dysentery.
   A. The organisms may be found in feces and vomitus.
   B. The organisms may be transferred directly by fecal material or vomitus, and indirectly by contaminated food and water. Flies are frequently responsible for indirect transmission.
   C. The portal of entry is the mouth.
   D. The organisms can live outside of the host for weeks and possibly months.
4. The *Vibrio comma* causes cholera.
   A. The organisms may be found in feces and vomitus.
   B. The organisms may be transferred directly by fecal material or vomitus, and indirectly by contaminated food and water.
   C. The portal of entry is the mouth.
5. Species of the genus Brucella cause brucellosis (undulant fever).
   A. The organisms may be found in cattle, goats and pigs.
   B. The organisms may be transferred directly by contact or indirectly by food products from the infected animals.

    C. The portals of entry are the mouth and the skin.

    D. The organisms can exist outside the host in milk and milk products or on the skins of animals. Pasteurization of milk and milk products is an important control measure.

6. *Pasteurella tularensis* causes tularemia.

    A. The organisms may be found in rabbits and other wild rodents and game birds In infected human beings the organisms are found in infected lymph glands.

    B. The organisms may be transferred directly by contact with the skins of infected animals, or indirectly by the bites of infected ticks, deer flies and other insects, and by infected meat.

    C. The portals of entry are the mouth and the skin.

    D. The organisms can survive for some time in water and in dead bodies.

7. *Pasteurella pestis* causes plague.

    A. The organisms may be found in rats and, in pneumonic plague, in the respiratory tracts, urine and feces of infected persons.

    B. The organisms may be transferred directly by respiratory discharges (in pneumonic plague) and contact with infected animals, and indirectly by rat fleas which are vectors.

    C. The portals of entry may be the respiratory tract, the mouth and the skin.

8. *Hemophillus pertussis* causes pertussis (whooping cough).

    A. The organisms are found in the upper respiratory tract and occasionally in the epithelium of the eye.

    B. The organisms may be transferred directly by respiratory discharges, and indirectly by air contaminated with droplets of respiratory discharges.

    C. The portal of entry is the respiratory tract (nose and throat).

    D. The organisms are not very resistant outside the host.

9. *Corynebacterium diphtheriae* causes diphtheria.

    A. The organisms may be found in the upper respiratory tract and the skin.

    B. The organisms may be transferred directly by respiratory discharges or from the skin, and indirectly by air or milk contaminated by the microorganisms.

    C. The portal of entry is the respiratory tract (nose and throat) and, occasionally, the skin.

    D. The organisms are strictly parasitic and are easily killed by heat and various chemicals.

10. *Neisseria meningitides* causes epidemic meningitis.

    A. The organisms are found in the nasopharynx, the blood, spinal fluid and skin petechiae.

    B. The organisms may be transferred directly by respiratory dis-

charges, blood or spinal fluid, and indirectly by air contaminated with droplets of respiratory discharges.
C. The portal of entry is the respiratory tract (nose and throat).
D. The organisms are fragile and can live only briefly outside of the host.

11. *Neisseria gonorrheae* causes gonorrhea.
A. The organisms may be found in the genitourinary tract, pelvic cavity, eye, heart or joints.
B. The organisms may be transferred directly by contact with infected areas or by discharges from the genitourinary tract, pelvic cavity or conjunctiva.
C. The portals of entry are the mucous membrane of the genitourinary tract and the conjunctiva.
D. The organisms are fragile and die quickly when exposed to the air or dried.

12. *Diplococcus pneumoniae* frequently causes pneumonia.
A. The organisms may be found in the respiratory tract.
B. The organisms may be transferred directly by respiratory discharges, and indirectly by air contaminated with droplets of respiratory discharges.
C. The portal of entry is the respiratory tract (nose and throat).
D. The organisms are strictly parasitic and easily killed by heat and various chemicals.

13. Species of Streptococci cause scarlet fever, septic sore throat, upper respiratory infections, erysipelas and puerperal fever. They may act as opportunists, causing wound infections and infections of many body tissues (e.g., ear, lungs or kidneys).
A. The organisms may be found:
   (1) In the respiratory tract during scarlet fever, septic sore throat, and various respiratory infections.
   (2) In the skin in erysipelas.
   (3) In the uterus in puerperal fever.
   (4) In the bloodstream if the organisms invade blood vessels.
   (5) In the drainage from infected wounds or infected body tissues.
B. The organisms may be transferred directly by discharges from infected parts of the body, or indirectly by air, milk, milk products and food that have been contaminated with discharges.
C. The portals of entry may be the respiratory tract (nose and throat), the skin or the mucous membrane of the reproductive tract in women.
D. Streptococci are fairly resistant to drying and can live in milk and food for some time.
E. Streptococci are pyogenic organisms.
F. Some streptococci are usually present in the upper respiratory tract.

G. Cows may be infected with streptococci (e.g., in the udders).

H. Rheumatic fever appears to involve allergic response to strepto-cocci that cause continued or repeated throat infections.

14. *Staphylococcus aureus* (*Micrococcus pyogenes* var. *aureus*) can cause many types of infection (e.g., wound infections, skin infections or respiratory infections).

A. The organisms may be found on the skin and mucous membranes or wherever the infection exists.

B. The organisms may be transferred directly by contact or through discharges from infected parts of the body.

C. The portals of entry may be the skin and mucous membranes, especially of the respiratory tract.

D. The staphylococci are hardy microorganisms. Many staphylococci become resistant to antibiotics.

E. The organisms are pyogenic.

F. Virulent strains of staphylococci produce an exotoxin that can cause severe enteritis if ingested in sufficient quantity. The production of exotoxin may occur in poorly refrigerated foods (e.g., chopped meats or cream foods) that have been contaminated with the organisms.

15. The toxin formed by *Clostridium botulinum* causes botulism.

A. The organisms are saprophytes found in the soil.

B. The toxin is ingested with canned fruits and vegetables (the organisms grow best in a weakly acid to basic pH environment).

C. The organisms are anaerobic, gas-producing spore-formers.

16. The toxin produced by *Clostridium tetani* causes tetanus.

A. The organisms are found normally in human and animal feces and in the soil, as well as in the infected wounds when the individiual has tetanus.

B. The organisms may be transferred by contaminated soil.

C. The portal of entrance is a wound in the skin (especially puncture wounds).

D. The organisms are anaerobic spore-formers.

17. Several species of Clostridium (including *Clostridium perfringens*) cause gas gangrene.

A. The organisms are normally found in human and animal feces and in the soil, as well as in infected wounds when the individual has gas gangrene.

B. The organisms may be transferred by contaminated soil.

C. The portal of entry is a wound in the skin (especially deep or lacerated wounds).

D. The organisms are anaerobic spore-formers.

18. *Mycobacterium tuberculosis* causes tuberculosis.

A. The organisms are obligate parasites and may be found:

(1) In man: in the respiratory tract (sometimes in the stomach

if swallowed), or in body tissues that have been invaded by the organisms (e.g., meninges, lymph nodes, joints or skin).

(2) In the cow: in the respiratory tract, the intestinal tract and in the udder.

B. The portals of entry may be the respiratory tract or the gastro-intestinal tract.

C. The organisms are capable of long survival inside or outside the host, particularly in sputum or pus. The organisms can remain encapsulated in the host (e.g., lungs or lymph glands) for many years.

19. *Mycobacterium leprae* causes leprosy.

A. The organisms grow within the cells of human living tissues.

B. Open nodules are believed to be a source of infection. Organisms may also be found in the respiratory tract.

C. The portal of entrance into the body is usually the respiratory tract, but the organisms may enter the body through the skin and mucous membrane.

D. Leprosy is not readily transmitted.

20. *Treponema pallidum* causes syphilis.

A. The organisms are obligate parasites and may be found:

(1) In the first stage of the disease, in the chancre.

(2) In the second stage of the disease, in lesions of the skin and mucous membranes.

(3) In the third stage of the disease, in various internal tissues.

B. The organisms may be transferred directly by contact (e.g., sexual intercourse, kissing); they may be transferred by an infected mother to an unborn child through the placenta.

C. The portals of entry may be the skin and mucous membranes.

D. The organisms are fragile and can live only very briefly outside the host.

21. Species of Borrelia and Fusobacterium cause Vincent's stomatitis, Vincent's gingivitis and Vincent's angina.

A. These organisms are normally found in the mouths of human beings and may be considered to be secondary invaders when resistance is low.

B. These organisms are not readily transferred from one person to another.

Some Pathogenic Rickettsia

1. Rickettsia are obligate intracellular parasites; they are natural parasites of arthropods such as fleas, lice, ticks, and mites.

2. Rickettsia are usually found in the alimentary canals of these arthropods. Rickettsia are generally introduced into the human host by injection into the skin (insect bites), or by rubbing or scratching the skin contaminated with fecal material from the infected arthropod.

3. The animal reservoirs vary.
   A. Epidemic typhus is louse-borne, and the animal reservoirs are human beings.
   B. Rocky Mountain spotted fever is tick-borne, and there are various wild animal reservoirs.
   C. Q fever is tick-borne, and the animal reservoirs are primarily cattle and sheep. In the transfer of these organisms, milk and air contaminated with dust from infected animals play important roles.

Some Pathogenic Viruses

1. Viruses are obligate intracellular parasites that cause specific communicable diseases, but may also cause infections in many tissues of the body following the specific disease process (e.g., encephalitis following mumps).
2. The virus of psittacosis is a natural parasite of many birds.
   A. The viruses can be found in bird droppings and dust containing bits of these droppings.
   B. The portal of entry is the respiratory tract (nose and throat).
3. The viruses of smallpox and chicken pox are found in the respiratory tract, in saliva and in the skin lesions.
   A. The viruses may be transferred directly by contact or by respiratory discharges and saliva.
   B. The portal of entry is usually the respiratory tract, but may be the skin.
4. The virus of herpes simplex is in the tissues of infected persons (the virus generally remains there for life), and may be activated by a lowered resistance in the tissues.
   A. The virus may be transmitted by direct contact.
   B. The portal of entry is the skin or mucous membrane (generally of the face).
5. The virus of measles (Rubeola) is found in the respiratory tract.
   A. The organisms are transmitted directly by respiratory secretions.
   B. The portal of entry is in the respiratory tract (nose and throat).
6. The virus of German measles (Rubella) is found in the respiratory tract.
   A. The organisms are transmitted directly by respiratory secretions.
   B. The portal of entry is the respiratory tract (nose and thoat).
7. The virus of infectious hepatitis is found in feces, blood, and, possibly, in urine and nasopharyngeal secretions.
   A. The viruses may be transmitted directly or indirectly by food and water contaminated by feces and, possibly, urine and nasopharyngeal secretions.
   B. The portals of entry include the gastrointestinal tract and possibly the respiratory tract.

8. The virus of serum hepatitis is found in the blood.
   A. The organisms are transmitted directly by blood.
   B. The portal of entry is usually the skin (through injection).
9. The virus of influenza is found in the respiratory tract.
   A. The organisms are transmitted directly by respiratory secretions, and indirectly by air contaminated with droplets of respiratory secretions.
   B. The portal of entry is the respiratory tract (nose and throat).
10. The virus of the common cold is found in the respiratory tract.
    A. The organisms are usually transmitted directly by respiratory secretions, or indirectly by air contaminated with droplets of respiratory secretions.
    B. The portal of entry is the respiratory tract (nose and throat).
11. The virus of the mumps is found in saliva.
    A. The organisms are usually transmitted directly.
    B. The portal of entry is the mouth.
12. Little is known about the virus that causes infectious mononucleosis, and the modes of transmission are unknown.
13. The virus of rabies is found in the saliva of infected animals (e.g., dogs, foxes, bats, skunks or cattle) and infected human beings.
    A. The organisms are transmitted directly by the saliva.
    B. The portal of entry is the broken skin (i.e., bites from infected animals).
14. The virus of poliomyelitis is found in the nasopharynx (early) and in the feces (from the onset of the disease up to a month or more).
    A. The organisms are usually transmitted directly by infective discharges, but contaminated food may provide an indirect means. Flies may be an important means of transmission.
    B. The portals of entry are the nose and throat.
15. The virus of encephalitis is found in birds and animals.
    A. The organisms are transmitted indirectly by arthropod vectors (e.g., mosquitoes).
    B. There is no evidence of person-to-person transmission.

Some Pathogenic Fungi

1. Fungi can cause disease in persons of normal health, but some of the common skin and mucous membrane fungous infections occur in people when tissues are injured by constant uncleanliness or abnormal moisture.
2. Saprophytic food-spoilage types and plant pathogens are only rarely associated with human disease.
3. The dermatophyte fungi causes dermatomycosis, and may be found in the skin, hair or nails.
   A. The fungi are usually transmitted directly by contact.
   B. Pet animals are sometimes a source of some types of ringworm.

4. *Candida albicans* causes moniliasis.
   A. The organisms are found, normally, in mouths and in the feces.
   B. The organisms tend to develop in tissues injured by malnutrition or irritation, in tissues kept abnormally moist or in tissues whose normal flora have been reduced (e.g., by antibiotics).
5. *Histoplasma capsulatum* cause histoplasmosis.
   A. Suspected animal sources include rodents and pigions.
   B. Spores can be found in water, air and in the soil around farm buildings.
   C. The organisms are not spread from man to man.
6. *Coccidiodes immitis* causes coccidiodomycosis.
   A. Rats, cattle, sheep and dogs may harbor the fungus.
   B. The fungus is present in soil and is spread by dust-borne spores.

Some Pathogenic Protozoa

1. *Endameba histolytica* causes amebiasis.
   A. The source of the organisms is the feces of infected persons.
   B. The cysts may be transmitted directly by feces, and indirectly by food, water, and flies.
   C. The trophozoites encyst in the intestines, and the cysts are passed in formed stool.
   D. The cysts become infective upon ingestion.
   E. Cysts can survive several weeks outside a host, but are fairly susceptible to cold and drying.
2. Species of the genus Plasmodia cause malaria.
   A. The sources of the organisms are the blood of man and the saliva of the infected female Anopheles mosquito.
   B. The organisms are transmitted by bites of the infected female Anopheles mosquito.
   C. Malaria may be transmitted by blood transfusions from infected persons.
3. *Trichomonas vaginalis* causes trichomonas vaginitis.
   A. The sources are the vagina or urethra of women or the urethra of man.
   B. The organisms may be transmitted directly by contact or by fomites.
   C. It is not certain whether this protozoan is a true pathogen or an opportunist.

Some Specific Helminths

1. The male and female pinworms live in the ileum.
   A. The gravid female migrates to the perineum, where she lays her eggs.
   B. If the eggs are ingested, they hatch in the intestines and develop into adult worms.

C. The eggs may be found on contaminated parts of the body, fomites, in dust particles and in the air.

2. The intestinal hookworms live in the small intestine.
   A. Eggs that are laid are passed in the feces.
   B. Larvae hatch from the eggs and grow in the soil.
   C. After approximately 7 days, the larvae are able to penetrate the skin of a new host.
   D. The larvae then pass through the blood to the respiratory tract, where they are swallowed. The adult forms develop in the small intestine.

3. The large intestinal roundworms cause ascariasis.
   A. The adult worms live in the intestinal tract.
   B. The female worm lays eggs, which are passed in the feces.
   C. After about 3 weeks, the eggs, if ingested (e.g., from contaminated food, drink or fingers), reach the intestines where the larvae are liberated.
   D. The larvae penetrate the intestinal mucosa and travel through the lymphatics to the blood vessels, and, by the circulation of the blood, reach the lungs.
   E. After reaching the lungs, the larvae migrate up the respiratory tract, are swallowed, and develop into adult worms in the small intestines.

4. The trichina worm causes trichiniasis.
   A. The adult worms live in the intestinal tract.
   B. The females produce larvae that are capable of encysting in muscle tissue.
   C. Man becomes infested by ingesting the flesh of carnivorous animals that contain encysted larvae (e.g., hogs).
   D. The ingested larvae develop in the intestines, and larvae produced by the female encyst in muscle tissue.

5. The source of tapeworms that infect man is man himself.
   A. The adult tapeworm lives in the small intestine and produces eggs, which are passed through the feces.
   B. If animals ingest these eggs (e.g., steer, hogs or fish), the eggs develop in the small intestines; the developed embryo passes through the blood to muscles where it encysts.
   C. Viable encysted forms, when ingested by man, develop to adult forms in the small intestine.
   D. One type of tapeworm that infests man needs no intermediate host; the eggs are immediately infective for the same or another person.

Immunity

1. Natural immunity seems to be due to the general defense mechanisms of the body.

2. Immunity to each specific disease of microbial origin is due to the presence of specific antibodies.
3. Active immunity may be acquired as a result of the development of specific antibodies from:
   A. The body's response to an actual attack of the disease.
   B. The body's response to the introduction of antigenic biologicals, including:
      (1) Living cultures.
      (2) Killed cultures.
      (3) Derivatives of cultures.
4. There is usually prolonged immunity to the following diseases:
   A. Cholera, plague, diphtheria, scarlet fever, typhoid fever and paratyphoid fever.
   B. Rocky Mountain spotted fever and typhus.
   C. Chickenpox, smallpox, rubeola, rubella, mumps and pertussis.
5. There is little if any immunity developed with the following diseases:
   A. Erysipelas, gonorrhea, syphilis and pneumonia.
   B. Common cold, herpes simplex and influenza.
6. Antigenic biologicals, which are generally available for immunization against specific diseases, include those for the following diseases:
   A. Smallpox. (Many state and local governments require vaccination.)
   B. Pertussis, tetanus, diphtheria, poliomyelitis and measles. Immunization is recommended early in life.
   C. Typhoid, parathyphoid, cholera, epidemic typhus, tuberculosis, Rocky Mountain spotted fever, influenza, some types of streptococcal infection and rabies.
      (1) Immunizations may be recommended (or required) when the possibility of infection is increased by such factors as occupation, environmental conditions and actual exposure.
      (2) BCG vaccine, available as immunization against tuberculosis, is believed to have some usefulness.
7. There are some biological preparations that can be used in the skin to test for immunity or hypersensitivity developed by previous exposure to certain diseases. These tests include:
   A. The Schick test and Maloney test for diphtheria.
   B. The Dick test for scarlet fever.
   C. The tuberculin test for tuberculosis (Mantoux test or Vollmer patch test).
   D. The Histoplasmin test for histoplasmosis.
   E. The Coccidiodin test for coccidioidomycosis.
8. Passive immunity may be acquired temporarily by the introduction of antibodies into the body. Gamma globulin may be injected to provide passive immunity against measles.

PATHOLOGY

1. Signs and symptoms of infections include those associated with inflammation. (See Chap. 14.)
   A. Local signs and symptoms may include:
      (1) Swelling, redness, pain, heat and loss of function. "Pain" may include such discomforts as a sore throat, burning with urination, painful respirations, intestinal cramping, headache.
      (2) Sneezing and coughing.
      (3) Lesions of the skin and mucous membrane (e.g., pustules, carbuncles). (See Chap. 13.)
      (4) Vomiting, diarrhea.
      (5) Inflammatory exudates.
      (6) Local enlargement of lymph nodes.
   B. Systemic signs and symptoms may include:
      (1) Lassitude, malaise, headache.
      (2) Anorexia, nausea and vomiting.
      (3) Lesions of the skin and mucous membrane (e.g., generalized rash). (See Chap. 13.)
      (4) Fever and associated signs and symptoms. (See Chap. 9.)
      (5) General enlargement of lymph nodes.
2. Signs and symptoms of specific infectious diseases vary with the tissues injured by the specific microorganisms (or their toxins), and the body's inflammatory responses to the specific microorganisms (or their toxins). (Because of effects upon particular body structures and functions, some of the specific infectious diseases and nonspecific infections have been included in the preceding chapters.)
3. Prodromal signs and symptoms of many of the communicable diseases include those listed under No. 1, B.

NURSING APPLICATIONS

1. Patients (as well as others) should be protected from infections and infectious diseases.
   A. The immediate environment (e.g., furniture, bedding, clothing, walls, floors, sinks, toilet seats) should be maintained free from dust, dirt, and organic materials such as food or body discharges.
   B. Air currents should be controlled, good ventilation promoted and adequate space provided for the number of persons in a given situation.
   C. Insects such as lice, flies, fleas and mosquitos should be eliminated or controlled adequately (e.g., with use of screens, netting, appropriate insecticides).

D. Provision should be made for the safe care and disposal of all organic wastes (e.g., urine, feces, vomitus, respiratory secretions, drainage from wounds or body cavities).

E. The skin, hair, nails and exposed mucous membranes (e.g., of nose, mouth, external genitalia and anal region) should be kept clean and free from excessive moisture.
   (1) Hands should be kept away from the nose, mouth, external genitalia and the anal region.
   (2) Frequent and effective handwashing should be encouraged and provided for; this is of particular importance:
      (a) Prior to eating.
      (b) Following any activity in which hands have come into contact with the external genitalia, the anal region, body discharges (such as respiratory secretions), or known "dirty" areas, such as floors.

F. Special cleansing techniques (e.g., scrubbing and/or application of a bacteriocidal agent) should be utilized in the preparation of the skin and/or mucous membrane prior to such procedures as surgical incisions, injections or catheterizations.

G. All objects used in or around the mouth should be clean (e.g., drinking glasses, straws, toothbrushes).

H. All equipment used in patient care should be clean (free from dust, dirt and organic material).

I. Equipment used for different patients should be properly disinfected or sterilized before use for each patient. Disposable equipment is desirable whenever possible.

J. Effective methods of disinfection and sterilization should be employed.
   (1) All organic material should be removed from equipment prior to disinfection or sterilization processes.
   (2) If heat (dry or moist) is used for disinfection or sterilization, the equipment must be fully exposed to the required temperature for the required length of time in order to destroy the particular type or form of microorganisms present.
   (3) If chemicals are used for disinfection, the equipment must be fully exposed to the required concentration of drug for the required length of time in order to destroy pathogenic microorganisms.
   (4) If ultraviolet radiation is used for disinfection, the exposure must be direct and for the required length of time in order to destroy pathogenic microorganisms.

K. Only sterile equipment and solutions should be used for patient care that involves parts of the body normally free from microbial growth.

L. Wounds should be protected from microorganisms and microbial growth.

(1) Minor superficial wounds (e.g., abrasions) may be treated using clean technique (if necessary), but wounds, in general, should be treated with strict aseptic technique.

(2) Accidental wounds should be thoroughly cleaned as soon as possible after their occurrence. When wounds are deep and/or difficult to clean thoroughly, medical attention should be obtained promptly (both for effective cleaning and tetanus precautions).

(3) The skin or mucous membrane around open wounds should be kept clean.

(4) Wounds should be protected from possible contaminants, such as hair, lint, dust, respiratory secretions or fecal material.

(5) Dressings (dry) should be reinforced or changed (if allowed by medical orders) when they become moist.

M. Excessive use of soaps for skin cleansing, or use of antiseptic solution for irrigations (e.g., mouthwashes, vaginal douches) should be discouraged.

N. Thorough handwashing or special cleansing of the hands should be done by nursing personnel:

(1) Before giving personal care to a patient.

(2) After giving personal care to a patient.

(3) After contact with infective (or potentially infective) organic material (e.g., respiratory secretions, saliva, feces, urine, blood or exudates).

O. Individuals who have infections that can be transmitted to others should not care for or visit patients.

2. Patients should be observed for signs and symptoms of infections and infectious diseases; these should be investigated, evaluated and reported appropriately.

3. Specific isolation (or precaution) techniques should be carefully followed as ordered (e.g., respiratory, enteric, contact) and/or indicated by a diagnosed disease condition. In some instances, precautionary measures to prevent the possible spread of microorganisms may be indicated by a patient's signs and symptoms prior to medical orders or a definite diagnosis.

A. Isolation requirements should be determined by:

(1) Where the causative microorganisms are in the host and their portal(s) of exit (e.g., lungs and respiratory secretions, intestines and feces, wounds and wound drainage).

(2) How the causative microorganisms can be transmitted from one person to another (e.g., directly and/or indirectly).

(3) How the organisms are able to enter the body (e.g., the respiratory tract, the gastro-intestinal tract, the skin or mucous membrane).

(4) The nature of the microorganisms (e.g., highly resistant or fragile, pathogenic or opportunist).

B. When a patient has a disease condition caused by microorganisms, the following must be considered contaminated and be cared for appropriately:

(1) Anything that has direct (or indirect) contact with the organs or tissues of the body that contain the causative organisms.

(2) Anything that has direct (or indirect) contact with organic substances that come from an infected part (e.g., exudates, feces, urine).

(3) Anything that has direct (or indirect) contact with organic substances associated with the portal(s) of exit for the pathogenic organisms (e.g., respiratory tract, urinary tract, alimentary canal).

C. Fomites should be burned whenever possible, but when contaminated articles must be reused, they should be kept separate, cleaned and properly disinfected (or sterilized, if possible, and always if spore-formers are involved). Fomites should be cared for as soon after use as possible.

D. The furniture and floors in the patient's area should be maintained free from dust, dirt and organic material at all times. Meticulous cleaning with disinfectant solutions should be done when the patient is no longer infective or has left the unit.

E. Infective (or potentially infective) body discharges should be wrapped and burned when possible (e.g., tissues, soiled dressings, uneaten food), or disposed of into the sewer system. In some instances, disinfection of excreta is necessary before its disposal into a sewer system. Body discharges should be properly disposed of as soon as possible.

F. Meticulous cleansing of the hands after patient care is absolutely essential.

G. When a patient has a disease condition caused by microorganisms that can be transferred to others, directly by respiratory secretions or saliva, and indirectly by air (e.g., as with active pulmonary tuberculosis, diphtheria, measles, mumps, pneumonias meningococcic meningitis), everything in the patient's immediate environment, including the air, must be treated as contaminated with microorganisms.

(1) Protective gowns should be used.

(2) Masks should be used. (Masks should be changed frequently, and always when moist.)

(3) A barrier to prevent the free circulation of air outside the unit (e.g., closed door) may be indicated in some airborne diseases.

(4) Adequate air movement within the unit should be promoted (to limit droplet nuclei).

(5) Careful tissue technique should be used for coughing and sneezing. Tissues and other objects that contain or have come in contact with respiratory secretions or saliva should be handled with special precautions.

H. When a patient has a disease condition caused by microorganisms that can be transferred to others, directly by feces and/or urine or vomitus, and indirectly by sewage, food, water or insect vectors (e.g., as with typhoid fever, paratyphoid fever, bacillary dysentery, amebiasis), everything that comes into contact with the patient or with his potentially infective discharges must be treated as contaminated with microorganisms.

(1) Protective gowns should be used when giving personal care.

(2) Gloves may be desirable when giving direct care involving the alimentary canal or the external genitalia.

(3) The patient's hands should be washed thoroughly whenever they have been in contact with the external genitalia or anal region.

(4) A barrier to prevent the circulation of flies (e.g., closed door, screening) may be indicated.

(5) Excreta should be handled with special precautions promptly after elimination.

(6) Utensils used for excreta should be cleaned thoroughly and disinfected (or sterilized if possible).

I. When a patient has a disease condition caused by microorganisms that can be transferred to others by direct contact with the infected area or infectious material from it (e.g., infected wounds, draining abscesses, ringworm, urethral or vaginal discharge of gonorrhea), everything that comes in contact with the infected area or exudate from it must be treated as contaminated with microorganisms.

(1) Protective gowns should be used when giving personal care and doing dressings.

(2) Gloves should be worn for wound care.

(3) Any soiled dressings should be promptly wrapped and burned.

(4) Any contaminated clothing or bedding should be handled with special precautions.

(5) The patient's activities should be controlled to prevent direct contact of infected part or material from it with other persons.

J. When a patient has a disease condition caused by microorganisms that can be transmitted by blood (e.g., serum hepatitis) special care must be taken of any equipment that comes into contact with his blood (e.g., needles, syringes, laboratory test tubes). Disposable equipment is preferable.

4. The spread of helminthic infections may be prevented by:
   A. The sanitary disposal of feces.
   B. Thorough cleansing of the hands after defecation and before eating.
   C. Wearing shoes in areas where hookworm is prevalent.
   D. Thoroughly cooking meat (primarily pork) and fish.

5. All food, water, milk and ice should be clean, prepared in a sanitary manner and properly stored.
   A. Thorough handwashing should precede the preparation or service of food or drink.
   B. No individual with known respiratory or enteric infections should be allowed to handle food, milk or water.
   C. Raw fruits and vegetables should be thoroughly washed before eating.
   D. Unpasteurized milk (or milk products) should not be used.
   E. Milk should be kept properly refrigerated at all times.
   F. Ice and ice equipment should be maintained in a clean condition.
   G. Foods that spoil easily or provide a good culture media (e.g., meats, poultry, creamed foods) should be kept properly refrigerated and should be discarded if not eaten within a few days.
   H. Home-canned foods that have a bad odor or those whose liquid contains bubbles should not be eaten.

6. Immunizations and dignostic tests for communicable diseases should be encouraged.
   A. Immunizations for smallpox, pertussis, tetanus, diphtheria, measles and poliomyelitis should be encouraged for infants and young children.
   B. Immunization for typhoid fever should be obtained whenever there is a possibility of water pollution.
   C. In general, immunizations for the above and other communicable diseases (for which vaccines are available) should be encouraged for all individuals (a few exceptions exist) when there is a likelihood of contacting the diseases.
   D. Children who have been exposed to measles and have not been immunized should obtain medical attention promptly (for passive immunization).
   E. Women should be encouraged to seek medical supervision early in their pregnancies (to provide for serological tests for syphilis).
   F. Skin tests for immunity or to determine exposure to certain communicable diseases should be encouraged whenever these tests are available.

Part III

Social Science and Nursing Applications

INTRODUCTION

Several points need to be emphasized before the reader gives consideration to the material presented in Part III. It cannot be stressed often enough that *this material is not a complete outline of social science principles important to nursing.* Although the revised edition does include much more complete science information, it still does not pretend to include every fact, principle or hypothesis that might be useful to the nurse in perfecting nursing care planning and implementation. For example, in Chapter 9, the "Sociocultural Influences on Behavior," the amount of possible information on relationships between sociocultural influences and behavior is almost limitless. However, the material included in this volume relative to cultural groups and subgroups is intended to be representative of the *types* of information the nurse needs to seek about individual patients, and to remind the nurse of the extent to which both the patient's and the nurse's behavior patterns are influenced by sociocultural factors.

In the revised edition, the author has attempted to keep the expanded material within reasonable bounds by avoiding theories, however currently popular, and by emphasizing concepts and principles demonstrated through organized research studies. Even with this limitation, certain areas have not been thoroughly developed. For example, very little has been included that is particularly aimed at the growing patient population in the older age group.

It is of particular interest to note that Chapter 7 (Primary and Acquired Needs), is the most extensively developed of the ten sections in the revised edition as it was in the original edition. This is due to the exceedingly large number of nurse-patient situations reported in the original study that described patient distress or satisfaction in the area of comfort and security, as associated with need satisfaction. Within this section of the study, the most important single factor was the patient's need to cope successfully with a current siuation—to know what was happening, what was expected of him and what action was required to resolve current problems. Second in importance was the patient's need for a situational definition—the need to know who and where he was, and how he and others fitted into the current environmental picture. These two needs were demonstrated repeatedly in the incidents reported, and the extensive development of substatements represent the wide variety of situations in which these needs were depicted.

The material in Part III is organized in ten major sections, with statements of science making up the major part of each section. At the end of each section, examples or guidelines for the application of science to nursing have been included. The nursing statements are examples intended to demonstrate how social science material can be used by the nurse to make judgments and decisions; they are not a complete reiteration of every statement of science in nursing principle form.

No attempt was made to designate the specific social science discipline or sub-discipline (i.e., psychology, sociology, anthropology) to which the concepts, principles, facts and hypotheses were most closely related. A cursory glance at the material would seem to indicate that the majority of the statements are most likely to be related to psychology. A closer look reveals the interrelatedness of all three major social science areas as they relate to nursing.

In the original study, certain assumptions and beliefs were used as a guide in the analysis of situations and the statement of principles. The major guiding assumptions or beliefs were as follows:

Assumption: That the human being cannot survive as a psychologically healthy social being (even though he may physiologically survive) unless certain required conditions prevail. It is further assumed that these conditions include both internal (psychological) and external (sociocultural) factors which have a reciprocal relationship.

Assumption: That the human organism functions as a total unit, implying that physiological homeostasis is affected by psychosocial factors, and that psychosocial homeostasis is affected by physiological factors.

Assumption: That the person who seeks medical attention and subsequently receives nursing care for a disturbance of physiological function, requires and has a right to expect attention and care in the area of psychosocial function if he is to receive maximum benefit from medical and nursing care.

It was further held that a person who is in the situation described by the above assumptions comes within the province of nursing responsibility. Moreover, the nurse must necessarily have the understanding and the ability to assist the individual patient in achieving psychosocial equilibrium whenever equilibrium is disturbed, or likely to be disturbed, as a result of the situation. Further, it is precisely in the area of care most closely related to the social sciences that the nurse is least likely to be guided by "doctor's orders" and medical or hospital policy. Probably the most uniquely *nursing* aspect of nursing care is the intelligent and creative application of social science principles.

Perhaps some discussion of the terminology used may offset negative mental sets about the particular wording consistently used throughout Part III. The terms "psychosocial equilibrium" and "psychological homeostasis" were used, even though they seemed to be in disfavor in current sociological literature. Equilibrium and homeostasis, when used in the natural sciences, can be defined with far greater scientific accuracy than when applied to social science material. But, relatively speaking, other terms would be equally difficult to define, would meet with equal disfavor from some readers, and would be much less useful. In Part III, the term "homeostasis" refers to the tendency of an organism to seek and maintain relatively stable conditions of existence. In the physical sciences, homeostasis has a restricted meaning, implying the *internal* stability of an organism as maintained by self-regulatory mechanisms. As used in Part III, the term has been expanded to include psychological and social factors that influence human stability, and the individual and collective actions that man may take to establish and maintain relative homeostasis. As for the term "equilibrium," the common dictionary definition was used. This definition implies a state of balance or even adjustment between opposing forces, influences or interests of any kind. As used in Part III, equilibrium and homeostasis are complementary conditions toward which the human being strives in his attempts to exist in relative safety, comfort and satisfaction.

In the original study and the current expansion of science and nursing material, the term "principle" was used, even though its use may be somewhat controversial. In common practice, this term has been used rather loosely to denote any currently believed "fact" or idea, with or without scientific validation. In the science fields, principles have a much more restricted meaning. In the area of social sciences, strictly scientific principles that have been proven by testing are few and far between! In order to avoid as much controversy and negative reaction to perfectly useful material as possible, the terms "facts," "principle" and "hypothesis" have been used to designate the social science material included. The term "hypothesis" refers to any tentative theory or supposition provisionally adopted to explain facts and to guide in the investigation of others, or something assumed or conceded for the purpose of guiding action. The science material in Part III includes statements at concept, principle or fact level, including hypotheses where necessary. At any level, the statements are used in terms of guides to action. Their validity has either been scientifically demonstrated or they represent man's best "educated guess" at this particular stage of human understanding of human behavior.

The balance of Part III contains the complete material resulting from the original study and later abstractions from science literature. It is presented in outline, simple statement form for the sake of clarity and brevity.

1

Perception

Psychological equilibrium (as well as physical survival) requires the ability to perceive and interpret internal and external data.

SOCIAL SCIENCE PRINCIPLES

1. Perception of a given person, object or event is unique to the individual, and depends upon a variety of factors:
   A. Perception is influenced by the nature of the stimuli.
      (1) A given stimulus tends to be more effective in shaping perception if it has one or more of the following qualities:
         (a) Intensity.
         (b) Repetitiveness.
         (c) Isolation from other stimuli.
         (d) Movement and change.
         (e) Novelty.
         (f) Incongruity.
      (2) Perception of a given object or event tends to be of better quality if aspects of the object or event occur or are arranged in meaningful, related groupings, to constitute a whole or pattern.
      (3) Perception is less adequate if various aspects of the object or event are so divided as to demand division of attention among the various aspects.
      (4) Adequacy of perception is decreased or delayed if the stimuli or stimulus pattern is ambiguous.
   B. Perception is influenced by the nature and condition of the individual's perceptual equipment.
      (1) Perception is influenced by the sensitivity of the individual's sensory equipment.
         (a) There is great individual variation (both constitutionally and developmentally determined) in sensory ability, with variation occurring among the several senses (e.g., one person may have particularly astute hearing but be less sensitive to taste or smell).

(b) A person who is hypersensitive in any given sensory area will tend to react to environmental stimuli, regardless of his need to rest or to attend to other stimuli.

(2) Perception is influenced by the individual's constitutional or developmental level ability to utilize congnitive equipment.

    (a) See Chapter 2.

(3) Perceptual equipment influences the automatic selection and organization of stimuli or stimulus patterns.

    (a) Perceptual equipment can tolerate an individually determined amount of stimulation at any given time.

    (b) When perceptual capacity is overloaded, attention shifts to less demanding aspects of a situation.

    (c) Perceptual attention to a given stimulus cannot be maintained indefinitely. When perceptual equipment becomes "tired" of a given stimulus, attention automatically shifts.

        i. Ability to maintain perceptual attention for longer spans of time increases with age and practice; the young child is much less able than an adult to concentrate attention over a long period of time.

    (d) When a given situation involves more separate parts than perceptual equipment can handle adequately, attention focuses on isolated aspects of the situation. (Unless later correction is made, recall of the perceived object or event may be distorted by such focusing of attention.)

    (e) Man has a natural tendency to organize perceptual data.

        i. Man organizes incomplete perceptual data by "filling in" with data to complete it.

        ii. Man tends to organize perceptual data by finding meanings and relationships that provide adequate interpretation of the data and influence perception of subsequent data.

        iii. Both the selection of data for attention and its organization are influenced by past experience and the current psychological and physical state of the perceiver. (See C following.)

        iv. In general, perception is more likely to be complete and adequate if more than a single sense is involved.

C. Perception is influenced by the individual's current physiological and psychological states and his past experiences.

(1) An individual's physical size influences perception of objects, persons or events. (A small person or a child perceives a large person differently than will a person of the same size).

(2) An individual's physical condition influences perception of objects, persons or events. (A physically handicapped person perceives objects in the environment in a different way

than a physically adept person; a person who is acutely ill perceives the environment in different terms than the person who is well.)

(3) Perception is influenced by the individual's current state of need. The most strongly felt need is most likely to shape or direct perception. (See Chap. 7.)

(4) Perception is influenced by the individual's current emotional state. (See Chap. 5.)

(5) Perception is influenced by the individual's attitudes, opinions, values and current interests. (See Chap. 2.)

(6) Preoccupation with personal matters or other distracting influences interferes with adequate perception.

(7) Past experience influences an individual's "perceptual set," or his tendency to organize and select perceptual data.

(a) Conflicting perceptual sets may interfere with adequacy of perception by causing inattention to some details, over-attention to some details, and distortion of some details or of the total situation in order to avoid unpleasant recognition of discrepancies.

(b) Perceptual set helps to determine what is perceived and how it is interpreted by setting up a state of anticipation of what will be perceived.

(8) The more ambiguous perceptual data is, the more its interpretation is influenced in the direction of need, desire or expectation.

(9) An individual's perceptual ability and characteristic ways of perceiving situations follow a pattern of growth and development.

(a) A certain amount of actual physical stimulation appears to be necessary to the normal maturation of sensory equipment, and the training of sensory equipment for use.

(b) In addition to physical stimulation, non-physical stimulation of sensory equipment is necessary for adequate maturation of sensory equipment and its training for use.

(10) A person may have perceptual experiences without corresponding stimuli (e.g., dreams, hallucinations).

2. An individual's perceptions influence his behavior.

A. An individual reacts to a situation or event as he perceives it, regardless of the reality of the situation or how the majority of other people see the situation.

B. Perception of persons, objects or events (thus behavior toward these persons or objects, or in the situation) is susceptible to a number of errors or distortions. Such errors may involve one or more of the following:

(1) Superficial observations.
(2) Preconceptions.
(3) Incorrect inferences.
(4) Faulty memory.
(5) Superstitions and prejudice.
(6) Incorrect premises.
(7) Rationalization.
(8) Projection.
(9) Certain errors in perception of people or events are particularly common. Such errors include:
(a) Tendency to oversimplify and reduce the total possible data about a person or event to the most quickly formulated generalizations (e.g., the use of stereotypes or categorizations made on the basis of one or two perceived characteristics, omitting other characteristics).
(b) Tendency to adhere to a stereotype or categorization once it is formed. Future data tends to be ignored or rationalized unless it fits the stereotype, in which case it tends to be overemphasized.
(c) Tendency to project onto others characteristics common to oneself. (Need to eliminate possibly threatening differences.)

NURSING CARE

The principles, hypotheses, and facts related to perception can be used by the nurse to help patients maintain adequacy of perception.

1. The nurse can increase her understanding of the processes involved in perception in order to better understand the patient and herself, and therefore guide her behavior toward wiser judgments.
2. The nurse can increase her knowledge and understanding of the individual patient and his life circumstances, in order to anticipate how he will perceive a specific situation. She can attempt to determine through observation:
   A. The patient's general sensory ability, by comparing and contrasting his ability to expected norms, in order to detect any deviations from those norms. (She notices such things as photosensitivity, poor eyesight, hypo- or hypersensitivity to auditory stimulation, hypo- or hyperasthesias, decreased ability to taste or smell, or hypersensitivity to odors.)
   B. The patient's general developmental level as it might affect perception (e.g., intellectual ability in general, typical cognitive styles as demonstrated by the patient, educational level which

might indicate concept development, age as an indication of possible perceptual level).

C. The patient's current physical and psychological state (e.g., emotional state, type of illness and/or physical disability, current need state insofar as it can be determined, currently demonstrated attitudes and opinions).

3. Using her knowledge of the processes of perception, the nurse can guide her observations of the patient and his situation to determine any errors, omissions or distortions of perception, and/or any ways in which data may have been presented that would decrease adequacy of perception.

4. After observation of the patient and his situation, the nurse can use information gained in order to make decisions for action that will increase or ensure adequacy of perception. For example, she can:

A. Control her own behavior in the presence of patients who are small (e.g., children) or physically handicapped, in order to avoid behavior that might be perceived as threatening, or that might be distorted because of handicap.

B. Regulate perceptual data presented to the patient in accordance with his ability to attend to details or to specific kinds of data (e.g., adjust for confusion, preoccupation, gross need states, hyper- or hyposensitivity in any given area, and so forth).

C. Regulate perceptual data presented to the patient in accordance with his emotional state (e.g., decrease demands on attention if the patient is particularly tense or anxious; introduce necessary new information when he is less tense; manipulate the environment to avoid depressing perceptions if the patient is already depressed; attempt to avoid anger-producing situations when they would interfere with perception).

D. Control or influence the presentation of stimuli for most effective perception by:

(1) Regulating the quality of the stimuli (e.g., providing adequate amount of information, with optimal degree of intensity, repetitiveness, novelty).

(2) Presenting perceptual data in organized forms most conducive to adequate perception and interpretation (e.g., showing meaningful relationships and whole patterns rather than bits of isolated information; reducing the number of diverse parts of a situation needing attention).

(3) Avoiding ambiguity and vagueness in the presentation of perceptual data.

(4) Avoiding the "overloading" of stimulus patterns beyond the patient's ability to be attentive.

E. Either avoid the introduction of perceptual data that will cause increased conflict or tension because of pre-existing attitudes and beliefs, or do not pressure the patient to change his ideas simply because he has been presented with "facts."

   F. Obtain feedback from the patient to determine his adequacy of perception. Using feedback to plan the correction of errors, fill in gaps in data, attempting to correct distortions.

   G. In working with infants and young children, especially if they are isolated from parents and other children, the nurse should plan for adequate physical contact and/or sensory stimulation.

   H. In working with adults who must be isolated for long periods, the nurse should provide sensory stimulation through such means as reading, radio or television, handcrafts, conversation with hospital personnel, and so forth.

   I. Be alert to any indications that perceptual experiences are not based on objective stimuli, and regulate behavior accordingly. (Avoid ridiculing the patient; see that protective measures are taken if hallucinations may cause irrational behavior; decrease environmental stimuli that may promote illusions.)

5. The nurse should, in her observation of patients and interpretation of their behavior, be alert to clues regarding perceptions that might influence behavior. For example, she can:

   A. Obtain feedback from the patient regarding exactly how he sees a situation.

   B. Obtain any necessary additional information from the patient that might indicate perceptual set or errors in perception that may be influencing his behavior (e.g., superstitions, preconceptions, lack of information, past experiences, use of stereotypes).

6. The nurse must be alert to her own behavior, including her perceptive behavior, in order to determine how she may be perceived by the patient, how her perceptions may influence her actions in relation to the patient, and how she can alter her behavior to the best interests of the patient.

2

Cognition, Attitudes and Beliefs

Psychological equilibrium is influenced by and complexly related to cognitive function, including opinions, beliefs and attitudes.

SOCIAL SCIENCE PRINCIPLES

1. Psychological equilibrium is influenced by cognitive function.
   A. In general, psychological equilibrium is enhanced if the individual is able to think clearly and rationally.
      (1) For an individual who is confused, frequent re-orientation is necessary to decrease confused behavior and prevent or decrease fear caused by the confused state.
      (2) The attention span of the confused person is usually short and easily interrupted.
      (3) Extremes of emotion and tension may interfere with rational thinking and behavior.
      (4) Extremely distorted thinking, such as occurs in delusion, may result in a corresponding illogical behavior.
         (a) An individual who has delusions acts on the basis of those delusions, regardless of the apparent reality of a situation or any attempts to convince him of the falsity of his ideas.
   B. An individual's psychological state, including cognitive function, ideas, beliefs and attitudes, influences his physiological function.
      (1) Conscious and unconscious cognitive processes, in conjunction with other aspects of psychological function, can cause the subjective experiencing of physiological symptoms where no physiological pathology can be demonstrated (e.g., pain, anesthesia, paresthesia).
      (2) Conscious and unconscious cognitive processes, in conjunction with other aspects of psychological function, can have

268

substantial influence on physiological functioning (e.g., paralysis, convulsive seizures, blindness, nausea and vomiting, increased pulse rate).

(3) There is some degree of general muscular tension always present during thinking.

    (a) The more vivid the imagery of thinking, the greater the muscular tension.

    (b) Thinking about certain kinds of activities causes muscular tension in those muscles involved in the activity being imagined.

2. Cognitive function is influenced by a variety of factors.

  A. The physical environment has a substantial influence on individual cognitive function (e.g., distracting features in the environment; events or objects that focus attention and direct the train of thought).

    (1) Through the process of developmental experience, an individual may learn to think better under certain environmental conditions (e.g., presence or absence of certain kinds of sounds or certain visual situations; varieties of physical position).

  B. An individual's physiological state has an influence on cognitive function (e.g., thirst, hunger, physical discomfort, pain, endocrine balance).

  C. The cognitive process of remembering is subject to the same influences as perception.

    (1) Remembered material tends to be systematized, organized and reinterpreted in relation to the individual's unique fund of percepts, past knowledge, current needs and interests.

    (2) In the process of remembering, actual events frequently become so reorganized and reinterpreted that they are only vaguely literal and may be substantially distorted.

3. Development of cognitive ability follows a systematic pattern of maturation, based on both constitutional ability and maturational experiences.

  A. The adequate development and functioning of cognitive equipment requires varied perceptual stimulation.

  B. Some cognitive styles develop in the process of maturation and experience.

    (1) An individual may develop rigid patterns of thinking, making it difficult for him to change ideas, attitudes, beliefs and concepts even when objective conditions demand it.

    (a) The person who utilizes primarily rigid thinking patterns most often was subjected to restrictive, punishing experiences during formative years.

    (b) The person with rigid thinking patterns seems to have

other personality characteristics which either promote rigid thinking, correspond to rigid thinking, or are reinforced by rigid thinking. These characteristics include: little initiative, excessive submission to authority, poor personal insight, feelings of insecurity, low self-esteem and self-acceptance, greater dependence on support from others, and greater susceptibility to threat.

(2) An individual may develop flexible patterns of thinking, making it easier for him to adapt to new ideas and to change concepts when objective conditions warrant change.

    (a) The person who utilizes primarily flexible thinking patterns most often was subjected to permissive, autonomous experiences encouraging independence during formative years.

    (b) The person with flexible thinking patterns seems to have other personality characteristics which either promote flexible thinking, correspond to flexible thinking, or are reinforced by flexible thinking. These characteristics include: unrestricted use of initiative, ability to organize, self-reliance, goal direction and motivation, relatively good personal insight, acceptance of self but with ability to control impulses, adequate sense of self-esteem and of personal adequacy, less susceptibility to threat and ability to tolerate ambiguity.

(3) Some individuals tend to develop thinking patterns that make it easier for them to conceptualize in concrete, specific, literal terms, and others develop thinking patterns that make it easier for them to conceptualize in abstract terms.

C. Ability to conceptualize develops relatively slowly. (For example, the child usually attributes life to nonorganic objects.)

  (1) The development of conceptualization requires communicative contact with others.

  (2) Concrete concepts are more easily grasped, both in the child and the adult. The development of concrete concepts precedes the development of abstract concepts.

  (3) Abstract conceptualization is either interfered with or impossible in some forms of mental handicap (e.g., mental retardation, brain damage, and apparently in schizophrenia).

4. Attitudes, beliefs and opinions seem to have certain characteristic features.

A. It is unsafe to assume that people having the same attitude or opinion regarding a given object, person or event have the same cognitive content to support that attitude or opinion.

B. Attitudes, opinions and beliefs may not always be supported by systematic reasoning; they may be vague, poorly defined or not consciously based on logical reason.

C. All the attitudes, opinions and beliefs of a given person may not be consistent with each other. Some attitudes may conflict, but be held in isolation from each other. (See Chap. 8, 2.)

D. Attitudes, opinions and beliefs are more likely to give force to behavior motivation and be resistant to change if:
    (1) The reasoning behind the attitude, opinion or belief is clearly defined.
    (2) The feeling or emotion associated with the attitude, opinion or belief is extreme.
    (3) The attitude, opinion or belief is consistent with the individual's other attitudes, opinions or beliefs.
    (4) The attitude, opinion or belief is approved of by the groups with which the individual identifies.

E. An individual's attitudes, opinions and beliefs exert substantial influence on his behavior.
    (1) Attitudes, opinions and beliefs that consistently guide or motivate behavior are most resistant to change.
        (a) A person whose attitudes, opinions and beliefs have strong emotional overtones, resists suggestions for change, including "not hearing or seeing" data that would suggest change. There is a tendency to avoid contact with new or opposing ideas.
        (b) When a person consciously commits himself to an attitude, opinion or belief, the commitment itself serves as a further barrier to change.
        (c) When a person receives support for his attitudes, opinions and beliefs from others he perceives as significant, he is less likely to change.
    (2) Attitudes, opinions and beliefs may be used to organize experience and give meaning to behavior.
    (3) The expression of attitudes, opinions and beliefs may be used to gain position in desired social groups.
    (4) Attitudes, opinions and beliefs influence perceptual experience by directing attention, shaping the interpretation of data to fit the attitudes, opinions and beliefs, and guiding the "selectiveness" of perceptions.

F. Attitudes, opinions and beliefs are formed in the process of growth and development.
    (1) Most attitudes, opinions and beliefs are culturally determined, the earliest and strongest determinants being the family group and child-rearing practices of parents.
    (2) The growth and change of attitudes, opinions and beliefs occurs slowly as a result of several factors:

      (a) Change in group identity.

      (b) Enforced changes in behavior.

      (c) New learning through information or different experiences with the object, person or event in question.

      (d) Perceived changes in the object, person or event in question.

      (e) Use of reason in the presence of one or more of the above factors.

NURSING CARE

Constructive nursing care in relation to cognition, attitudes and beliefs can be achieved by the nurse in the following ways:

1. The nurse should increase her understanding of cognitive function and the relationship of opinions, beliefs and attitudes to physiological and psychological well-being.

2. The nurse should orient her observations of the patient to determine the patient's:

    A. Clearness and rationality of thinking.

    B. Deviations from accepted "normal" cognitive function.

    C. Emotional states that might influence thinking.

    D. Environment as it might influence cognitive function.

    E. Physiological state as it might influence or be influenced by cognitive function.

    F. Individual thinking habits or styles of thinking.

    G. Age in relation to thinking and attitudinal behavior.

    H. Demonstration of attitudes, opinions and beliefs as they relate to illness, care and treatment, hospitalization.

    I. Factors in the environment that might influence or be in conflict with opinions, ideas, attitudes and beliefs.

3. The nurse must use her knowledge of cognitive function and the formation of attitudes, opinions and beliefs, and their influences on behavior, as well as her observations of the individual patient, as a base for planning nursing approach and intervention.

    A. When nursing a confused person, avoid ambiguity and multiplicity of stimuli; do not demand immediate responses involving reasoning and/or prolonged attention; provide frequent reorientation; make simple directive statements or requests; provide environmental support to orientation (such as written signs, objects the person may recognize); allow the patient frequent contact with calm, supportive people.

    B. When nursing a person under emotional strain or in an exaggerated emotional state, avoid demands on reasoning abilities; avoid increasing tension or the exaggeration of emotion; provide emotional support when problem-solving is unavoidable; create distractions from emotions or tension-causing factors while problem-solving is in progress; give clear and simple directions requiring less work in thinking.

C. If the patient is delusional or irrational, avoid arguing with or ridiculing his ideas; do not introduce problems or environmental factors that would come into direct and open conflict with delusional content; do not attempt prolonged reasoning or expect that reasoning is possible while the person is irrational; provide adequate observation and other safety measures to prevent the patient from harming himself or others; provide unobtrusive reminders of reality that do not demand choice between delusional content and reality; give kind, firm, simple direction when direction is necessary, but may be in conflict with delusional or irrational ideas.

D. When the patient demonstrates functional physiological states or subjective symptoms unsupported by pathology, avoid such things as drawing attention to the symptom or state, showing rejection, hostility or ridicule, or providing secondary gains by giving sympathy and attention to his symptoms or state. Provide opportunity for the patient to function normally without drawing attention to any inconsistency between his symptoms or state and normal function; give emotional support while the patient mentally and verbally works through problems related to his symptoms or state; give good physical nursing care to relieve discomfort regardless of cause of symptoms; give attention and emotional satisfaction for behavior or achievements not related to his condition.

E. If a person is acutely ill and/or in need of large amounts of rest for recovery, avoid demands on cognitive function, and do not expect that he will be able to function at optimal cognitive level.

F. Provide the best possible climate for cognitive function:

(1) Keep the environment conducive to optimal cognitive function (e.g., control distracting factors; avoid thought-directing events that interfere with the problem at hand; introduce thought-directing events conducive to the problem at hand).

(2) Reduce physiological discomfort or need states that interfere with adequate cognitive function (e.g., do not ask the patient to concentrate on an important problem if he is hungry, thirsty or in pain).

(3) Provide needed information; ask thought-provoking questions; provide a supportive and non-judgmental attitude while the patient verbally works through problems.

(4) Act as a sounding board, asking helpful questions and providing information as the patient attempts to remember and correct his memory for greatest accuracy.

(5) If the patient is isolated from others for long periods, or is

a child away from family and peers, provide the opportunity for development and adequate function of cognitive faculties by planning varied perceptual stimulation; allow him communicative contact with others and the opportunity to assist in planning his own care and solving his own problems. Adjust demands on cognitive function to the patient's developmental level and/or handicap state.

(6) Avoid conflicts with the patient's particular style of thinking.

(a) Avoid demands on the person who demonstrates rigid thinking patterns (and associated personality characteristics) to adjust to new ideas and routines unnecessarily, particularly if the person is in an unusually stressful situation.

   i. Increase emotional support when illness and hospitalization place increased demands on the patient for adjustment to new ideas, situations or circumstances.

   ii. Provide for successful experiences with new ideas, situations or behavior, and for ego-building experiences in general. (Avoid actions that would lower self-esteem and the ability to use flexible thinking patterns.)

   iii. Prevent reinforcement of rigid thinking habits and associated personality characteristics by avoiding punitive and/or restrictive attitudes and practices.

(b) Avoid demands on the person who demonstrates flexible thinking habits and associated personality characteristics to conform to rigid rules and regulations, unless absolutely necessary. The nurse can foster flexible thinking habits by:

   i. Allowing maximum participation of the patient in planning his own care.

   ii. Providing reasons and information regarding actions that must be required.

   iii. Providing non-judgmental supportive attitudes as the patient thinks through problems caused by illness or hospitalization.

   iv. Avoiding rejective or hostile attitudes if the patient finds solutions to problems that do not necessarily fit with the nurse's preconceived ideas.

(c) Avoid demands for abstract thinking if the patient has a "concrete" orientation to problem-solving. (Provide concrete, specific and literal information and interpretations, avoiding ambiguous and highly abstract generalizations.)

(d) Expect that the person who is very ill or very threatened may regress and need more specific information coming from the environment. Also, expect a greater need for specifics among those who are mentally retarded, schizophrenic or suffering from brain damage.

G. Make use of the patient's existing attitudes, opinions and beliefs whenever possible to effect optimal therapeutic care.
 (1) Avoid assumptions about the patient's attitudes, opinions and beliefs until they have been assessed through communication with the patient.
 (2) Avoid criticism or rejection of the patient whose attitudes, opinions and beliefs are different from one's own.
 (3) Avoid, unless necessary for optimal health care, increasing tension or conflict for the patient by avoiding the pointing out of conflicts among his attitudes, opinions and beliefs or behavior.
 (4) Avoid, unless necessary for optimal health care, demanding behavior of the patient that would be in conflict with his existing attitudes, opinions and beliefs.
 (5) Attempt to show relationships between new behavior necessary for the patient to acquire, and his existing attitudes, opinions and beliefs.

H. When new attitudes, opinions or beliefs are necessary for optimal physical and/or mental health, the nurse should make use of what is known about attitude, opinion and belief formation to effect change with the least amount of psychological discomfort. For example, she should:
 (1) Provide adequate information upon which to base changes.
 (2) Promote the reasoning process in relation to change.
 (3) Point out the relationship of changed attitudes, opinions and beliefs to valued goals or known motivations.
 (4) Provide contact with persons the patient may hold in high esteem who have the desired attitudes, opinions or beliefs. (Contact may be through reading, movies, etc., as well as actual contact.)
 (5) Provide supportive and pleasurable or rewarding experiences that reinforce the new attitude, opinion or belief.

4. The nurse should examine her own thinking habits, attitudes, opinions and beliefs, in order to determine how they may influence patient care, or her own development as an increasingly effective professional person.

3

Integrative Function: Development of Ego and/or Self-concept

Psychological equilibrium requires adequate integration of all aspects of the individual's psychological processes.

SOCIAL SCIENCE PRINCIPLES

Integrative processes are usually seen as a function of the "ego" or "self." Such terms as "ego integrity" and "personality integrity" are frequently used to denote the individual's total psychological integrative processes.

1. The "self" is experienced by the individual as an organized and enduring perception, involving integrated processes of perceiving, feeling and thinking.
   A. Included in the concept of self is the concept of body image. (Body image is one of the earliest self-concepts to be developed.)
   (1) When body image must be changed as a result of physiological changes (surgery, injury), the total concept of self is threatened, resulting in psychological tension or anxiety.
   (2) Body image is usually so firmly established that any necessary changes are accomplished slowly (e.g., after amputation, imagined body image still retains the absent limb for some time, including the physical sensation of its presence. A person who has been very heavy for a long time and has lost much weight continues to walk, act or use mannerisms appropriate to his previous weight.)
   B. The concept of self exists in relation to one's total psychological environment, including what one sees as the world or worlds in which he may function.
   (1) Changes in one aspect of a person's psychological environ-

276

ment necessitates readjustment to total concept of self and self-function.

    (2) Gross changes in self-concept necessitated by changes in psychological environment are usually accompanied by increased stress, tension, uncertainty and loss of a sense of direction.

C. The concept of self includes a culturally determined self or ego ideal—the concept of what one ought to be—against which the individual measures his own behavior and achievement.

2. The concept of self is acquired through the process of growth and development.

    A. Development of self-identity follows a characteristic order of development:

        (1) Sense of bodily self.

        (2) Sense of continuous self as separate from others and from the environment.

        (3) Sense of self-esteem.

    B. The infant has no sense of "self" as separate from the environment. Sense of self develops slowly over the first five to six years of life, the most rapid growth occurring after the acquisition of language.

    C. During the early stages of development of self-identity, fantasy and reality merge and separate on an uneven course. By the age of four to six years, the child still occasionally merges fantasy with reality (as with imaginary playmates), but can identify other "selves."

    D. During the first few years of self-identity development, the child is ego-centered, seeing the world as for his benefit and without any purpose separate from himself.

    E. Between the ages of four to six, the child develops the concepts of:

        (1) Self extension (e.g., "I" as a separate person, with "my" as object of ownership).

        (2) Self ideal (e.g., what "I" should or ought to be and do).

    F. Between the ages of six and twelve, the child gradually develops the ability to use self as a mediating instrument to cope with the world rationally (e.g., he learns to think and to think about thinking).

    G. Further development of adequate integrative function during adolescence is marked by:

        (1) Increased efforts at conscious self-identity, characterized by the demonstrated need to be a separate self, apart from the peer group.

        (2) Confusion and contradiction, particularly in some societies, caused by the need to become a definite separate self and at the same time retain identification with peer groups.

(3) Increased efforts to be an autonomous self, able to function without parental direction.

H. The development of conscience as a part of total self and integrative function follows a characteristic pattern.

(1) The first stages of development of conscience are characterized by nonreasoned "oughts," "musts," "must-nots," and "shoulds" directly incorporated from parental edict. Reasons for conformity are based on fear of damage or withdrawal of valued objects or events.

(2) Further development of conscience depends upon separation of self from others as a controlling and reacting agent, together with testing reality to determine consequences of behavior.

(3) During adolescence, the individual has acquired enough knowledge of the world and self to look for reasons for behavior as a basis for conscience. If ego development has progressed with stability, the adolescent:

(a) Tests previously accepted authoritarian dictates of conscience.

(b) Uses rational recognition of consequences when making choices of behavior.

(c) Experiences considerable anxiety if reasoned consequences deviate too much from previously acquired parental edicts, necessitating either blind conformity or open opposition to previous learning.

(4) Failure to develop a "reasoned conscience" usually leaves the individual under the control of nonautonomous, rigid rules of conduct derived in the first stages of development. He will be most likely to experience nonrational guilt when conscious and unconscious wishes and desires run counter to dictates of conscience.

(5) The development of conscience proceeds faster when parental attitudes demonstrate love and warmth, than when punishment without love and warmth is used to control behavior.

(6) The development of conscience proceeds more slowly and with less consistency if parental behavior is inconsistent with their verbalized rules or codes of conduct.

I. Development of integrative function (self-concept and/or ego function) is also influenced by the following factors:

(1) Self-identity is partly acquired through experiencing other people's reactions toward one's self.

(2) Nonconstructive experiences in growth and development may result in unstable self-concept, or in contradictory or multiple "selves."

(3) Prolonged sensory deprivation may result in disturbance of self-concept or the sense of self.

    (a) Ego identity requires constant reminders that self is separate from others, as provided by contact with the environment (e.g., being referred to by name, being reacted to as a separate and autonomous organism, experiencing reactions from the environment that indicate other, separate individuals and objects).

(4) Adequate personality integration requires some degree of satisfaction of basic primary and acquired needs. (See Chap. 7.)

(5) Adequate personality integration and/or ego function requires that an individual participate with and be accepted by other individuals and groups of individuals.

    (a) Ego integrity requires that an individual be able to identify with other individuals.

        i. One of the methods by which individuals learn the sociocultural limits for ego function is through identification with other individuals.

    (b) Adequate self-concept requires that the individual have the opportunity to learn and subsequently achieve satisfaction in practicing sociocultural roles.

(6) One of the methods by which the individual learns the socioculturally acceptable limits for ego-determined behavior is through "reality testing."

(7) A person who has acquired flexible methods of adaptation adjusts to life situations with greater ease and satisfaction than one whose methods are rigid and uncompromising.

3. If self-concept or ego integrity is disrupted, disorganization of personality results. (See Chap. 8.)

NURSING CARE

The nurse can increase and maintain effectiveness of nursing care in relation to integrative function in some of the following ways:

1. She can increase her knowledge of human psychological integrative processes in order to understand patient behavior and needs, and to understand her own behavior as it relates to patient care.

2. The nurse can guide her observations of patients and their environment to determine:

A. How the patient sees himself, particularly in relation to his illness and/or hospitalization. (Observe for expressions of self-doubt, self-assurance, autonomy, orientation toward family, friends, hospital personnel, work role, ability to adapt to hospital experiences and health promoting procedures.)

B. Any indications of disturbance of integrative function, particularly if illness and/or hospitalization requires changes in self-concept (e.g., evidences of increased anxiety, confusion and doubt, depression, refusal to participate in necessary therapeutic procedures that will alter either body image or social image, regression to earlier forms of integrative function).

C. Indications of the individual's stage of growth and development of ego structure and function. (In working with children, is the child's integrative behavior appropriate to chronological age?)

D. Factors or situations in the environment or caused by illness and/or hospitalization that might disrupt integrative function (e.g., experiences the patient might be subjected to, such as attitudes of hospital personnel, family and friends; therapeutic procedures that might lower self-esteem and/or sense of individuality and autonomy; isolation procedures that might be destructive to self-concept).

3. The nurse should use both her knowledge and observations to guide nursing care planning in order to maintain integrative function at optimal level, and/or assist in further development of integrative function. She can, for example:

A. Provide opportunity for the patient who is sustaining a change in body image or social image to talk with supportive, non-judgmental, informed persons, in order to gradually incorporate change and its implications for future living (e.g., allowing questions and discussion of possible future behavior, expression of feeling about changes).

(1) If possible or necessary, provide positive experiences in relation to changes (e.g., observation of others who have benefited from similar changes; opportunity to experiment successfully with "new" self in protected environment).

(2) Avoid unnecessary demands for adjustment to life situations until the individual has had an opportunity to "get used to" altered self-concept. (Don't push the patient faster than he is able to develop.)

B. Through attitudes, information and positive experiences, provide opportunity for the patient to adjust changes in self-concept to previous concept of ideal self (e.g., if changes are in conflict with previous ego ideal, provide positive experiences to help the patient alter his concept of "ideal").

C. Adapt nursing care of children and adolescents to provide for maximum growth and development of integrative processes.

(1) Allow maximum autonomy consistent with age level and physical or psychological safety.

(2) Provide consistency in attitudes of hospital personnel toward the patient, including attempts to avoid conflict with paren-

tal attitudes, unless parental attitudes are deemed actually harmful.

(3) If appropriate to age level, provide reasons for nursing actions and required patient behavior, requesting cooperation rather than blind compliance with rules.

(4) Provide adequate sensory experiences and contact with the environment.

    (a) In direct contact with the child, communication should point out "self-hood" and extensions of self, as well as relationships of self to environment.

    (b) Provision should be made for maximal opportunity to interact with other children and objects, consistent with health requirements.

(5) Avoid punitive, rejecting and rigid attitudes and behavior in general, particularly when the child or adolescent experiments with limits of self-direction.

(6) Alter attitudes and behavior to the most constructive, reflecting respect for the individual, approval of self-directed actions and variations in adaptive behaviors, showing warmth, caring, and patience with uncertainty, fear and inconsistent changes in direction.

(7) Increase contact with parents or known and trusted persons, who can affirm ego identity, particularly when self-concept is threatened by illness and/or hospitalization. (Attitudes should reflect faith in the *continuous* existence of the child as a cared for and esteemed person, regardless of permanent or temporary disruptions of usual existence.)

D. Provide supportive nursing care whenever integrative function and structure is threatened. For example, the nurse can:

(1) Increase efforts to help the patient retain individual indentity and sense of worth.

(2) Increase positive contacts with hospital personnel, family and friends (e.g., assign the patient to the most "person oriented" staff rather than the most "task oriented" staff).

(3) Increase efforts to permit verbal expression of fears, uncertainties and disturbing emotions, in the presence of warmly supportive people, who can accept the patient's feelings without needing to deny the validity or necessity of such feelings.

(4) Increase efforts to avoid additional demands for change and/or conformity to behavior that might be inconsistent with the patient's self-concept.

(5) See Chapter 8 for additional nursing actions.

4

Communication

Psychological equilibrium requires that the individual have an adequate means for communication with others and/or for self-expression.

SOCIAL SCIENCE PRINCIPLES

(Note: Most of the information pertinent to communication is included in other chapters. For example, an understanding of communication processes would be impossible without first understanding perception—the first step in message reception is, after all, perception. At the same time, the learning and use of language symbols is central to the development of cognitive function, but language symbols cannot be learned apart from cognitive function. And, the complex relationships developed in the satisfaction of human needs would be literally impossible without communicative interaction. Therefore, in a sense, all the material in other chapters is a part of the human communication process. This chapter contains only those few generalizations not already included in other chapters, or those generalizations needed to show relationships between the concept of communication and concept statements included in other chapters. It does not include either validated principles or current theories about abnormal patterns of communication found in mental illness.)

1. Communication between individuals takes place in a variety of ways:
   A. Every culture provides a symbolic means for communication between individuals and groups of individuals.
   B. In order for symbols to be used effectively in communication, they must be mutually understood.
   C. Nonverbal behavior is an essential part of the communication process.
   D. The total complex of interactive and interrelationship behavior constitutes continuous communication between individuals and groups of individuals (i.e., an understanding of communication processes requires an understanding and analysis of all interactive behavior).

2. Communication is influenced by a variety of internal and external factors:
   A. Communication between individuals is influenced by the relationship that exists between them (i.e., communication is influenced by the perceptions that the message sender and the receiver have of each other).
      1. The more a person is trusted or viewed as a prestige person, the more likely others are to accept his communication as valid and acceptable without alteration.
      2. Messages received from persons perceived as less trustworthy or of less prestige tend to be discredited or distorted.
      3. If the communicator is liked but the message has negative or unpleasant connotations, the message tends to be distorted or "rationalized" to fit with the opinion held about the communicator.
      4. Reception and intepretation of a given message is influenced by the degree of expertness assigned to the message sender.
      5. Reception and interpretation of a given message is influenced by what the recipient believes to be the intent of the message sender (e.g., persuasion, evasion, kindness, harm).
      6. Message sending and receiving is influenced by stereotyped categorization or perception of each other by sender and receiver (e.g., a patient's stereotyped perception of "social worker," or a nurse's stereotyped perception of "Negro").
   B. In addition to the relationship of the communicators, reception and interpretation of messages is influenced by a variety of factors such as:
      (1) The situation in which communication takes place, which includes:
         (a) What the recipient perceives as expected behavior in response to the communication (i.e., what the message requires him to do, such as act in support of the message, or reinterpret the message to others in his own words).
         (b) The presence of others in the situation (e.g., when other people are present who might inhibit response, or cause response to be altered because of known attitudes or later consequences of response to communication).
         (c) Concentration of attention on environmental events, and distracting influences in the environment.
         (d) The general tone or atmosphere of the environment (e.g., a school room as opposed to a kitchen).
      (2) The individual's internal state, personality characteristics

and other factors relative to the individuals involved in communication.

(a) Preoccupation with personal matters and/or the presence of thoughts regarding emotionally charged subjects may interfere with an individual's ability to receive, interpret, respond to and send messages.

(b) A message is more likely to be received if its content is personally desired or pleasing, or if it fits existing attitudes, ideas and beliefs.

(c) A message is more likely to be either ignored or distorted if its content has negative connotations for the recipient, or if it does not fit pre-existing attitudes, ideas and beliefs.

(d) The educational level of the recipient of messages influences the effectiveness of various types of communication media.

   i. An individual with a higher level of education tends to make more adequate use of written communicative material.

   ii. An individual with a lower level of education tends to respond more efficiently to aural and visual communication media, less efficiently to printed words alone.

(e) Message reception and interpretation is subject to the same processes as perception in general (i.e., to undergo the same organization, omission of data to simplify complex messages, selective attention to details, filling in of data to complete percepts or concepts in order to form whole patterns).

(f) Message reception and interpretation is influenced by the appeal of the message to emotion versus cognition (i.e., if the message has elements evoking fear, the reception and interpretation of the message is different than if it appeals primarily to reason).

(g) The interpretation of communicative symbols is limited to meanings made possible by the experience of the recipient, regardless of any possible meanings those symbols might have for others.

(h) Message reception and interpretation is influenced by the individual's need, interest or motivation state (e.g., a message relative to a need state is more likely to be attended to if the need exists prior to the message).

(i) Message reception and interpretation is influenced by social and personality characteristics of recipients and senders (e.g., a chronically anxious, insecure person attends to and interprets messages differently than an individual who has a stable self-concept, characterized by high self-esteem and ability to tolerate threat). Studies, although inconclusive for women, indicate that:

    i. Men who are consistently hostile and aggressive, or who are consistently withdrawn from interactions with others, are less easily influenced by persuasive communication.

    ii. Men who are capable of vivid imagery tend to respond empathically.

    iii. Men who have lower self-esteem and higher dependency levels are more easily influenced by persuasive communication.

  (j) Communication is altered by an individual's physiological or psychophysiological state (e.g., state of consciousness, ability to hear or see, reaction to medications such as sedatives, toxic states).

  (k) Communication is influenced by the perceptive and cognitive ability of the individual, his current emotional state, his integrative abilities, and so forth.

  (l) A reciprocal relationship exists between learning and communication (i.e., much of human learning is not possible without adequate communicative ability, and adequate communication depends on learning).

 (3) Reception and interpretation of messages is influenced by the way a message is organized for presentation (i.e., the order of presentation of parts of the message, the relationship of the message to environmental events).

3. Problems in communication frequently arise because of inattention to certain characteristics of message sending and reception. For example:

  A. The content and intent of messages as well as reception and interpretation of messages depends upon the frame of reference of the individuals involved.

  B. Difficulty in transmission and reception of messages may be increased if the participants in communication use specialized verbal symbols, form a personal compression of complex ideas into single symbols, or use vague symbols or ambiguous generalizations.

  C. Difficulties in communication occur because of individual assignment of values to symbols used, and the assumption that others involved in communication assign the same values to those symbols.

D. Problems in communication often arise because participants in the communication process draw inferences from inadequate data.

E. Difficulties in communication are increased because a given communicative symbol usually has both a denotative meaning and a connotative meaning. Although the denotative meaning may be the same for all individuals, the connotative meaning may vary widely from individual to individual (e.g., a cross may be, in the dictionary sense, the same to several people, but have quite different emotional or evaluative meanings for people with different religious backgrounds and experiences).

F. Difficulties in communication are increased because messages may have both a literal meaning, and an underlying or subtle meaning not obvious in interpretation of the actual symbols used. (A mother, while visiting a neighbor, may observe her own child doing something that displeases her. She may say, "Johnny, I think it's about time we went home." The message may have both literal meaning in terms of time of day and length of visit, and subtle meaning such as "You, Johnny, have committed a social error and you're going to catch it when you get home.") The same characteristic of messages or symbolic conventions may facilitate communication and interpersonal relationships. For example, "Good morning, how are you?" is usually a symbolic communication that does not require a literal answer, but carries with it the intent to convey interest in the individual and desire to begin communication.

G. Difficulties in communication (and therefore in responsive relationships) occur if the verbal message is not consistent with the nonverbal message, regardless of the intent of the communicator.

H. Difficulties in communication occur if the message is overloaded (carries more content than the recipient can take in), disorganized, ambiguous or has too many diverse elements. (Communication is subject to the same difficulties as perception in general.)

NURSING CARE

Effective nursing care depends largely upon the nurse's effective use of communication skills and knowledge.

1. The nurse should increase her knowledge and understanding of the process of communication, and the relationship of communication processes to all other psychological functions.

2. A nurse can guide her observation of the patient and his environment, and obtain feedback from the patient, in order to determine:
   A. The individual patient's personality characteristics, sociocultural background, and educational and intellectual developmental level as they influence communication in general.

B. Factors in the environment that may influence specific communication.

C. Frames of reference of the patient in relation to specific communications.

D. Current physical and psychological states that might influence specific communication.

E. Characteristics of various relationships that might influence specific communications (e.g., nurse-patient relationships, patient-doctor relationships).

F. Indications that problems exist in communication in general, that specific communication processes are ineffective, or that the patient's communication patterns deviate from normal.

3. The nurse can use her knowledge of the communication process and her observations of a specific patient to plan nursing interventions. She can:

A. Avoid use of specialized language symbols, vague referents, or language symbols outside the patient's experience in communicating with the patient.

B. Be careful to obtain feedback from the patient to determine the actual message he has received.

C. Attempt to correct misinterpretations and distortions of messages, as determined through feedback.

D. Be alert to nonverbal communicative behavior of the patient, and of her own nonverbal behavior that might have unintended meaning for the patient.

E. Avoid discrepancy between verbal and nonverbal messages.

F. Attempt to establish a relationship of trust that will facilitate effective communication.

G. Avoid communicative responses to the patient based on stereotyped perceptions (i.e., get to know the patient as an individual, not as a typed representative of some sociocultural group).

H. Use her knowledge of the role of emotion, perception, and motivation in the organization and presentation of communication to allow for maximum communication effectiveness.

I. Avoid giving important messages when the patient is in an unreceptive state (e.g., when the patient is upset, semiconscious, sedated, highly distracted).

J. Alter communications to fit the patient's current state and current environmental situation.

K. Alter the environment when possible or necessary in order to achieve maximum benefit from communication efforts.

L. Plan for patient learning experiences that will increase communicative ability when necessary or appropriate.

5

Emotional Behavior

Emotion is a basic psychological experience common to man; it has a wide variety of effects, both constructive and nonconstructive, on total psychological equilibrium.

SOCIAL SCIENCE PRINCIPLES

1. Emotion is demonstrated or reflected in subjective feeling states, emotion-generated behavior and adaptive changes.
   A. Emotions are related to situational events. Certain situations tend to evoke certain feelings, and are usually sought or avoided, depending upon the total physical and psychological state.
      (1) Joy is a desired and usually sought emotional experience accompanying tension release or goal achievement.
      (2) Anger is an uncomfortable and usually avoided emotional experience accompanying the accumulation of tension or goal frustration.
      (3) Fear is an unpleasant and usually avoided emotional experience accompanying danger to the life of the organism, or damage to it, especially when the individual perceives himself as unable to avoid or eliminate the threat.
      (4) Grief is an unpleasant and usually avoided emotional experience accompanying loss of something valued.
      (5) Pride is a pleasant and usually sought emotional reaction to goal achievement in accord with ego-ideals.
      (6) Shame is an unpleasant and always avoided emotional reaction to goal failure, when the goal is important to the maintenance of self-esteem.
      (7) Embarrassment or self-consciousness is an unpleasant and therefore avoided emotional reaction to perceiving oneself as an actual or potential object of criticism, dislike or ridicule.
         (a) Criticism is usually interpreted and felt as a sign that one is inadequate, incompetent or unworthy.
         (b) Embarrassment or self-consciousness may interfere with the clarity of rational thought and action.

(8) Loneliness is an unpleasant and usually avoided emotional experience accompanying real or perceived isolation from other human beings.

    (a) Identification of oneself with other individuals or groups of individuals is necessary to decrease or eliminate loneliness.

(9) A given group of similar or related emotions sustained over time is referred to as "mood" (e.g., sadness, happiness, anxiety).

B. The expression of feeling or emotion may be achieved through a variety of behavior and adaptive reactions. In addition to commonly recognized vocal and nonvocal expressions, and the psychological and physiological manifestations of emotion:

(1) Energy generated by emotion that must be repressed tends to be expended in disguised, indirect ways.

    (a) Feelings that cannot be directly expressed toward the object or the individual engendering the feeling may be displaced onto other symbolic or convenient objects or individuals.

    (b) Illness and/or physical symptoms (physiological phenomena) may be used as a method of expressing unconscious feeling.

(2) Crying may be an effective form of behavior for relieving tension or expressing emotion that cannot be otherwise expressed.

(3) The presence of strong emotion alters cognitive function (e.g., anger may interfere with rational problem-solving; various emotions may lead to impulsive rather than reasoned behavior; exaggerated fear may lead to confusion and irrationality).

(4) A prevailing mood influences all other psychological experiences, including perception, cognition and motivation.

(5) Emotional experience is related in complex ways to total physiological and psychological function. In addition to the previous statements:

    (a) Experiencing emotion to any degree requires expenditure of energy.

    (b) Emotional reactions influence and are influenced by nervous system function, and physiological correlates to emotion can be demonstrated. (See Part II.)

    (c) Emotional reactions and their physiological correlates, when sustained over a period of time, can result in physiological structural changes (e.g., hypertension, ulcerative colitis, gastric ulcers).

    (d) The experiencing of unpleasant emotion or mood

usually has negative effects on total physiological and psychological function (e.g., promotes disequilibrium—profound and prolonged depression may be accompanied by general metabolic retardation, cognitive confusion and dullness).

(e) The experiencing of pleasant emotion or mood usually has positive effects on total psychological and physiological function (e.g., promotes equilibrium—a state of joy or happiness tends to be accompanied by a feeling of physical well-being, energy, motivation toward constructive action, ability to sustain problem-solving efforts).

(f) The more consistently the individual experiences the pleasant emotions, the more likely he is to adapt to frustrations and unpleasant adaptations with flexibility.

2. Emotional experiences are influenced by a variety of circumstances.

A. Environmental situations or changes influence emotion. In addition to situations cited under No. 1:

(1) Emotion may be controlled or manipulated by diverting attention from events causing the emotional reaction.

(2) Emotional states may be altered by environmental stimuli, such as object colors and arrangements, introduction of pleasant or unpleasant sounds, introduction or removal of objects having pleasant or unpleasant associations.

B. Emotion or feeling may be altered by changing perception of an object or event (e.g., introducing new elements, pointing attention to isolated aspects of an event, fostering mental rearrangement of data, seeing examples of different reactions to the same event by different people).

C. Emotional reactions are influenced by ideational content and cognitive processes.

D. Any given emotion tends to be blunted or decreased if sustained over time (e.g., fatigue occurs with over-stimulation and sameness).

E. Emotion tends to be contagious—to be transmitted to others in the environment.

F. Emotion is influenced by the individual's physiological state (e.g., in addition to statements under No. 1, exhaustion and malnourishment are usually accompanied by depression).

G. Verbalization of problems causing tension and emotion, in the presence of a nonjudgmental but receptive listener, may temporarily or permanently reduce the degree of emotion or tension.

3. Some varieties of emotional experience are learned in the process of growth and development, and others are thought to be basic or primitive emotions.

A. Anger, fear and a general sensation of pleasure are thought to be basic or primitive emotional reactions to appropriate stimuli.
B. Self-appraising emotions are thought to be learned through interaction with others and the experiencing of approval or disapproval. (Such emotions are shame, pride, guilt.)
   (1) Self-appraising emotions tend to be influenced by the reactions of others, even after the basic emotion has been learned, along with the learning of attitudes and values used for self-appraisal (e.g., the expression of criticism, disapproval or disgust by others tends to arouse shame or guilt, even when the adult, through conscious self-appraisal, may know that the attitudes are unjust or not well-founded).
   (2) Negative self-appraising emotions may be generated by internalized attitudes and values when behavior fails to be consistent with such values, regardless of external approval.
   (3) Experiencing vague or ambiguous disapproval may result in a feeling of guilt unattached to a specific object or event. As a result, the individual tends to feel that he is a "bad" person, rather than that he has committed a wrong act.
      (a) If the child, in the process of growth and development of self-concept, is continuously subjected to ambiguous attitudes that label him as a "bad" person, he will be less able to function with self-assurance, autonomy and freedom from restrictive unattached guilt.
C. Differentiation of basic primitive emotional reactions into specifically identifiable subcategories occurs as a result of interaction with others (e.g., general pleasure is differentiated as joy, love, sensory pleasure, and so forth, through identification with others and the variety in experience causing the reactions).

NURSING CARE

In order to plan nursing care that is consistently therapeutic, the nurse can implement her knowledge of emotional behavior.
1. The nurse should increase her understanding of emotional processes and their relationship to health and well-being.
2. The nurse can guide her observations of the patient and his environment in order to determine:
   A. The patient's current emotional state, either as related to a specific event, as part of a prevailing mood, or as emotional reaction patterns typical of the specific patient.
   B. The effect of events necessitated by illness and/or hospitalization on the patient's emotional state.
   C. Aspects of the environment that will be most likely to cause specific emotional reactions.
3. Utilize both her knowledge of emotional processes and her observa-

tions of the individual patient to plan nursing interventions. For example, she should:

A. Promote situations, experiences or events that increase pleasurable emotions.
B. Attempt to control or eliminate unnecessary situations, experiences or events that increase unpleasant emotions.
C. Intervene if a specific emotion is detrimental to health care. For example:
   (1) Avoid emotion-producing actions if the patient needs total energy for physical restorative processes.
   (2) Use distraction or environmental manipulation to alter existing undesirable emotions or moods.
   (3) Introduce new ideas and accompanying discussion that will alter mood or emotional reaction, eventually altering the patient's perception or emotion- or mood-producing life situations.
   (4) Decrease anger or other undesirable emotion before the patient is required to take rational action or make problem-solving decisions.
   (5) Actually control impulsive or irrational behavior caused by emotion, if the emotion cannot be reduced and rationality restored in time to prevent harm to the patient or others.
   (6) Through her knowledge of the nervous system and physiological correlates of emotion, attempt to prevent the experiencing of emotions detrimental to specific health conditions (e.g., avoid anger for hypertensive patients, excitement for coronary patients).
D. Attempt to induce the mood or emotional reaction most consistent with the achievement of other desired goals (e.g., help the patient to feel comfortable, pleased with himself and his surroundings, oriented toward pride-producing action, before introducing a new idea or action that will require effort; reduce or prevent the experiencing of disgust, anger, fear, embarrassment before meals or in relation to elimination procedures).
E. Provide for adequate expression of emotion in the most direct fashion, consistent with patient safety and well-being (e.g., allow the patient to express anger, fear and frustration, without guilt, punishment or retaliation).
F. Avoid demonstrating emotional reactions that might negatively influence the patient, but attempt to demonstrate moods and emotional reactions that might positively influence the patient.
G. When planning patient care, take into account and be aware of the patient's physical condition (including reactions to medications) that might influence mood or emotional reaction (e.g., the patient who has been physically exhausted by therapeutic

procedures and who has been without food for several hours will be in no "mood" to assimilate new information about sodium-free dietary restrictions).

H. In caring for children, organize nursing care to promote healthy experiences and the expression of emotion.

   (1) Avoid demonstrations of ambiguous, generalized disgust, criticism or rejection. If criticism is deemed necessary, it will be most constructive if specifically related to isolated behavior that is objectionable and can be changed.

   (2) Allow and promote a full range of emotional experience and expression consistent with health and well-being, including social well-being (e.g., anger can be safely expressed in some ways, but it must be controlled to prevent destruction. Any emotion and its expression can be considered "normal" and/or permissible, if the expression is consistent with safety of others and goals of self).

   (3) Plan for experiences that will elicit expressions of approval from others (thus, stimulate pride and self-assurance).

   (4) Avoid experiences that cause unnecessary shame and embarrassment; make provision for supportive attitudes when shame and embarrassment cannot be avoided.

4. The nurse should examine and evaluate her own emotional reactions to determine possible effect on nursing actions.

6

Growth and Development, Learning and Adaptive Problem-solving

Maintenance of psychological equilibrium requires that the individual have the opportunity for positive growth and development experiences, for learning in general, and for the acquisition of adaptive problem-solving behavior in particular.

SOCIAL SCIENCE PRINCIPLES

(Note: Where appropriate, growth and development principles have been included in other sections. For example, growth and development aspects of perception, cognitive function, and integrative function have been included in those sections. Therefore, only minimal additional material has been included in this section as a matter of the most expedient organization.)

1. Patterns of behavior are learned in the process of growth and development.
   A. The development of behavior reflects maturation through growth, as well as the cumulative effects of learning through experience.
      (1) Over-all physical and mental growth curves run parallel courses, with the rate of growth showing a drop at puberty.
      (2) Growth and development follows an uneven course; not all aspects of function mature at the same rate at the same time.
      (3) Gross, general patterns of behavior precede differentiated behavior, with structure and function becoming increasingly differentiated (e.g., the infant demonstrates total organismic reaction, rather than differentiated emotional response, to situations normally calling for such differentiated response).

294

  (4) In cortical development, sensory and motor areas develop first, with association areas developing later. (Simple conditioning may be possible at relatively early ages, while complex pe_ epts and problem-solving functions are impossible until later.)

  (5) At adolescence, physical and intellectual growth decelerates, except for the accelerating development of the sexual system.

B. According to the best of current knowledge, various emotional experiences seem to have certain effects on growth and development.

  (1) Evidence collected to date indicates that single or isolated traumatic events do not usually result in major or lasting effects on personality.

  (2) Excessive degrees of anxiety and insecurity experienced in connection with need satisfaction and training practices seem to result in the belief, as an adult, that people cannot be trusted.

  (3) Parental attitudes seem to have substantial influence on subsequent adult behavior.

   (a) The child who receives little affection, satisfaction of dependency needs, warmth and tenderness is likely to progress toward maturity more slowly, to experience more problems in adjustment, to be more apathetic and less able to exercise independent action, and to have a more slowly developed and less definite sense of self.

   (b) Rejection by parents seems to cause insecurity and self-devaluation.

    i. Rejection-induced insecurity and self-devaluation may result in hostile, negativistic, rebellious behavior.

    ii. Rejection-induced insecurity and self-devaluation may result in apathy, indifference and withdrawal from relationships in general.

    iii. Rejection-induced insecurity and self-devaluation may result in inability to give and receive affection freely.

   (c) Maternal overprotection seems to produce behavior that interferes with adult adaptation.

    i. Indulgent maternal overprotection may cause selfishness, egocentrism, irresponsibility and low frustration-tolerance levels.

    ii. Dominating maternal overprotection may cause submissiveness, obedience, inadequacy, lack of initiative and passive dependence.

(d) Excessively severe discipline may cause an overde-veloped need for social approval, feelings of self-con-demnation, displaced hostility from parents to society in general.

(e) Inconsistent or insufficient discipline may cause inade-quate development of self-control, vacillation in decision-making, inability to work within authority-led social institutions.

(f) Excessively strict moral standards may cause rigidity, guilt-producing conflicts, or generalized rebellion against moral restrictions.

(g) When parental demands for achievement are started early, and the rewards for achievement are in the form of parental affection rather than material objects, the child is more likely to develop strong and lasting drives toward achievement.

(h) Parental attitudes of consistent warmth and openness are more likely to help the child develop ability to relate to peers in a friendly, responsive way.

(i) Greater dependency needs may be experienced in both early and subsequent stages of development if parental attitudes are rejective, overly-rigid and restrictive dur-ing feeding and weaning phases of development.

(j) Parental imposition of independent behavior before the child is ready to move toward independence is likely to produce anxiety and overconcern regarding independence as an adult.

(4) Prolonged separation of the child from parents and home (as in hospitalization) produces different effects on differ-ent children, depending upon the child's age and his rela-tionship to his parents.

(a) Prolonged separation is more likely to produce emo-tional and intellectual retardation in development if the child is between three months and five years, than at other ages (e.g., less satisfactory peer or extra-family relationships, delayed ability to express or experience affection, slower speech and cognitive development).

(b) Up to the age of five, the child who has had a better and closer relationship with his mother seems to suffer most from prolonged separation.

(c) After the age of five, the child who has had a better and closer relationship with his mother seems to suffer less from separation (e.g., can tolerate it better).

C. Prevailing cultural attitudes may either impede or accelerate growth and development in several areas.

(1) For the adolescent, inconsistencies in social attitudes and demands may cause increased conflict, retarding adequate adjustment (e.g., society encourages the adolescent to accept adult attitudes and responsibilities, and at the same time, disapproves of any attempts at adult sexual behavior and independent life decisions).

(2) Identical child training practices favored by different cultures may have different effects on children (e.g., the particular practice seems to have less definite effect than the significance of the practice for the child—that is, his perception of what the practice means in terms of relationship to parents).

(3) Role diffusion in a complex society may cause inability to develop, without anxiety or conflict, a clear self-concept.
    (a) Conflict due to role diffusion may be particularly acute during adolescence, when the individual must identify and harmonize a variety of sociocultural roles to form a coherent self-identity.

(4) In order to live comfortably within sociocultural limits for behavior, the individual must have the opportunity to learn accepted roles, rules and codes of conduct.
    (a) One of the methods by which individuals learn sociocultural limits for behavior is through testing and exploring the environment to determine results of specific behaviors (i.e., "reality testing").
    (b) Individuals learn sociocultural limits for behavior through identification with others.
    (c) Individuals learn sociocultural limits for behavior by having authority figures impose and enforce the limits.
    (d) Personal definition and acceptance of a social role is learned through contact with the social environment in which the person has the opportunity to see and practice the designated role.

2. Psychological equilibrium requires that the individual have and be able to utilize the ability and opportunity for learning.
  A. Learning is influenced by a variety of internal and external factors.
    (1) Learning is most likely to be effective if the learner has the opportunity to try out the new behavior.
      (a) For task-involved learning to be effective, practice should include as many sense experiences as possible.
      (b) For ego-involved learning to be effective, practice should include behaviors that are motivated by goals, motives, interests and self-concept.

(2) Disturbing emotional factors may interfere with effective learning.

    (a) In extremely tense or traumatic situations, an individual may need frequent repetition of what is to be learned, or repeated successful experiences before learning can take place.

(3) A behavior that obtains an adequate response in one situation is likely to be repeated in similar situations.

    (a) Once a person has learned a response to a given situation, he tends to generalize that response to other situations (e.g., if the situation or certain parts of the situation are similar, the first response will be in accord with past learning).

    (b) When a behavior no longer obtains expected results, the behavior tends to disappear.

        i. An unreinforced behavior disappears slowly or rapidly, depending on the strength of the original stimulus and the amount of emotion involved in original learning.

(4) First impressions are likely to be the most lasting impressions, tending to shape or influence subsequent impressions.

(5) In complex learning, acquisition is more effective if separate parts of a whole are studied intensely, and later put together to form a whole made up of related parts.

(6) Acquisition of knowledge (memorization) is influenced by a variety of factors.

    (a) Boredom, fatigue, exaggerated emotional states and negative motivation decrease efficiency of acquiring knowledge.

    (b) Information encountered at the beginning and end of a learning period is more likely to be learned with ease than information encountered in the middle of a learning period.

    (c) Information that has meaning in the life context of the individual is more efficiently learned.

    (d) Acquisition of knowledge generally proceeds more rapidly if practice is distributed and spaced over time, rather than practice in long, uninterrupted sessions.

    (e) Active participation or motion by the learner assists the process of memorization (e.g., speaking, writing, moving objects, as opposed to reading alone).

    (f) Acquisition of knowledge is facilitated if material is grouped into meaningful units.

(7) The changing of concepts or perceptions may be facilitated

by the separation of parts from a whole for concentrated attention.

(8) The changing of concepts or perceptions may be facilitated by the addition of new information or experience that necessitates reinterpretation or reorganization of originally held concepts or perceptions.

(9) The learning of motor skills or cognitive skills is influenced by a variety of factors, including:

    (a) Repeated performance, necessary to the acquisition of a complicated motor skill.

    (b) The opportunity to practice many variations of the basic skill (e.g., concentrated repetition of a single aspect of a skill, or one basic variation of a skill, tends to limit future adaptation of the skill to different situations).

(10) What a person learns in a given situation depends upon what he perceives.

B. Retention of learning is influenced by a variety of factors.

(1) Retention of information or other learning is more stable if the original learning experience was efficient.

(2) Retention of learning is more stable if ego-involvement was high in the original learning (e.g., if learning was consistent with beliefs, values, ideals, or accompanied by high motivation).

(3) In general, recent learning tends to take precedence over remote learning, as far as recall of details is concerned.

C. Motivation is prerequisite to optimal learning.

(1) Learning is facilitated when an individual sees the relationship between what he is learning and his personal needs and problems.

(2) If an individual is able to recognize or experience for himself what he is able to do, learning is likely to be more effective.

(3) Comfort in the learning situation is increased if motivation for learning is positive (rewarding) rather than negative (punishing).

(4) Change in behavior may be motivated by the anticipation of desirable conditions that will result from the behavior.

D. Learning is influenced by the individual's stage of growth and development.

(1) Individual differences in maturation, experience, and constitutional capacity have a substantial influence on learning (e.g., what is learned, rate of learning).

(2) The acquisition of new behavior partially depends upon the individual's physiological and psychological readiness to learn.

    (a) Attempts to learn by going through learning steps (even when the individual is not yet "ready" to learn) may increase the speed of learning, because learning is itself a skill procedure.

    (b) Conversely, forced and repititious attempts to learn before the individual is physiologically or psychologically ready, may set up resistance to the future learning of a particular skill.

    (c) With advanced age, sensory abilities are less acute, and complex perceptual capacities are decreased, influencing the ability to learn and the efficiency of learning.

    (d) It is believed that older people may have more difficulty in learning new tasks because they interfere with the security of long-practiced habitual patterns.

       i. Older people will be aided in learning new skills if these skills are related to or incorporated in well-established habit patterns.

3. Psychological equilibrium is directly influenced by the ability to adapt to a variety of life situations, which involves both conscious and unconscious problem-solving processes.

    (Note: As with growth and development, most of the material related to adaptive behavior has been incorporated in other chapters—particularly Chap. 7 and 8. The following statements are mostly generalizations relevant to creative problem-solving.)

    A. Creative problem-solving usually runs an erratic course, including changes and shifts in perception and discontinuity of conscious effort.

    B. Ego-involvement tends to increase the amount of effort sustained in problem-solving activities.

    C. Problem-solving is influenced by the individual's ability to utilize imagery (e.g., the more ability a person has for vivid mental imagery, the more likely he is to "see" relationships and to visualize alternatives without having to experiment with actual materials).

    D. The way in which a problem is presented may determine the way in which it is solved (e.g., initial presentation may provide a perceptual "set" that directs thinking, either promoting or preventing possible alternatives.)

    E. Successful problem-solving requires a fund of previously acquired knowledge and/or experience.

    F. Previous problem-solving patterns may interfere with new approaches to current problems.

       (1) Problem-solving tends to be more difficult when solutions require the application of the familiar in an unfamiliar way.

       (2) When a given solution to a problem has been learned to be

associated with a specific situation, the individual will have
more difficulty in adapting that solution to other situations.

(3) Preconceptions and previously learned concepts, or ways
of relating concepts, tend to limit novel interpretations of
data and creative solutions to problems.

(4) If previous learning has been generalized and/or abstract,
it is less likely to inhibit new approaches to problem solutions (e.g., if learning has been in the form of specific
procedures or formulas, it will be less useful in creative
problem-solving).

G. A person who cannot tolerate ambiguity will have more difficulty with creative problem-solving.

(1) The more rigid the person is, the less he can tolerate
"unknowns" and unexplained phenomena (e.g., he will tend
to generalize or categorize too quickly, to organize material
with insufficient data, or to draw hasty conclusions in order
to have the problem "solved").

(2) The more rigid the person is, the more he tends to avoid
new and novel ideas and interpretations of data and untried
solutions that might fail.

(3) A person who is otherwise flexible, but who is currently
under unusual threat or discontinuity of life-style, may
react with greater rigidity in problem-solving situations
than would be usual for him.

H. Highly creative problem-solving, although dependent upon adequate levels of intelligence and a fund of knowledge and experience, equally depends upon certain personality characteristics.

(1) The individual who is secure in his self-concept, who is less
dependent upon authority and more independent in arriving at decisions and judgments, who is less likely to perceive
situations in predetermined ways and has a sense of humor,
usually demonstrates a better ability to arrive at creative
solutions to problems.

(2) The more creative person tends to be less afraid of being
wrong or of being criticized for his problem solutions.

(3) In general, the person who demonstrates creative ability
tends to show more evidence of psychological well-being
than the less creative person.

NURSING CARE

The nurse can increase her knowledge and understanding of processes of growth and development, learning and adaptive problem-
solving in order to accomplish optimal nursing care. For example:

1. A nurse can make observations of the patient and his environment
in order to determine:

A. The patient's growth and development level, particularly when he is a very young child.
B. Any apparent problems or incongruities in the growth and development process.
C. Individual learning needs necessitated by illness and/or hospitalization.
D. Individual problems requiring adaptive problem-solving.
E. Environmental or circumstantial influences that may interfere with growth and development, learning and/or adaptive problem-solving.
F. Child-parent relationship patterns that will influence growth and development, learning and problem-solving.

2. A nurse should plan nursing care in accord with both her knowledge of processes, and her observations of the patient and his environment. She can:
   A. Gear expectations for behavior of the individual (child, adolescent, adult and older adult) to his particular level of development, including allowance for regression during stressful illness and/or hospitalization.
   B. Prevent or avoid situations that would increase negative effects on growth and development of the child or adolescent. For example, she can:
      (1) Plan nursing intervention to avoid increasing anxiety and insecurity in relation to need satisfaction and training practices.
      (2) Avoid demonstrating attitudes that the child might interpret as rejective.
      (3) Provide, if possible, sources of counsel for parents who demonstrate nonconstructive or actually destructive attitudes and childrearing practices.
      (4) Avoid open conflict (in front of the child) with parents regarding differences in beliefs and attitudes regarding childrearing practices and attitudes.
      (5) Avoid judgmental behavior toward parents regarding childrearing practices based on inadequate data or superficial observations (e.g., if any specific practice differs in result from culture to culture, or subculture to subculture, the practice itself may not be detrimental).
      (6) Avoid the exaggeration of conflict for the adolescent (e.g., allow maximum desired autonomy consistent with safety without making demands for performance based on the nurse's preconceived expectations for behavior).
      (7) Avoid punitive or rejective attitudes when the adolescent attempts to test social attitudes and role behaviors, providing a rational, nonjudgmental and reasoned sounding-board

for testing ideas and behaviors (e.g., provide a climate accepting adolescent inconsistencies in behavior, which vary from childlike to adult behaviors while under stress).

C. Plan nursing interventions in accord with growth and development principles relative to other aspects of behavior. (See other Chapters, such as 1, 2, 3, etc.)

3. The nurse should plan nursing care in accord with both her knowledge of learning principles and of the individual patient, his circumstances, needs for learning and environmental influences on learning. (See Principles, No. 2. These are explicit enough to be directly applicable, provided the situation has been adequately analysed).

4. The nurse should plan and implement nursing actions that promote adaptive problem-solving whenever possible, or that prevent interference with adaptive problem-solving. She can:

A. Increase supportive behavior for the patient who is faced with problems to be solved under stress.

B. Avoid excessive demands for problem-solving by the patient under extreme stress.

C. Avoid any interference with the patient's adaptive problem-solving efforts by remaining nonjudgmental, patient and non-rejecting of novel solutions that might not have occurred to her (e.g., the patient is most likely to find solutions suitable to his total life situation, regardless of how desirable other solutions may seem to the nurse, who has different life circumstances).

D. Assist the patient less likely to see alternative solutions to visualize possibilities (e.g., if the patient lacks needed information or has been restricted to narrow ranges of choice, discussion with informed but supportive persons may help increase possible alternative solutions).

E. Organize the presentation of problems in such a way as to maximize use of previous experience and minimize problems associated with previous learning (e.g., present problem in a novel way if previous learning will interfere; relate problem to past experience if relationship will promote problem-solving).

F. Present problems in such a way as to draw on maximum motivation and ego-involvement.

5. The nurse can utilize principles of learning to guide the development of her own professional and personal competence.

6. The nurse can utilize principles of learning and of adaptive problem-solving to guide leadership activities and interactions with auxiliary staff for improvement of patient care.

7

Primary and Acquired Needs

There are some psychological and psychosocial needs that may be considered common to all people, for which there must be some degree of satisfaction if the individual is to maintain psychological or psychosocial equilibrium.

SOCIAL SCIENCE PRINCIPLES

1. In order to achieve and maintain psychological equilibrium, man must have satisfying relationships with other human beings, both individually and in groups.
   A. The feeling of being cared for or about by another person or persons is necessary for psychological homeostasis.
      (1) The attitudes and actions of others that indicate that the individual is worthy of attention, assistance or concern, contribute to a feeling of being cared for or about.
      (2) The physical presence of those who are affectionally close reassures the individual that he is cared for.
   B. The awarness that one is not alone is basic to psychological homeostasis. The feeling of aloneness is decreased by:
      (1) The sharing of experiences with others.
      (2) The knowledge that one's behavior, experiences or feeling are not unique, but are common to or shared by others.
      (3) Effective interaction and communication with other individuals.
      (4) The feeling that one is understood by others.
   C. The approval of others in one's sociocultural environment is necessary for the psychological homeostasis of the average person.
      (1) Approval from others may be elicited by contributing valued actions, materials or beliefs, or otherwise by conforming to group standards.
      (2) A feeling of being approved by others is achieved by being regarded or reacted to with positive, as opposed to negative,

attitudes. The value of the attitude is determined by the culture in which one lives.

(3) A feeling of being approved by others is increased if one's presence or participation in social groups is sought.

(4) Assurance of approval by others is achieved by conforming to social conventions established for interpersonal relationships.

D. Acceptance by others of one's self and one's individual differences is necessary for psychological homeostasis for the average person.

E. In order to experience satisfying relationships with others, the average individual must be able to feel that he will not be harmed as a result of the relationship.

(1) If an individual experiences a feeling of acceptance and esteem in relation to other individuals or groups of individuals, he is better able to tolerate criticism or correction with a minimum of discomfort.

(2) In general, opportunities for satisfying relationships with others are increased if the individual is able to see others as trustworthy and capable.

(a) Trust and confidence in others is acquired through experiences in which the individual is not harmed, or by which he has benefited.

(b) Trust and confidence in others is enhanced by the demonstration of concern and interest of others in the individual's welfare.

(3) An individual who is suspicious, fearful or distrustful of others may be threatened by interpersonal relations, and may be unable to experience security and satisfaction in group relations until fear is decreased.

(4) Individuals who are threatened by interpersonal relations may be able to achieve satisfaction and comfort in group relations by learning through experience that they will not be harmed in such situations.

F. The achievement of satisfying relationships with others is influenced by the psychobiological structure and function of the organism. These factors include the following:

(1) Perceptual ability and learned patterns of perception, which involves:

(a) Perception of one's own role and the role of others in relationships.

(b) The ability to examine and evaluate one's own behavior in relation to others.

(c) The ability to perceive oneself correctly; of knowing one's own capabilities and limitations.

(2) Self-concept and ego-function.
   (a) Positive self-esteem contributes to the achievement of satisfactory relationships with others.
   (b) The ability to accept one's self and one's own capabilities and limitations contributes to the achievement of satisfactory relationships with others.
   (c) Any mutilation or basic change in body structure will influence the individual's concept of himself and his relationships with others.
(3) The ability to communicate effectively.
(4) Behavior in relation to thinking patterns, attitudes, opinions and beliefs.
(5) Ability to experience and appropriately control emotion.
G. The achievement of satisfying relationships with others is influenced by sociocultural factors.
   (1) If satisfactory interpersonal relationships are to be achieved and maintained, there must be a mutual recognition of culturally established roles, with behavior appropriate to those roles. (See Chap. 9.)
   (2) In every society or culture there are established rules and codes of conduct to which the individual must adhere, in order to be approved and accepted by others. (See Chap. 9.)
   (3) In order to live comfortably within a given sociocultural structure, an individual must have the ability and opportunity to learn the accepted roles, rules and codes of conduct. (See Chap. 6.)
   (4) A single individual may function satisfactorily in a variety of roles.
   (5) An individual is likely to respond to others in a social situation in a manner similar to the one by which he is approached.
2. The achievement and maintenance of psychological equilibrium is enhanced if the individual has a sense of self-esteem.
A. Satisfying relationships with others are necessary to the development and maintenance of self-esteem.
B. The development and the maintenance of self-esteem depend upon one's ability to function in accordance with the internalized standards, beliefs and values that have been acquired from the sociocultural environment.
   (1) In our culture, self-direction and independent action are highly valued forms of behavior.
   (2) In some cultures, maintenance of individuality is necessary for a sense of self-esteem.
   (3) A sense of self-esteem may be increased or decreased, depending upon one's identification with a particular socio-

cultural group and the status of that group within the total social structure.

C. Repeated failures tend to decrease self-esteem and foster development of the expectation that one will fail or be inadequate.

3. In order to achieve and maintain psychological equilibrium, the individual must have an adequate means of self-definition and situational definition (i.e., he must know, to his own satisfaction, who he is, where he is, and what his goals are).

A. A sense of personal identity may be enhanced by the recognition (by oneself and others) of the person's individuality in relation to others.

B. Adequate personal and situational definition requires a knowledge and understanding of what the individual perceives to be the facts about himself and the situation.

  (1) Knowledge of the facts about a situation requires adequate perception of factors in the situation.

  (2) In addition to factual knowledge about a situation, an individual may be helped to achieve an adequate personal and situational definition through beliefs and convictions. (For some individuals, a belief in a supreme being or deity provides a means of personal and situational definition.)

C. Adequate self-definition is partially achieved through identification with and sharing of experiences with other individuals and groups of individuals.

D. Adequate personal and situational definition requires clarity of perception of one's role and status in relation to others.

E. Adequate situational definition requires that the individual be aware of the behavioral limits in a situation.

F. Development and maintenance of an adequate personal and situational definition requires the establishment of familiar and consistent sociocultural patterns.

G. For some individuals, the possession of material objects provides a symbolic means of identification.

4. In order to establish and maintain psychological equilibrium, the average individual attempts to achieve a feeling of safety and comfort in life situations.

A. A feeling of safety and comfort is engendered if the individual feels he is able to cope with life situations sucessfully (i.e., control the situation and himself in such a way as to prevent harm).

  (1) The ability to handle life situations in a socially approved manner requires a knowledge of and ability to act within the sociocultural limits of the situation.

  (2) The ability to handle life situations with success is most probable when there is a clear perception of the factors inherent to each situation, including the goal to be reached.

(a) One of the factors contributing to the clarity of perception of a situation is the possession of factual knowledge.

(b) Clarity of perception is increased if one is able to identify one's own feelings, attitudes, limitations and capabilities.

(c) Clarity of perception may require the opportunity to experience the actual situation, in addition to or rather than hearing a verbal description of the situation.

(d) Clarity of perception may be increased by verbal exploration of the situation in the presence of an informed and supportive person.

(e) Inconsistency, confusion and multiplicity of demands may contribute to a lack of clarity of perception.

(3) An individual is more likely to achieve a feeling of comfort and safety in coping with life situations if he has an understanding of action to be taken, and possesses the skills and abilities necessary for the action.

(a) Security in life situations is likely to be increased as the individual gains more experience (skill) in coping with specific situations or variations of a situation.

(b) The acquisition of skills necessary for successful action requires the opportunity for adequate learning experiences.

(4) For some individuals, or in some situations, a feeling of comfort and safety requires that the individual maintain control of himself and the situation, regardless of the actual necessity for such control.

(a) Most individuals in our culture experience anxiety if deprived of the opportunity or right to make decisions regarding self and personal property.

(b) Frustration of one's efforts toward a specific goal constitutes loss of control over the situation.

(c) Dependence upon others imposed by illness constitutes loss of control.

(d) For some individuals a feeling of comfort and safety is achieved through controlling or manipulating the environment and the people in it, above and beyond self-control.

(5) A feeling of comfort and safety in handling life situations may be achieved by the establishment of familiar routines, behavior patterns and environmental circumstances which have been previously experienced as safe and comfortable.

(a) A feeling of comfort and safety in coping with life situations is enhanced if the individual has had previous similar experiences in which he has not been harmed.

(b) Any interference with or change in normal physiological and/or psychological functioning is likely to cause psychological disequilibrium, because: it may be perceived as a threat to life; it may require new, unknown patterns of behavior; unknown consequences may be feared.

(c) Illness or hospitalization disrupts previously established behavior patterns.

(6) A feeling of safety and comfort in a specific situation may be increased by positive preparation before the situation occurs, which may include:

(a) Increasing one's knowledge about the event.

(b) Changing one's perception of the event. (See Chap. 1.)

(c) Verbalization about the event in the presence of a supportive person.

(d) The opportunity for vicarious successful experiences, through discussion with someone who has lived through the event successfully.

(e) An opportunity to learn skills that will be needed for mastery of the situation.

(7) Disturbances of physiological or psychosocial equilibrium that result in exaggerated emotional reactions or mental dysfunction decrease the individual's ability to cope successfully with life situations.

(a) Internal and external confusion interferes with an individual's control of his own behavior.

(b) In extremely threatening situations, an individual may need constant repetition of successful experiences before tension can be decreased sufficiently to allow successful coping with a situation.

(c) A high degree of apprehension may interfere with the ability to successfully cope with a situation.

(d) Clarity, simplicity and lack of threat in the way others approach a confused person facilitates cooperation between the confused person and others in the environment, and gives the feeling of comfort and safety to the confused person.

B. A feeling of comfort and safety in a situation may be increased by identification with others who have experienced the situation without harm.

C. Comfort and safety in a situation may be increased by the possession of material objects that symbolically represent safety and comfort.

D. A feeling of comfort and safety may be achieved through relationships with others.

(1) A feeling of comfort and safety may be achieved through feeling able to depend upon and/or cooperate with others.

(a) Cooperation between individuals depends upon adequate communication between the individuals involved.

(b) In a situation where the individual must depend upon others, a feeling of safety and comfort is based on the assurance that help is available for the satisfaction of basic needs of self and dependents.

(c) An individual may be helped to feel safe and comfortable in a dependent situation if he receives a positive interpretation of on-going events. (The feeling of safety and comfort is further increased if the positive interpretation is unsolicited.)

(d) The achievement of a feeling of comfort and safety through dependence upon or cooperation with others requires that the individual be able to trust and have confidence in others.

Confidence in others is likely to be increased if:

i. The individual receives assurance that important matters pertaining to self will be considered confidential.

ii. The individual is assured that others are competent to carry out tasks assigned or entrusted to them.

iii. The individual is assured that others have a genuine concern for the health and welfare of persons dependent upon them.

iv. There is consistency of attitude and behavior demonstrated by those on whom the individual must depend.

v. An individual has had repeated experiences involving trustworthy and honest people.

vi. The suspicious or doubtful person receives a realistic interpretation and encouragement from someone outside the situation whom he trusts.

(e) The person who is suspicious, doubtful or fearful will react with increased suspicion and fear if others in the environment show doubt and lack of control.

(2) A feeling of comfort and safety may be achieved through mutually sharing responsibility with others whom one trusts or for whom one cares.

(a) The inclusion of an individual's family in a situation may increase the feeling of safety and comfort by the sharing of responsibility within the family group.

(b) In a threatening situation, an individual may receive the greatest support from a member of the family or from some individual with whom a close affectional bond exists.

(3) A feeling of safety and comfort may be achieved through relationships with others who realistically indicate that the individual will not be harmed or allowed to come to harm.

  (a) Psychological support and assistance may be given through the attitudes and behaviors of others in the situation.

   i. The suspicious, doubtful or fearful individual can frequently be helped to feel safe and comfortable in a situation if others are, or appear to be, calm, self-assured and in control of the situation.

   ii. An attitude of objectivity on the part of others in a situation may help the individual to feel safe and comfortable.

   iii. In some situations, setting limits or giving firm directions will be helpful in assisting a person to feel safe, comfortable and competent.

   iv. A feeling of comfort and safety may be enhanced by the presence of a warm, understanding person.

   v. Realistically based approval and the encouragement of others contributes to one's feeling of safety and comfort in a situation.

   vi. An individual's feeling of security may be increased if he is made to feel welcome in strange or unfamiliar surroundings.

   vii. Physical care procedures may be used as a means of giving emotional support, and may help in the establishment of positive interpersonal relations.

  (b) Actions by others, motivated by the anticipation of an individual's needs, tend to increase one's feeling of safety and comfort.

  (c) If an individual experiences a feeling of acceptance and esteem in relation to other individuals, he will be better able to tolerate criticism, correction or guidance from those individuals with a minimum of discomfort.

(4) A feeling of comfort and safety in life situations requires that the individual experience a feeling of approval and acceptance by others.

(5) For most individuals a feeling of comfort and safety in life situations requires that the individual experience a feeling of relatedness to others.

E. The ability to communicate one's needs is prerequisite to a feeling of safety and comfort.

    F. A feeling of safety and comfort may be achieved through religious beliefs and practices.

    G. A feeling of safety and comfort requires the absence of threat to the life and integrity of the organism.

       (1) The presence of persons who are in ill health or who are diseased may constitute a threat to the life of other individuals, either through fear of contracting the illness or through the symbolic implications the illness may have.

       (2) The presence of hostility in the environment may have implications of potential danger.

       (3) Any interference with or change in normal physiological and/or psychological function is usually perceived as a threat to the life or integrity of the organism.

       (4) Any use of physical force by one person upon another may constitute (symbolically or realistically) a threat to the integrity or life of the organism.

       (5) Illness and hospitalization realistically or symbolically imply an existing or potential threat to the life and integrity of the organism.

       (6) The presence of dead or dying persons in the environment usually produces anxiety, particularly if the individual is himself in a state of impaired health.

5. Above and beyond basic or primary needs and the most strongly inculcated secondary or acquired needs, man seems to be motivated toward "self-actualization" (e.g., he demonstrates drives in the direction of adaptation, reproduction, creative invention, growth toward whatever potential he may have).

    A. The individual tends to seek new experiences, to explore environmental or personal possibilities, and to know and understand that which is not necessary to merely survive comfortably.

6. Above and beyond basic or primary needs and the most strongly inculcated secondary or acquired needs, man seems to be motivated toward seeking stimulation and novelty.

    A. The individual exhibits interest in mental and physical exercise and stimulation (e.g., he shows interest in puzzles and problems, games requiring physical and mental challenge, and other activities that are experienced as pleasurable above and beyond mere necessity).

    B. The individual tends to respond to novel or changing stimuli as opposed to familiar stimuli.

    C. The individual tends to spend energy seeking varieties of experience, even in relation to otherwise satisfactory situations.

7. Above and beyond basic or primary needs and the most strongly inculcated secondary or acquired needs, man seems to be motivated toward activities that are experienced purely as pleasurable, including that which is referred to as aesthetic appreciation.

  A. The individual who is provided with (or able to acquire) a reasonable amount of purely pleasurable experience, tends to exhibit a more positive outlook on life in general and is better able to tolerate necessary unpleasant experiences.

8. The needs of an individual at a given time vary according to internal and external factors, such as the following:

  A. The constitutional and life-experience altered nature of the organism.

  B. Membership in a specific sociocultural group.

  C. Past experiences, particularly those associated with growth and development.

  D. Current life situations:

    (1) Illness or hospitalization disturbs the individual's total pattern of need satisfaction.

    (2) Certain needs of the individual are intensified by physical illness.

    (3) Certain needs of the individual are more difficult to satisfy if he is physically ill or hospitalized, and the frustration of needs adds to the problems of adjustment to illness and/or hospitalization.

    (4) Inherent in illness or hospitalization are potentially traumatic elements or problem situations, to which the individual must make some form of adaptation.

    (5) At any given time, those needs which are most intense take priority over those creating less tension. Those needs most closely related to actual survival and to survival of ego-integrity usually take precedence over other needs.

    (6) All human needs are interrelated; a disturbance in one area of function causes reactions in other areas of function.

      (a) Persistent lack of satisfaction of psychological needs appears to be correlated with physiological reactions, and vice versa.

      (b) Psychological comfort and well-being are partially dependent upon physiological comfort and well-being, and vice versa.

  E. A behavior that obtains an adequate response (reduces a need) in one situation tends to be repeated in similar situations.

NURSING CARE

To plan for and implement therapeutic nursing interventions effectively, the nurse can use her knowledge of primary and acquired needs.

(Note: As with the chapter on learning, unnecessary reiteration of each principle has been avoided. The following statements are examples directing the nurse's attention back to science content.)

1. The nurse should increase her knowledge and understanding of

human needs and their relationship to physiological and psychological equilibrium.

2. The nurse can guide her observation of patients, in order to determine:

   A. Needs the patient may be experiencing but which he cannot satisfy by independent action under circumstances of illness and/or hospitalization.

   B. Factors in the environment that are actually or potentially interfering with need satisfaction.

   C. Evidences of unusual need states (e.g., behavior that might indicate chronic unmet needs for acceptance and approval or satisfying relationships with others).

   D. Individual patterns of and preferences for behavior and activities that satisfy specific needs.

   E. Evidences that frustration of need satisfying behaviors not specifically related to illness and/or hospitalization is interfering with therapy goals.

3. The nurse can use both her understanding of the function of human needs as they relate to total equilibrium and her observations of the patient to plan individual patient care. For example, she will use basic principles regarding needs and need satisfaction to:

   A. Plan care to increase the patient's feeling of being genuinely cared for, particularly by those upon whom he must depend.

   B. Organize care to prevent exaggeration of feelings of aloneness.

   C. Demonstrate attitudes of approval and acceptance.

   D. Regulate her relationships with patients to increase the feeling of comfort, safety and satisfaction in the relationship, thus allowing the patient to make maximum use of the relationship for therapeutic purposes.

   E. Adapt nursing care to accommodate the individual patient's abilities and limitations in relation to need satisfaction.

   F. Avoid activities that tend to decrease or disturb the patient's stable concept of self and his self-esteem; increase activities that foster the development of a stable and constructive concept of self and maintenance of self-esteem.

   G. Provide opportunities for adequate situational and self-definition by patients under her jurisdiction; encourage others involved in patient care to do likewise.

   H. Avoid activities that increase fear regarding safety, integrity and discomfort, and plan activities that increase feelings of safety and comfort.

   I. Use her knowledge of need as a motivation for behavior to effect therapeutic goals (e.g., present necessary but unpleasant therapy procedures or desired activities in such a way as to capitalize on need motivation).

J. Devise comprehensive plans for care that include satisfaction of the individual's need for self-actualization, stimulation and pleasurable experiences.
4. Examine, evaluate and regulate her behavior in relation to her own needs and methods of need satisfaction, in order to avoid nontherapeutic activities while implementing patient care.

8

Disturbances of Equilibrium

The human so organizes and integrates his world as to prevent destruction or disruption of function. He develops elaborate systems of behavior (thinking, feeling and acting) to preserve ego-integrity and thus his ability to cope successfully. Severe disturbances of equilibrium may result in noticeably deviant and/or nonconstructive behavior systems.

SOCIAL SCIENCE PRINCIPLES

1. Frustration of efforts toward goals evokes a number of responses.
   A. Moderate or tolerable frustration may have a constructive effect.
      (1) Tolerable frustration serves to intensify goal-directed behavior.
      (2) Successful efforts to eliminate frustration-creating barriers tends to increase one's sense of adequacy and ability to cope.
      (3) Tolerable frustration tends to focus attention and organize problem-solving behavior.
   B. Intolerable and/or continuous frustration may have destructive effects.
      (1) Continuous failure to remove frustration-creating barriers tends to cause a sense of inadequacy and failure.
      (2) Ambiguous frustration (when the barrier is unidentified) tends to cause diffuse or random reactions, generally unsuccessful.
      (3) Continuous frustration usually leads to anxiety. (See No. 3.)
   C. Objectified frustration-creating barriers (causes outside of self) tend to provoke less anxiety than barriers arising internally.
   D. Frustration accompanied by punishment tends to produce rigid, nonadaptive behavior, which may endure as a chronic reaction when the frustration-creating barrier no longer exists.

316

E. When goal-directed behavior is accompanied by or results in inconsistent reward or punishment, neurotic behavior may result.

F. When goal-directed behavior is accompanied by both reward and punishment at the same time, neurotic behavior may result.

2. Psychological equilibrium requires the development of and ability to utilize psychological mechanisms for warding off anxiety and for adapting adequately to life situations.

A. Any disturbance of psychological equilibrium causes a primary reaction of anxiety, fear, apprehension or tension.

(1) Anxiety is commonly accompanied by physical reactions, such as tremor, loss of appetite, perspiration, sleeplessness, increased pulse rate, and so forth.

(2) Gross or continuous anxiety may be accompanied by disturbances of physiological function, such as endocrine system changes, alterations of autonomic nervous system responses, or circulatory system reactions.

(3) Some forms of behavior are nonspecific indications of threats to psychological equilibrium, the causes of which must be determined by further investigation.

(a) Attempts to manipulate or control the external environment (in excess of control necessary for safety) may be an indication of an individual's attempt to dissipate or alleviate anxiety.

(b) An individual may rely on hostility, dependence or withdrawal as methods for handling anxiety-producing and/or problematic situations.

(c) Regressive behavior is a common reaction to threatening situations.

(d) An attitude of suspicion, doubt or mistrust may be an indication of underlying anxiety or insecurity.

(e) Excessive demands for attention may indicate psychological disequilibrium.

(f) Excessive complaints or dissatisfaction in a situation may be an indication of underlying anxiety.

(g) Hostility may be a general indication of threats to ego-integrity, frustration or emotional stress.

(h) Withdrawal may be a general indication of frustration, traumatic experiences in interpersonal relations or threats to ego-integrity.

(i) Illness and/or physical symptoms may be used as a method of gaining attention, responding to a crisis situation, or expressing unconscious feeling or conflict.

(j) Activities that are primarily used to meet physical needs (e.g., eating) may be used as a symbolic means for attain-

ing emotional satisfaction, resolving unconscious problems or relieving general tension.

(k) Atypical or, to the observer, unexpected behavior may
indicate disequilibrium in some area of the organism's
function.

(l) Continuous states of anxiety, even though unconscious,
may result in physiological pathology because of the
effect on nervous system function (e.g., ulcers, hypertension).

(4) Some forms of behavior are more specific indications of
psychological disequilibrium, leading to easier determination
of the specific cause.

(a) An individual who is threatened by interpersonal situations tends to withdraw from social interaction in order
to prevent or avoid greater psychological discomfort.

(b) An individual who is in a state of gross disequilibrium
is more likely to experience an exaggerated emotional
response to minor environmental disturbances than an
individual whose equilibrium is relatively stable.

(c) An individual experiences feelings of inferiority or
inadequacy if he is unable to live up to personal or
social expectations.

(d) An abrupt change of subject usually indicates an area
that is either emotionally charged or that the individual
is fearful of exposing.

(e) Undesirable forms of behavior often indicate an individual's need for and attempts to obtain a positive response
from others.

B. Any given activity or adaptive mechanism may be considered
normal or healthy in one situation, and abnormal or unhealthy
in another, depending upon circumstances and cultural definition.

C. Adaptive mechanisms are not usually consciously selected, but
occur as a result of growth and development experiences.

(1) In general, there are no specific mechanisms for specific situations; the individual "selects" the mechanisms best adapted
to his situation and his general pattern of adaptation.

(2) Adaptive mechanisms, when not used to excess, have constructive benefits.

(a) Adaptive mechanisms decrease or alleviate anxiety, leaving ego-integrity intact.

(b) With anxiety under control, the individual is able to live
with conflict or threat while he seeks realistic solutions
to his problems.

(c) Creative and/or socially constructive work may result
from the use of some mechanisms.

(d) Excessive use of mechanisms to avoid anxiety or frustration may prevent the development of the ability for constructive problem-solving.

(3) A number of adaptive (defensive) mechanisms have been identified and described.

(a) Negativism: A person who fears loss of individual identity or loss of autonomy may react continuously and automatically with counter-suggestions or negative responses, even when the suggestion is in accord with his best interests or his own original beliefs and ideas.

(b) Displacement: If the original object of a feeling, thought or action is seen as too powerful or socially disapproved of as an object, or if the real object is unconsciously obscured, a person may direct the feeling, thought or action toward another (permissible) object.

(c) Somatization and Conversion: A person's ideas and convictions can cause him to experience subjective physiological symptoms where no physiological pathology can be demonstrated. Unconscious conflicts may give rise to physical manifestations, such as functional paralysis or blindness.

(d) Projection: Unpleasant or anxiety-producing impulses may be avoided by literally transferring such impulses, ideas, feelings or actions to others. Such cognitive distortion leaves the person unaware of the trait in himself, thus keeping free of anxiety, guilt or shame.

(e) Identification and Incorporation: The process of seeing oneself as similar to or like another, or of idealizing another and wishing to emulate, has several functions. (a) Identification may help a person to successfully relate to others without anxiety. (b) Identification is extensively used in learning one's role and function in life situations. (c) Identification can be used to dilute the intensity of one's own guilt or negative reactions by providing an acceptable climate for his reactions. (d) Identification is extensively used to reduce feelings of loneliness and isolation. (e) The incorporation of ideas, attitudes and attributes of others may reduce the threat of others, provide a way of "possessing" others, or help to retain a sense of autonomy while conforming.

(f) Rationalization: When a given thought, feeling or action is seen as unacceptable, cognitive distortion of facts may occur to allow acceptable reasons for the thought, feeling or action. Two forms of rationalization are "sour grapes" and "pollyanna." One constructive side-effect of rationalization may be the production of new or original perceptions of situations not ordinarily stimulated by nonthreatening situations.

(g) Insulation and Isolation: When two or more ideas, feelings, attitudes or necessary actions are conflicting, a person may separate them into logic-tight compartments without recognizing their discrepancy. One form of insulation is "intellectualization"—the process of separating emotion from ideational content, as though the understanding of an event strips it of any threat to the person. Another form is the attributing of feelings and thought to ambiguous "others," thus separating self from responsibility. This mechanism helps other mechanisms, such as projection, repression and fantasy, to be effective.

(h) Repression: Undesirable, unpleasant or painful thoughts, feelings or experiences may be completely erased from consciousness, unamenable to conscious recall, but still functioning as motivating forces or energy.

(i) Reaction-formation: Unacceptable impulses, ideas, feelings or desired actions may be first repressed, then transformed into actions in direct opposition to the original. This form of denial of the original impulse tends to result in exaggerations of behavior beyond what is reasonable for the circumstances.

(j) Fantasy and Autism: A person who cannot cope with reality because of threats to self-esteem or ego-integrity may withdraw from actual situations, substituting ego-enhancing and self-defensive fantasy. Fantasy may also be self-destructive in nature if the individual is experiencing guilt. Fantasy and autism may provide substitute satisfaction through wish-fulfilling imagery. Fantasy may be constructive if it leads to the creation of original approaches to problem situations.

(k) Compensation and Over-compensation; Substitution and Sublimation: An individual who experiences a sense of inadequacy may overcome the inadequacy by directly concentrating on the development of a specific skill (compensation), or by over-developing a particular ability (over-compensation). An individual who experiences inadequacy in one area or frustration of impulse or desire in one area may develop compensatory skill in a substitute area (substitution), or dissipate energy through some activity that has social approbation or significance (sublimation). Thus, ego-integrity is maintained, guilt and inadequacy are avoided, and satisfaction is experienced.

3. The removal, destruction or weakening of an individual's psychological defenses against anxiety by external forces or circumstances
   causes an increase in the anxiety experienced by the person and an
   intensification of his attempts to restore equilibrium.
   A. When defenses are threatened and tension increases, aggressive
      outbursts may serve to decrease tension and allow the person to
      direct his energy toward rational problem-solving or strengthen-
      ing the defenses.
   B. When defenses are threatened, the individual usually demon-
      strates over-actions and exaggerations of emotion rather than
      flexible attempts to use rational problem-solving.
   C. When defenses are threatened by anxiety-producing situations,
      distraction of attention may temporarily relieve the anxiety or
      allow the person to direct energy toward rational problem-solving.
   D. When defenses are threatened, the individual experiences a
      decreased ability to tolerate ambiguity.
   E. If adaptive mechanisms are unsuccessful, personality or ego-
      disorganization may result.
      (1) Disorganization or disintegration of the ego is manifested by
          such general behaviors as incoherence of thought and com-
          munication, confusion, random and unrelated ideation,
          inability to adapt or to cope with situations, lack of control
          of behavior and emotion, illogical and irrational behavior,
          emotional agitation and exaggerated outbursts, loss of sense
          of self or ego-identity.
      (2) Impending disorganization or disintegration of the ego may
          result in the development of patterns of behavior aimed at
          controlling the anxiety, but which leave the individual
          unable to participate normally in society (e.g., severe neurotic
          and psychotic behavior patterns, such as conversion reactions,
          schizophrenic reactions, hypo- or hyper-reactive states).
      (3) Impending disorganization or disintegration of the ego may
          result in the development of patterns of behavior that control
          the anxiety temporarily and allow the person to retain
          appearance of rational control, but are destructive in nature
          (e.g., alcohol and drug addiction, sociopathic behavior).

NURSING CARE

The nurse can be of therapeutic assistance to the patient if she has a
knowledge of principles related to disturbances of equilibrium. For
example:
1. The nurse should increase her knowledge and understanding of
   processes relative to preventing disturbances of equilibrium and
   attempting to restore threatened integrity.
2. The nurse can guide her observations of the patient in order to
   determine:

    A. Evidence of intolerable frustration, anxiety, defenses against anxiety and threats to adaptive defenses.

    B. The individual patient's particular behavior patterns for controlling threats to integrity.

    C. Environmental or circumstantial factors that would be likely to threaten ego-integrity or disrupt adaptive defenses.

    D. Evidence of ego or personality disorganization and/or psychotic and neurotic behavior patterns.

3. The nurse should use her knowledge and her observations as a guide to planning constructive patient care. She can:

    A. Introduce or allow only that amount of frustration that would serve as positive motivation for problem-solving.

    B. Attempt to eliminate or control intolerable amounts of frustration.

    C. In working with children, avoid use of punishment and inconsistent reward in relation to patient behavior directed toward need or goal satisfaction.

    D. Avoid destruction of the patient's consistently used adaptive mechanisms.

    E. Provide for the relief of uncomfortable or painful symptoms associated with anxiety.

    F. Assist the patient to use rational and flexible problem-solving methods of adaptation whenever possible.

    G. Provide substitute behavior or mechanisms to control anxiety whenever a particular mechanism must be interfered with or disrupted.

    H. Avoid criticism, rejection, punishment or negative attitudes and judgments when the patient uses adaptive behaviors which she personally sees as undesirable.

    I. Provide external control when patient behavior indicates disorganization of personality or behavior that will be dangerous to himself or others.

    J. Support or strengthen constructive mechanisms, and assist the patient to develop constructive mechanisms when development of mechanisms is necessitated by situations under her jurisdiction.

    K. Attempt to control the situation (including her own behavior), in order to prevent increasing threats to integrity or equilibrium.

    L. Seek consultation as necessary for herself in planning nursing interventions and for the patient when patient behavior indicates uncontrollable or intolerable anxiety, nonconstructive adaptive mechanisms used to excess, and impending or actual personality disorganization.

4. The nurse should examine and evaluate her own use of adaptive mechanisms in order to provide the patient with healthy examples for behavior and to avoid nontherapeutic nursing actions.

5. Record and report evidences of disequilibrium that may require medical intervention.

9

Sociocultural Influences on Behavior

Social and cultural institutions exist as a result of the needs of man (individually and collectively) and are maintained for the preservation of man's psychosocial and psychobiological equilibrium. The individual tends to seek satisfaction of his needs within his culture, through the channels that that culture has established for satisfaction of individual needs.

SOCIAL SCIENCE PRINCIPLES

1. The society or culture in which an individual lives, grows and develops helps to determine the ways in which his needs are met and the direction some of his acquired needs will take. A culture may provide alternative ways of satisfying a specific human need.
   A. Socialization takes place more rapidly in the process of growth and development if socializing agencies (home, school, peer groups) are consistent and in accord with one another.
   B. If there is a wide discrepancy or conflict between the socializing agencies, the individual tends to completely renounce one agency in favor of the other, renounce both agencies, or exhibit maladaptive behavior.
2. Man, as a social animal, tends to seek approval and acceptance by society. He is required to behave in a prescribed manner, within given limits, in order to be approved or accepted.
   A. In the process of growth and development, many cultural values become internalized to the extent that they are no longer regarded as sociocultural requirements, but experienced as subjective ideas, attitudes, beliefs and needs.
   B. Social role and socially acceptable behavior is learned through contact with the environment in which the individual is given the opportunity to see and practice the designated role.
   C. Any given activity may be considered normal, healthy or permis-

323

sible in one situation, and abnormal, unhealthy or unacceptable in another situation, depending upon cultural definition.

D. Every society or culture has established rules and codes of conduct governing major aspects of social interaction.

(1) Cultures differ in their conduct requirements regarding relationships of members of the same sex and members of the opposite sex. For example, physical exposure, even when necessitated by illness or hospitalization, in the presence of a member of the opposite sex is not condoned except under specific circumstances. In some subcultures, physical exposure is not permitted in any case.

(2) Cultures differ in their requirements of conduct regarding roles of authoritative, subordinate and peer positions.

(a) Every known society demonstrates some form of behavioral differentiation regarding status or dominance role positions and activities.

(b) In our culture, doctors are usually seen in a role of authority.

(c) In our culture, authority figures are usually regarded with respect, awe, sometimes fear, frequently suspicion and resentment.

(3) Every known culture has some culturally organized form of behavior associated with religion.

(a) The importance of religious beliefs and practices tends to be increased during times of stress and/or uncertainty.

(4) Societies having more than one racial and/or religious group will have some systematized codes for behavior regarding role, status and intergroup relations between the groups. In addition, subgroups within the society as a whole develop additional customs, attitudes and practices regarding race and religious differences.

(a) In a society where there are multiple racial and religious groups, satisfactory interpersonal relationships may be interfered with because of preconceived ideas, misconceptions, and lack of knowledge of one group for another.

(b) Individuals who belong to minority or fringe groups within a society usually experience some feeling of insecurity or inadequacy by reason of belonging to a group that is not accepted as part of the major group.

(c) Behavior resulting from stereotyped prejudice is more likely to decrease when members of ethnic groups interact on a personal basis of equality, while sharing a common task or activity that does not emphasize ethnic differences.

(5) Every society or culture has established rules and codes of

conduct governing the roles and relationships of family members.

   (a) In every society, certain types of parental behavior in childrearing practices are either condoned or disapproved.

(6) In every society or culture, there are established rules and codes of conduct governing voluntary physiological functions and physical appearance.

   (a) In our culture, the control of eliminative processes and associated procedures is governed by comparatively rigid standards.

   (b) In our culture in general, physical cleanliness and a neat appearance are socially approved attributes.

   (c) Some subgroups within our culture place less emphasis on physical cleanliness and neat appearance.

(7) In every society or culture there are established customs and beliefs governing attitudes and behaviors regarding illness and death.

   (a) In some cultures, attendance at the bedside of a dying person by specified other individuals is socially approved or mandatory.

   (b) In every culture, there are some physical conditions, states of health or disease processes that have negative connotations.

   (c) Every organized religion has specific attitudes, beliefs and ritual practices associated with death.

(8) Every society or culture places positive or negative value on certain general attitudes, ideas, beliefs and their attendant actions, and gives or withholds approval of the individual according to how he conforms to those standards.

   Generally speaking, in our culture:

   (a) Personal adequacy in handling problems, independence and self-control are highly valued attributes.

   (b) Self-direction and independent action are considered basic human rights.

   (c) Any action that is perceived by the individual as a threat to independence or freedom (right to select action by free choice) is most likely to be resented and/or resisted.

   (d) Respect and consideration are considered basic human rights.

   In some cultures and subcultures:

   (a) Personal privacy is highly valued.

   (b) The suppression of overt hostility is required.

   (c) Individual possession, ownership and subsequent disposal of material objects has significance and is governed by customs and laws.

(d) Expression of emotion before strangers and/or demonstration of pain or unhappiness is disapproved.

(9) In the development of the above culturally determined attitudes, ideas, beliefs and practices, some that originally arose from a basic need have attained a significance sufficient to guide behavior even though the original need may no longer exist.

3. Changes in a society or culture may cause diverse reactions.

A. When social changes are perceived by the individual or group as threatening to traditional values, change will be resisted, or the individual or group will experience disequilibrium and/or disorganization.

B. When social changes occur slowly, or are seen as related to other existing values, there is less resistance, disorganization or disequilibrium.

C. When social change is attempted by an agent, there will be more conflict and resistance if the communication between members of the society and the agent effecting the change is inadequate.

D. When social change is caused by rapid industrialization, there may be a number of predictable results.

(1) Family relationships may be disrupted because of changes in social roles of family members.

(2) The individual may experience increased tension if the social change necessitates an increase in the number of social roles for which he has not been adequately prepared.

(3) Possibilities for social mobility increases, furthering the disruption of family relationships and individual uncertainty and tension.

4. Every known society has some system of establishing membership in social class; mobility between classes is usually governed by certain rules or codes, and such mobility may result in a variety of reactions.

A. In societies with a designated lower class, the motivation to move upward (improve standard of living) seems to be less among members of the lowest possible class or classes.

B. An individual learns, in the process of growth and development, to identify himself with a given social class and to conform to the practices peculiar to that class.

C. In our culture, lower class members tend to accept physical and psychological suffering with resignation and less motivation to eliminate or avoid such suffering.

D. Parents of lower class children tend to discourage more than minimal education.

E. Childrearing practices tend to differ from social class to social class within a society.

   (1) In our culture, lower class parents tend to be more authoritarian, use more physical punishment and less reasoning, provide less supervision, permit greater ranges of expression of feeling, permit less freedom of interaction between parents and children, and put less stress on achievement.

   (2) In our culture, middle class parents tend to place more importance on publicized "popular practices" in childrearing, be less authoritarian but more concerned about conformity to social standards, permit greater freedom of interaction between parents and children but less freedom of expressions of emotion and more stress on achievement.

   (3) When parents change social class (move upward in social placement), they tend to exhibit greater tension, strictness, and demands on conformity to class behaviors in childrearing practices.

F. Sudden or rapid shifts in social class membership tends to increase the general insecurity of family members because of uncertainty about how to behave in multiple new social roles.

G. In our culture, members of the middle class tend to place greater importance on joining and being active in organizations; there is less motivation for such activity among members of the lower class.

H. In our culture, members of the lower class tend to have a narrower range of interests and activities, not including hobbies or aesthetic experiences, than do members of the middle and upper classes.

NURSING CARE

The nurse can organize and implement nursing care in accord with sociocultural requirements for behavior. For example:

1. The nurse should increase her knowledge of the influence of sociocultural requirements on behavior in general, her knowledge of the cultures and subcultures to which her patients might belong.

2. The nurse can guide her observations of the patient and his environment to determine:

   A. Evidences of the patient's identification with any specific sociocultural group or groups.

   B. Evidences of the intensity of the patient's need to adhere to specific socioculturally determined behavior or codes of conduct, even though health requirements might indicate a departure from that behavior or code of conduct.

   C. Patient behavior that indicates conflict between social role requirements of different groups to which the patient might belong.

    D. Environmental influences or circumstances that might put the patient in a position of conflict with socioculturally determined values and practices (i.e., be a source of tension, embarrasment, loss of self-esteem).

    E. Experiences necessitated by illness and/or hospitalization that will be difficult for the patient to adjust to, because of previously acquired sociocultural attitudes or codes of conduct.

    F. Ways in which the patient's membership in sociocultural groups influence health practices and adaptation to altered states of health.

    G. Evidences of difficulty in learning necessary role behavior in relation to group membership.

    H. Indications that the patient is confused, uncertain or insecure about role expectations while in the hospital.

3. The nurse should utilize her knowledge and her observations to plan and implement nursing interventions for optimal physiological and psychological well-being. She can, for example:

    A. Avoid conflict whenever possible between the patient's established socioculturally determined requirements for behavior and the requirements of health agencies (e.g., arrange for required dietary practices, religious practices, the maintenance of family interaction patterns).

    B. Avoid disruption of the patient's identification with sociocultural groups, unless such identification is obviously detrimental to health and well-being (e.g., avoid demonstrating rejective attitudes, such as criticism, belittling or disgust when the patient demonstrates attitudes not in accord with the nurse's group identification).

    C. Provide the patient with the opportunity to practice sociocultural roles, when the learning of those roles is necessary for psychological equilibrium (e.g., in child care, promote the practice of behavior consistent with future role behavior).

    D. Avoid placing patients in close proximity to other patients if such proximity will arouse negative feelings and tension (e.g., if the patient retains strong prejudice regarding some racial or religious group).

    E. If prejudice or stereotyped reactions are detrimental to health and well-being, provide experiences to help decrease and eliminate such prejudice or stereotyping.

    F. Avoid placing the patient in distressing or embarrassing positions relative to socioculturally acquired behaviors (e.g., avoid physical exposure, provide privacy for eliminative functions and the expression of emotion, if these are in accord with the patient's expectations for behavior).

G. Provide the patient with clear definitions of expected role behavior *as a patient*, whenever role requirements differ from his usual practices or whenever role requirements are unfamiliar to the patient.

H. Avoid hasty stereotyping of patients upon superficial observations.

I. Avoid pressuring patients to conform to a certain sociocultural role behavior, simply because the nurse favors those roles by virtue of her own identification.

4. The nurse should examine and evaluate her own sociocultural identification, role behavior, and expectations in order to avoid nontherapeutic nursing actions.

10

Small Group Behavior

Within organized groups, certain phenomena have been observed to occur predictably.

SOCIAL SCIENCE PRINCIPLES

1. In the development of any group, if it is in association long enough, there occurs a differentiation of social roles of individual members.
   A. Eventually, if none is appointed by external influences, a leader will emerge who will be perceived by the group as the person most likely to further group goals.
      (1) The particular member selected as leader depends on predominant personality types in the group, capabilities existing among members of the group, and the group goal.
         (a) A group in which authoritarian personalities predominate will tend to select a strong, directive leader.
         (b) Groups in which low-intelligence members predominate will tend to reject a leader of high intelligence.
         (c) In less formal groups not requiring designated leadership, leadership may tend to rotate, depending on the activity at any given time.
      (2) Leaders of groups functioning under a higher authority (such as individual hospital unit groups under nursing service administration authority) tend to experience greater conflict because of conflicting perceptions of what constitutes "good" leadership (e.g., higher authority has one set of expectations of the leader, and group members have another set of expectations).
      (3) In democratic cultures, there tends to be a general suspicion and resentment of leadership dominance.
      (4) "Authoritarian" leadership (where leader directs but remains somewhat apart from membership in general) tends to produce group behavior that is:
         (a) Either more aggressive or more apathetic than "democratic" leadership groups. The aggression is usually directed outward toward other groups or toward scape-

goats in the group, but not at the group leader directly.
  (b) Demanding of attention from the leader.
  (c) Disruptive and non-productive when the leader is absent
      or does not assign tasks.
  (d) Indicative of lower group morale.
(5) "Democratic" leadership (where action arises as a result of
    group discussion and decision with the leader fully partici-
    pating) tends to produce group behavior that is:
  (a) Less demanding of attention from the leader.
  (b) Productively active in solving problems when the leader
      is absent or does not assign tasks.
  (c) More supportive of group members in general, with less
      nonspecific aggressiveness and little need of scapegoats.
  (d) Indicative of higher group morale.
2. In addition to the type of leadership, group morale, motivation and
   interaction is influenced by a number of factors.
   A. If group morale is low in general, the group tends to disintegrate
      under stress (e.g., form antagonistic subgroups; openly and subtly
      demonstrate hostility toward each other and the leader; be unable
      to concentrate on problem-solving or productive activity).
   B. If group members are predominantly individually competitive,
      group action tends to be less consistently productive.
   C. If group members are predominantly oriented toward coopera-
      tion, group action tends to be more consistently productive.
   D. If group members, including the leader, are predominantly inter-
      ested in instigating innovations, differences or original adapta-
      tions, group action tends to be more consistently creative and
      productive in solving problems.
   E. If group members, including the leader, are predominantly rigid,
      rejecting newness, differences and untried ideas, group action
      tends to maintain the status quo, or to look for ready-made solu-
      tions to problems.
   F. Individual and group morale is enhanced when there is a clear
      perception of the goal to be reached and the steps necessary to
      reach that goal. Demoralization results when ambiguity or con-
      fusion are excessive.
   G. When group interaction under conditions of equality are in-
      creased, individual members tend to increase shared values and
      norms, and to like each other better, thus raising the level of
      morale and group unity.
   H. Group morale tends to be higher when group membership is
      stable.
     (1) Stable groups tend to reject the introduction of new mem-
         bers, with rejective behavior increasing in proportion to the
         number of new members introduced.

I. The less communication and interaction between related but separate groups, the greater the tendency toward conflict between those groups.

J. When small group actions are imposed from outside, there tends to be less development of norms by the group; when actions of the group are determined through group discussion, there tends to be the creation of ideal goals, with higher motivation to work toward those goals.

K. Group motivation toward changing goals or activities will be higher if potential changes are discussed freely in the group rather than imposed from outside or by an authoritarian leader.

L. Group activity is more likely to be stimulated if group effort produces demonstrably valuable results (i.e., if there is realization of accomplishment).

M. Effective group action is influenced by a number of environmental and practical considerations.

   (1) Noise, interruptions, distracting movements and visual stimuli, and physical discomfort decrease group efficiency.

   (2) Physical proximity and the position of members in relation to each other influence group interaction and efficiency (e.g., group interaction tends to be less effective if distance or position makes hearing difficult, if members are not facing each other, if members are crowded together in a small space, if the leader sits apart from the group).

   (3) The environment for meetings of small groups can be arranged for conduciveness to goal-directed activity (e.g., if writing or written materials are required, tables with materials can be present when members enter; if group action consists primarily of discussion, chair arrangement can suggest conversation and distracting materials can be removed).

   (4) Group members are likely to be irritated and thus less productive if prearranged meetings begin and end later than anticipated.

   (5) Effective group action is likely to be decreased if prearranged meetings coincide with other activities that members perceive as more important than group goals.

3. The actions of an individual within a group are influenced by a variety of factors.

A. In face-to-face group actions, the opinions, behavior, verbal and nonverbal expressions and prestige of each individual member will affect all members.

B. The reaction of group members (feedback) to an individual influences his subsequent behavior.

C. An individual who perceives himself as a member of a group (or desiring to be recognized as a member of a group) will have a stronger motivation to conform to group pressure than to deviate from it.

(1) Within a group, an individual member will be more likely to retain individuality (demonstrate independent thinking and resist group pressure to conform when his own ideas and attitudes are not consistent with the group) if he has certain characteristics, such as:

    (a) A higher than average level of intelligence.

    (b) A predominantly original or creative approach to personal problem-solving.

    (c) A high level of self-confidence and freedom from anxiety.

    (d) A tendency to approach other people and events with tolerance, responsibility and comfort in relationships.

    (e) An absence of such characteristics as passivity, dependence, and vagueness or instability in perception of self.

(2) Conformity or nonconformity to group pressure is influenced by:

    (a) The individual's perception of the group and the group's position in the total cultural structure.

    (b) The nature of the problem to be solved or task to be accomplished.

    (c) The strength of the individual member's own convictions and what he foresees as the results of conforming or nonconforming actions.

    (d) Rewarding or punishing actions of the group toward conforming and nonconforming behavior (e.g., the group will provide support, reinforcement, security, encouragement, protection and rationale for behavior that is acceptable to the group, and will provide punishment for deviant behavior by ridicule, dislike, shame and threat of expulsion).

(3) An individual who cannot tolerate authority tends to be a nonconformist in group behavior at all times, rather than only when his ideas conflict with group ideas (i.e., he tends to automatically reject group suggestion or pressure to conform, even when the desired behavior is in accord with his own original convictions).

4. Groups tend to stay in existence and to be consistently of benefit to individual members and to the purpose for which the group was formed, if certain conditions exist.

    A. A basic factor in the continued existence of a group is that the interaction of group members continues to satisfy the desires and needs of its members.

    B. Effective communication among group members is prerequisite to effective interaction and group continuity.

C. Effective group action requires that members be mutually compatible, or that individual members be able to control behavior to avoid disruption (e.g., occasionally a group will be unable to function effectively unless a disrupting member is removed).

D. Cooperation and effective group action are facilitated if individual members feel mutual trust and good will.

E. Efforts to reach a given goal are more likely to be stimulated if individual members and the group as a whole feel that their efforts are appreciated or that they are contributing something of value.

F. Group stability is greater and interaction increased if members experience a sense of unity or cohesiveness. Conversely, group stability is decreased and interaction is less when there is dissention and/or individual competitiveness.

G. Group stability and effectiveness tends to increase when group activities are consistent with both necessary task goals and personal goals of individual members.

H. When an individual member of a group feels threatened by either group activities or other members of the group, that member will be less effective, tending to decrease the effectiveness of the group as a whole.

I. In task-oriented groups, a certain amount of personal-social discussion and interaction tends to relieve tension produced by task-oriented discussion, and allows the group to return to work with greater comfort.

NURSING CARE

The orientation of this book has been toward basic sciences and their application to basic nursing care. There has been no attempt to include material appropriate to nursing specialization, such as, for example, psychiatric nursing. The chapter on small group behavior is therefore kept within the limits of appropriateness for actions of the average first-level nurse, and does not pretend to include principles relative to psychotherapeutic patient groups. Rather, the content of this chapter includes statements about behavior important to the nurse as she participates in work or professional groups.

The average nurse finds it necessary to actively participate in an increasing number of work-related groups. She almost certainly will be required to act as "team leader" in planning, organizing and implementing direct patient care. She will probably be required to serve on task-oriented committees, such as procedure or policy committees, and she will most likely participate in in-service education discussion groups. It is to be hoped that she will also belong to and be active in professional organizations and serve on committees for those organizations.

She may also be called upon to work with community agency groups interested in various aspects of health promotion.

The principle statements in this section are applicable to nursing action in groups of the type described. Nursing care implications for this chapter have not been outlined in the same manner as for other chapters, since these nursing actions are not directly related to individual patient care. The student or graduate nurse reader can find ready application of principle statements through observation and analysis of groups encountered in daily experience. For example, can the reader, in remembering the last daily nursing care planning conference, evaluate the environment and the interaction to determine either interferences with group effectiveness or factors which increased group efficiency? Can she, by reviewing principle statements, think of ways in which the meeting could have been made more conducive to effective action?

Part IV

Potential Usefulness of the Science and Nursing Material for Nursing Educators

During the process of developing the science content and nursing care presented in Parts II and III, and during the study of teaching and evaluation methods in the first three years of the Commonwealth Project, a number of ideas emerged about how the material could be of value to other instructors of nursing or, possibly, to science teachers who work with nursing students. One of the most exciting features of identifying the important science and related nursing care was the imagination shown by persons who participated in the original study in considering various ways in which this material might be utilized in teaching.

Although we offer the following suggestions, it is hoped and expected that instructors will discover many other helpful functions for the material contained in Parts II and III. In the discussion that follows, natural and social sciences have been separated to some extent to allow for differences in content, and combined to some extent because both underlie comprehensive nursing care.

For the sake of organization and readability, the authors have selected in this section a recognized method of curriculum development as an outline for content. The method advocates the following:

1. Definition of objectives, including content and behavior.
2. Planning of learning experiences to attain these objectives.
3. Selection and organization of learning experiences.
4. Evaluation of attainment of the objectives.

DEFINITION OF OBJECTIVES

It sounds ridiculously simple to say that one major objective of any nursing curriculum has to do with the ability to perform effectively the nursing care of patients. But finding an answer to the automatically

337

implied question "What is effective nursing care?" is anything but simple. Nowhere in nursing literature does there exist a comprehensive, universally agreed upon—and simple—statement that defines nursing or its effectiveness at various levels of practice. An attempt to answer this question leads naturally to a qualitative analysis of nursing care—an analysis that takes into consideration the major aspects of nursing, as well as the means for accomplishing nursing care to the desired end of patient well-being.

Because the life of an individual depends upon the maintenance of a constant internal environment (physiologic homeostasis), and because in disease that internal environment is threatened and/or changed, the maintenance and the restoration of homeostasis are primary nursing goals. Similarly, the well-being and adequate adjustment of man to life situations depends upon the maintenance of psychosocial homeostasis. Because illness and hospitalization, whether due primarily to a disturbance of physiologic function or not, disturb the total pattern of the individual's satisfaction of psychosocial needs, the nurse must be concerned with the maintenance and the restoration of psychosocial homeostasis. The analysis of the nursing care of patients in terms of requirements of physiologic homeostasis is essentially the material found in Part II. Part III contains statements of nursing action related to the identified social science facts, principles and hypotheses that have direct bearing on the achievement and maintenance of psychosocial homeostasis. If the statements of nursing care in these two sections actually do present major aspects of nursing care, one should be able to use them in the process of defining objectives—objectives related to: (1) providing physical and psychosocial comfort; (2) providing essentials of life, such as oxygen, fluid balance and emotional security; (3) providing protection from traumatic chemical, physical, microbial or psychological injury; and (4) providing for the observation of deviations from normal physiologic and psychosocial function and the appropriate communication of these deviations to other members of the health team.

It has been pointed out that completely-stated student objectives contain two essential components: some indication of the behavior that is desired on the part of the nurse, and some indication of an area of knowledge to which that behavior is related. Objectives concerned with the physical and psychosocial nursing care of patients can be stated readily in this manner. Following are two examples of the development of unit objectives. In the examples, a major objective was identified and analyzed to ascertain specific objectives inherent in it.

NATURAL SCIENCE: MAJOR OBJECTIVE

To perform nursing care that serves to maintain the body temperature within a normal range.

Preliminary Analysis

1. To be able to make observations of signs and symptoms of abnormal body temperature.
2. To be able to communicate effectively with other members of the health team relative to the signs and symptoms of abnormal body temperature.
3. To be able to perform specific nursing activities to:
    A. Measure the body temperature.
    B. Lower an elevated body temperature.
    C. Elevate a low body temperature.

Continued Analysis

1. To understand normal regulation of body temperature (heat production, heat loss, physiologic temperature-regulating mechanisms).
2. To understand possible causes of deviation in body temperatures (disease conditions that may affect heat loss, heat production, or the temperature-regulating mechanisms).
3. To understand observable body responses to abnormal body temperature (e.g., peripheral vasoconstriction or vasodilatation, changes in heart action, chills and fever, sweating, delirium, convulsions, loss of consciousness).
4. To be able to recognize signs and symptoms associated with abnormal body temperature and to understand when patients should be observed especially closely for those signs and symptoms.
5. To be able to apply scientific knowledge in:
    A. Using equipment for measuring the body temperature.
    B. Adjustment of external environment conditions.
    C. Adjustment of insulating materials.
    D. Adjustment of physical activities.
    E. Application of external heat.
    F. Removal of body heat.
    G. Administration of drugs to lower body temperature.
6. To be able to report and record appropriately information about body temperature.

It will be noted that the major objective involves an essential factor of homeostasis; namely, that "there is a definite temperature range for efficient cellular functioning and proper enzymatic activity." The science and nursing applications related to this requirement of homeostasis can be found in Part II, Chapter 9.

SOCIAL SCIENCE: MAJOR OBJECTIVE

To take action that will assist the patient to acquire or maintain the approval of others, or to prevent disapproval from others, in his sociocultural environment.

Preliminary Analysis
1. To make observations regarding:
   A. Patient behavior that indicates that he receives adequate approval from others.
   B. Patient behavior that indicates a disturbance of psychological equilibrium due to lack of approval or to disapproval.
   C. Patient behavior that demonstrates the patient's attempts to acquire approval in satisfactory or unsatisfactory ways.
   D. Patient behavior that might cause disapproval or lack of approval.
   E. Factors in the patient's life situation that influence the receiving or withholding of approval or the demonstration of approval.
2. To analyze and interpret the observed data to determine:
   A. The relative satisfaction or dissatisfaction of the patient's need for approval in his current life situation.
   B. The sources of disturbance or interference with the satisfaction of the patient's need for approval.
   C. The necessity and/or feasibility of nursing action to help the patient satisfy his need for approval in his current life situation.
   D. The extent of nursing responsibility in assisting the patient toward satisfaction of his need for approval.
   E. The necessity and/or feasibility of referring the patient to other sources of assistance.
3. To take specific nursing action aimed at:
   A. Removing, eliminating or changing factors in the current situation that cause the patient to feel disapproval or lack of approval.
   B. Providing an environment and/or experiences that will contribute to the patient's feeling of being approved.
   C. Providing the patient with psychological support as he works through adjustive problems relative to receiving approval or avoiding disapproval.
   D. Helping the patient to change behavior that interferes with receiving approval or causes disapproval.
4. To communicate with other members of the health team regarding:
   A. Patient behavior that indicates a disturbance of psychological equilibrium due to lack of approval or to disapproval from others and the causes of the disturbance.
   B. A plan of care that will assist the patient in the satisfaction of his need of approval.

Continued Analysis
1. An understanding of and ability to recognize human behavior that indicates a state of psychological disequilibrium due to lack of approval or to disapproval from others in one's sociocultural environment.
2. An understanding of the dynamics of human behavior relative to the satisfaction of this particular need.

3. An understanding of the relationship between psychological equilibrium and physiologic homeostasis, as demonstrated by lack of satisfaction of this need.

4. An understanding of the sociocultural influences on the satisfaction of this need in general and in specific situations.

5. An understanding of personality growth and development patterns that influence the satisfaction of this need.

6. An understanding of and ability to function within the nursing role in the satisfaction of this need.

7. A knowledge of additional sources of assistance in satisfying the patient's need and how to utilize these sources when necessary.

8. An understanding of and ability to apply sociopsychological principles in establishing an environment that will:

   A. Eliminate or reduce sources of disapproval.

   B. Provide or encourage opportunities for the patient to receive approval from others.

   C. Provide the patient with psychological support and encouragement when he is working through potentially traumatic problems relative to approval or disapproval.

   D. Assist the patient to learn new behaviors or modify behaviors that will contribute to a feeling of approval or the elimination of disapproval.

It will be noted that the major objective involves one of the subconcepts relative to psychosocial homeostasis: "The approval of others in one's sociocultural environment is necessary for psychosocial homeostasis." The nursing care and underlying principles related to this subconcept can be found in Part III, Chapter 7.

In each of the primary analyses of the above examples, major skills (observational, technical and communicative) involved in the nursing care were identified along with a general description of the nursing content. The more specific objectives stated in the continued analyses not only include reference to these major skills, but also contain some degree of information about the knowledge that underlies the effective performance of these skills, and a more complete description of nursing activities involved in attaining the major objective.

The skills, the knowledge and the specific nursing activities included in the foregoing examples are either stated or implied in the material contained in Parts II and III. It can be seen that this material does not provide complete and final answers to the questions of *what* skills and *what* knowledge should be taught to nursing students. It does, however, provide a basis for determining some of the behaviors and some of the knowledge toward which clinical nursing instructors should be guiding their students. Other objectives similar to those presented here can be identified from the analysis of the natural and social science material.

PLANNING LEARNING EXPERIENCES

The determination of possible learning experiences that could be developed to attain desired objectives stems quite naturally from a careful examination of the objectives. If understanding is involved, the nursing student must have access through such media as lectures, laboratory sessions, informal discussions, textbooks and guided observations of the facts that are essential to the understanding. The same is true if the objective concerns the application of scientific knowledge. The student should be given an opportunity to learn the science material before or during the teaching of the nursing care that involves the application of that material.

The scientific content identified in this study as being important for a nurse to understand and be able to apply can be used as a partial answer to the question of which science should be taught. Identification of additional facts can be accomplished through the analysis of specific observational and technical skills involved in physical nursing care, and through the analysis of specific diagnostic tests and therapeutic procedures in which the nurse participates or which she should be able to interpret. Additional facts also can be identified through the analysis of specific patient problems in the area of social and psychological adjustment, when such problems are encountered in the nurse-patient situation.

The ability to observe signs and symptoms, the ability to apply facts and principles of science in the performance of nursing care, and the ability to perform tasks with some degree of manual dexterity can be developed only through practice. This implies that one responsibility of the clinical instructor is the planning of student experiences so that problems involving these skills are provided. Discussion of teaching methods for the development of knowledge and skills is not within the scope of this book. However, some general considerations of the selection and organization of learning experiences utilizing the identified science material and associated nursing care is included.

One type of decision facing every clinical instructor in nursing concerns the choice of patients for students to care for during clinical practice. There are many factors to be taken into consideration in this selection process, as for example: the individual learning needs of each student; the theoretical preparation of the student; and the need for new learning pertaining to a particular type of nursing problem. Now that the trend in nursing education is toward decreasing the time that students spend in the bedside practice of patient care and increasing the depth of any single experience, this selection process has become increasingly significant. The use of more effective teaching methods, with emphasis upon specific, selected learning goals, has shown that it is possible to shorten the length of time a student devotes to clinical experiences. The objectives for such learning experiences must be clearly defined, and the experiences themselves must be carefully planned. Following are some examples of how the principles contained in Parts II and III can be used in the identification, selection and organization of learning experiences.

Natural Sciences

The nursing applications contained in Part II can be helpful in the selection of patients for the purpose of teaching physical nursing care. At the beginning of each nursing section (with the exception of Chap. 20) there is a list of specific kinds of physical conditions that may result in problems related to the body functions or requirements under consideration (e.g., adequate oxygen, adequate nutrition, fluid balance, sensory processes). For instance, upon examining conditions that may interfere with an adequate oxygen supply, it will be noted that patients with many different conditions are likely to have problems in this area; these patients can provide good learning experiences for students. The instructor might select a patient who is unconscious, or one who has a lung tumor, pneumonia, asthma, ascites or a patent ductus arteriosus. Which patient the instructor selects should be decided not only on the basis of the type of respiratory problem involved, but also on the basis of any other problems that the patient has, and how well the student is prepared in the nursing care of patients with these other problems.

The care of a patient with an acute, uncomplicated attack of bronchial asthma probably would involve positioning and the administration of certain types of drugs, and possibly oxygen. The care of a patient with pneumonia might involve the administration of antibiotic drugs and oxygen, special positioning, isolation techniques and the management of fever. The care of a patient with ascites might involve special positioning, the administration of specific drugs, various nutritional problems, problems of fluid and electrolyte balance, and assisting a doctor with a paracentesis.

Obviously, the more problems a patient has the more complex the nursing care becomes. The more serious the problems are, in terms of the immediate requirements of life (e.g., maintenance of an adequate oxygen supply, maintenance of the volume and pressure of circulating blood within certain limits), the more demanding the nursing care and, usually, the more complex. The more a patient depends upon others for meeting basic needs, such as elimination and locomotion, the greater the demands for nursing care.

Would it be good judgement to have a beginning student care for a patient with a severe head injury? The patient may well have problems that involve circulation, respiration, nutrition, fluid balance, acid-base balance, temperature regulation, elimination, motor and sensory functions as well as his mental faculties. In the same vein, how fruitful would it be, for the purpose of learning physical nursing care, to have a student nearing graduation care for a patient who was having an uneventful convalescence following uncomplicated minor surgery?

The science material presented in Part II can be used in nursing studies. Bruno[1] has experimented with a method for determining levels of complexity in nursing care as revealed by the analysis of nursing care into specific activities and the scientific knowledge involved in them. In her study she chose two functional areas of nursing care: the positioning of patients and providing for their physical activities. Bruno divided the nursing care and related science into different categories determined by the extent to which a patient was able to meet his own needs for positioning and physical activity. The degree of complexity of nursing care was considered to be indicated by: (1) the number of nursing activities involved in achieving certain goals relative to positioning and physical activity; and (2) the amount of scientific knowledge that was basic to the effective performance of those nursing activities. Some of the material contained in Part II was used by Bruno in the course of the study.

Social Sciences

For several reasons, the social sciences as applied to general nursing practice are less amenable to consistent selection and organization of learning experiences than the natural sciences. With the exception of neuropsychiatric or psychiatric illness, the patient's primary presenting problem is physiologic in nature, so that at all times, in health agencies used for teaching, one can find problems relative to the material outlined in Part II. Since the patient asks for help with his physiologic problems, the diagnosis or identification of the problem area is made by the physician, and the nursing instructor can locate patients who will provide suitable experience for learning physical care at all levels of complexity. Although every patient has some psychosocial disturbance by virtue of being a totally reacting organism, the nature and the severity of the disturbance varies with each individual patient, regardless of his presenting problem. This does not encourage the use of a predetermined organizational pattern for the selection of learning experiences according to major psychosocial needs. Furthermore, identification of the patient's problems in this area, being secondary to his presenting complaint, is not a part of the formal diagnosis; and such identification occurs, if at all, during the ensuing process of physical nursing care. Unless the problem is outstanding, the identification of such problems

[1] Bruno, Pauline: A Determination and Examination of Nursing Measures and Related Science Principles Which Pertain to Positioning of Patients and Providing for their Physical Activities. (Unpublished post-Masters research investigation supported by a Research Fellowship [NF-7641] from the Division of Nursing Resources of the Public Health Service.) Univ. Washington, 1958.

usually is left to the discretion of the nurse and seldom receives medical attention or orders for care.

In some ways, the selection of learning experiences in the social science areas is helped rather than hindered by these factors. If we can assume that all patients have some degree of disturbance of psychosocial equilibrium as a result of physical illness and hospitalization, then we also can assume that every patient can provide the student with an opportunity to learn and to apply social science principles. If this is so, the instructor's problem is not so much one of selection and organization, but of identification and effective utilization of constant opportunity and careful guidance of the student in successive learning experiences. The successive experiences provide natural opportunity for increasing the depth of understanding and the skill in meeting problem situations concerning the patient's psychosocial adjustment.

The authors believe that, where patients are concerned, it is impossible to avoid *potential* learning experiences at all levels of complexity involving social science principles, regardless of the rationale for the selection and organization of learning experiences. It is in the failure of the instructor to recognize and utilize experiences that we encounter an uneconomical use of student learning time and capabilities. For example, let us consider the patient's need for satisfying relationships with others. Whatever the patient's reason for seeking medical care, his need for satisfying relationships is not left at home. He will, if he is hospitalized, experience some feeling of separation, of being alone. Unless health team members make attempts to prevent it, or unless it can be achieved through good physical care, he will feel uncared for. Because he is in an environment that includes many other people, usually strangers, he will have an increased need for the acceptance and approval of those people upon whom he must depend for his continued health and well-being. Since every patient has had different growth and development experiences, each demonstrates individual differences in the way he attempts to meet these needs; and since every patient is a member of some sociocultural group, his behavior indicates the influence of his particular group in meeting these needs. Further, the patient is in a new social situation where he has to learn the roles and functions of those around him, and how he fits into the social structure of hospital life.

Unless the instructor deliberately avoided patients who demonstrated intensified, chronic or exaggerated needs in these areas, the law of averages would make it impossible for the student not to encounter patients who demonstrate a range from highly satisfactory to acutely unsatisfactory relationships with others. The only problem in the deliberate selection of experiences for learning increasingly complex psychological nursing care is encountered when there are extreme degrees of psychosocial need. If the student is only beginning to learn the principles involved in, for example, helping the patient to achieve and maintain satisfying relationships with others, it is easy enough to avoid assignment to patients whose disturbances in this area are so great as to cause behavior that deviates widely from normal. Such experiences can be planned for later in the program, when the student may be assigned to a psychiatric unit, in which the patient's presenting problem is in this area. Similar examples could be given for all of the identified social science material in Part III. The crucial factor in guiding the student's learning of skill in applying social science principles is in the instructor's recognition of constant opportunity and in her deliberate plans to capitalize on natural resources. It seems quite reasonable to say that learning under such circumstances would be most effective, because it would help the student to recognize the interdependence of all aspects of human function, regardless of the specific acute problems.

If the instructor feels that it is necessary to have an organized outline or plan, she could utilize the identified principles to formulate a check list for herself, together with a more formalized plan for teaching according to the kinds of problems that students are most likely to encounter at various stages in their growth and development as nursing students. For example, the young student encounters her first problem in human relations when she meets a patient face to face and must communicate with him both for purposes of observation and comfort for herself and the patient. Emphasis on learning in this first experience, together with formal classes or ward conferences, might well be directed toward acquiring a beginning skill in communication. As the student is able to be comfortable in simple verbal communication with a patient, further guidance and conference time could be planned to increase her understanding of the total communication process and to use communication for therapeutic purposes. This implies the need for additional understanding of the dynamics of verbal and nonverbal communication, the use of symbols in communication, the dynamics of perception and some understanding of specific problems that can be solved through effective communication.

In addition, by reviewing the plan for the teaching of physical care, the instructor can foresee other problems that are likely to occur with regularity. For example, while students are having clinical experiences related to the maintenance of an adequate supply of oxygen, it is almost certain that they will encounter acute fear on the part of the patient because of the threat to his life. At this time, the instructor can plan to help the students learn some of the dynamics of behavior related to fear and some of the skills, based on principles, that the nurse needs in order to minimize fear. This method of organization has the advantage of being based on the student's motivation to solve the problems with which she is immediately faced.

The foregoing has covered a few ideas pertaining primarily to the identification, selection and organization of learning experiences in clinical nursing practice. Perhaps a few additional suggestions can be made regarding the selection and organization of learning experiences that are largely theoretical in nature. The following discussion has been limited to suggestions for helping nursing students to learn or to apply scientific knowledge. It is the sincere belief of the authors that a professional nurse should base nursing care on scientific facts, principles and hypotheses. The ability to apply such knowledge in giving nursing care enables the nurse to interpret and to follow medical orders intelligently, to perform and to adapt nursing activities effectively, and to be creative in the planning and the execution of the nursing care of the individual patient. This ability helps to prevent rigidity in thinking and acting; it frees the nurse from continual dependence upon others for solving her nursing problems; it frees her from the monotony of repetitive nursing activities which she might perform according to routine rather than reason. In short, this ability provides the nurse with one means of becoming a truly professional person.

It is usual to teach science to nursing students before they have had clinical practice; that is, before they have had direct contact with patients. A supposed advantage of this pattern is that the student comes to the clinical nursing instructor possessing the important facts of anatomy, physiology, physics, chemistry, microbiology, sociology and psychology, which she can then apply in learning and performing nursing actions. This seems to be an ideal method, but in actual practice it sometimes does not work, for which there are many possible reasons. The instructors in the various science fields may not be familiar with what aspects of the science are important in nursing; or they may be familiar with them but must teach a science course that cannot be directed toward the specific learning needs of nursing students. The clinical instructors may be weak in their own science preparation, causing difficulty in the integration of science into the teaching of nursing. A nursing instructor may not believe that the ability to apply scientific knowledge in solving nursing problems is an objective of nursing education, or she may not know what science content to integrate or what methods to use for successful integration. She may also be unaware of how much science content, or what specific science content, the student has had prior to her clinical experience. The students themselves may have learned relatively little science while taking the preclinical courses in an academic setting. They may have forgotten much of the memorized science content before they reach the clinical experience, or they may need to learn additional science content. Not infrequently they will need considerable guidance and practice in solving problems through systematic thinking, which requires the application of scientific facts and principles.

Let us look at a few of the possible ways in which the natural and social science material could be helpful in overcoming some of the difficulties mentioned in the foregoing paragraph. If the instructors of science courses are available for conferences with the clinical nursing instructor and are amenable to such conferences, the clinical instructor can seek information about the science course content. She could inform the science instructor of the nursing students' needs for specific science content. She also might work with the science teacher in determining discrepancies between the science content taught and the science content needed in nursing, and decide who will teach what science content in the future.

The material in Parts II and III could be used by clinical instructors to identify weak spots in their own knowledge of science, which they need to strengthen if they are to do integrative teaching. The material also might serve as a guide in thinking about how science can be applicable to nursing. It also seems possible that instructors could use the material in planning learning experiences for students that would help them in recalling important science content, learning additional science content and applying science content to nursing. Following are some examples of how the material can be used in helping students to recall or learn science content and to apply principles of science to the solution of nursing problems.

Review or Learning of Natural Science Content

Study guides can be prepared for students for use in the review of science content. These study guides can direct the student rather pointedly to specific knowledge that she should have readily available. There is a decided difference between suggesting that students review the anatomy and physiology of the cardiovascular system, and suggesting that they review such well-defined content as factors that affect blood pressure, how the circulation of blood is accomplished in the human body, and how the clotting of blood occurs. A student could study for a week with the first assignment and not be well-prepared for her clinical nursing experience. In the second assignment, she could focus her studying on science knowledge pertinent to her nursing care.

Class time can be planned for the express purpose of helping students to broaden and deepen their knowledge of science content in preparation for nursing classes. For instance, it is generally recognized that students tend to have a difficult time understanding the anatomy and physiology of the nervous system. While studying such a complex subject, it is not uncommon for a student to become so engrossed with details during her introduction to the content that the more general concepts that will be useful to her in nursing are lost by the wayside. Therefore, it may be desirable to devote class time to the discussion of important aspects of neuroanatomy and neurophysiology.

Formal classes and/or informal discussions that are planned to explore specific nursing problems also provide a means of helping students to recall science content. In this case, the application of knowledge is considered in addition to a review of the knowledge needed.

Study guides can be made specific enough to direct the student's study toward important new science content. Classes can be planned exclusively for the purpose of introducing new content. It may be desirable to ask resource people, such as science instructors, to teach this sort of class. Because many courses in general microbiology, required as part of nursing curricula, may not include some of the microbiology content most useful to a nurse, this type of class may be indicated to teach microbiology content relevant to nursing.

If the amount of new content to be taught is not extensive, it can be nicely integrated along with the usual classes and informal discussions. If the classes and the discussions are planned and conducted in such a way that the basic "whys" are an integral part of any discussion, new science content fits quite naturally into place. If going back to basic science for these reasons is not a common practice in teaching, such integration will require special attention.

Review or Learning of Social Science Content

One of the most effective ways for reviewing or learning social science content is through the use of references and questions pertaining to specific patient problems as the student encounters them in clinical practice. Theoretically, the most effective learning could be achieved if the individual student could be guided toward reference reading that would be in accord with the specific patient problem that she is concerned with at any given time. Practically, there is seldom a high enough ratio of instructors to students to make this entirely possible. The authors have found that group discussion of prepared problems, accompanied by reading assignments, has been useful for purposes of both review and new learning. These prepared problems, or cases, can be constructed on the basis of actual problems that one or more of the students in the group are having to deal with at the time. For example, we can refer to the area of communication as it was discussed in relation to the selection and organization of learning experiences. If one or several of the students are experiencing some difficulty in communicating effectively with their patients, a case could be constructed that would include the common and the specific elements of the actual experiential problem. References could be given for the students to review or read preparatory to the group discussion. If this method is used, there should be some designated time, such as weekly, or biweekly, for continuity in planning so that each case can build upon previous cases. The social science material as identified in Part III could serve as resource material for planning and constructing case materials and for selecting references.

Occasionally resource people, lectures or movies are helpful in acquainting the student with new facts and principles, or in helping the student to look at previous learning in a new light. For example, an anthropologist might be called upon to discuss some of the problems of acculturation, especially as it pertains to health practices.

In addition to group discussion of actual patient problems, the student may be asked to select a nurse-patient situation in which she is involved, to give a written description of the situation with particular emphasis on certain aspects of it, and to analyze the situation in terms of social science principles, supporting her analysis with reference materials. Some of the aspects she might be asked to emphasize are the forms of communication that took place, her own subjective feelings about the patient, behavior of the patient that indicated psychological disequilibrium, or the influence of the various team members on the patient's behavior.

Perhaps one of the most useful methods for helping students to learn social science principles important to nursing is the same method by which the principles and hypotheses in Part III were acquired. If students are helped to identify psychosocial problems of specific patients, and to analyze these problems in terms of underlying science principles, they would need to do less memorization of reference material, which might or might not be useful at some later date.

Whatever methods may be used for the introduction of new material or the review of previously encountered science content, the important element is pointing out or assisting the student to discover the relationship of the content to problems of nursing practice. Again, the material in Part III could be useful as a guide for helping students to look for such relationships.

Application of Scientific Knowledge

During the original study the authors found that the most effective method for teaching the application of scientific facts, principles and hypotheses in nursing was through the use of problem-solving techniques. As might be expected, the more practice the students had in using science to solve nursing problems, the more adept at the process they became. When the development of problem-solving abilities is an objective, it is important that instructors create an atmosphere, both in the classroom and in the clinical situation, that is conducive to the solution of problems by students. Encouraging students to look at situations analytically is essential. When an instructor volunteers a direct and positive answer to problems, the student's ability to solve problems is not allowed to develop.

It is believed that the natural science and the social science material can be helpful in planning learning experiences aimed at helping students to develop skills in problem-solving and in the use of science in solving problems. The nursing sections can be helpful in identifying specific nursing measures related to the kinds of psychosocial or physiologic problems that patients may have, and the science sections can be used to identify specific science content that is applicable in the nursing care. For example, suppose a clinical instructor wished to plan a class in which the nursing care of an unconscious patient was to be discussed. We know that an unconscious patient requires extensive nursing care because of the patient's dependence upon others for meeting his needs, both physical and psychosocial. One can readily identify the major needs of such a patient and the nursing measures designed to meet these needs through the scanning of the nursing material in all twenty chapters of Part II and the related nursing material in the ten chapters of Part III.

Are there problems related to blood pressure or blood volume? This may depend upon the reason for the comatose state. It may be that the patient has hypertension or hypotension. What nursing measures are important when a patient has an abnormally high or low blood pressure? Are there problems related to maintaining an adequate oxygen supply? What nursing measures are important in providing for an open airway or for optimum vital capacity? Are there problems related to maintaining a healthy skin or healthy skeletal muscles? What nursing measures are important when a patient is unable to move himself? Are there problems of communication? Does the level of consciousness permit sufficient awareness of surroundings to allow the patient to feel anxious regarding physical care? How do family relationships enter into the nursing care situation?

These are but a few examples of problem areas that could be identified. Following are a few of the statements from the science sections that can provide a basis for the selection of specific nursing actions that would be important in the care of an unconscious patient:

Natural Sciences

1. The horizontal position provides the most effective systemic circulation with the least demands upon the cardiovascular system.
2. Gravity is the force of attraction between two objects. The law of gravitation states that any two objects in the universe are attracted to each other with a force that is proportional to the product of their masses and inversely proportional to the square of the distance between them.
3. If the muscles that protrude the tongue are not functioning properly (e.g., as when there is loss of consciousness), the tongue is allowed to fall back into the pharynx.
4. Normally, pressure in the oropharynx causes swallowing.
5. Vital capacity is affected by movement of the rib cage and diaphragm.

6. Under normal conditions the blood supply to specific tissues is increased when there is an increase in the functioning of those tissues (e.g., the contractions of skeletal muscles during exercise causes an increase in the blood supply to the muscles involved).
7. Ischemia is a condition in which the blood supply to a part is decreased. A possible cause of ischemia is the mechanical occlusion of blood vessels (e.g., due to external pressure).
8. Possible consequences of ischemia include impaired function of the affected tissues and, possibly, atrophy.
9. When the blood supply to a part is decreased below the limits that the tissues can tolerate, the tissues become hypoxic, the blood vessels become atonic and congested with blood, and the tissues die because of anoxia and chemical injury.
10. Pressure applied over bony prominences shuts off the blood supply to overlying skin very quickly.
11. Muscles that hold the body erect or are involved with locomotion lose their tone very rapidly during prolonged periods of inactivity.
12. Injury to the peripheral nerves (e.g., due to trauma or an inadequate blood supply) usually causes paralysis.

Social Sciences

1. A feeling of comfort and safety in life situations may be achieved by the establishment of familiar routines, behavior patterns and responses from others that have been experienced as safe and comfortable.
2. Disturbances of equilibrium, which result in exaggerated emotional reaction and/or mental dysfunction, decrease the individual's ability to cope with a situation successfully.
3. A feeling of comfort and safety frequently may be achieved through dependence upon others.
4. Clarity, simplicity and lack of threat in the way others approach a confused person, or one who is easily confused, facilitates cooperation between the confused person and others in the environment and develops the feeling of comfort and safety in the confused person.
5. Actions of others motivated by anticipation of and attempts to satisfy an individual's needs tends to increase one's feeling of safety and comfort.
6. Nonverbal behavior is used frequently as a means of communication.
7. An individual whose conscious awareness is impaired needs protection from environmental stimulation that may be frightening.

Not only can the material in Parts II and III be useful in the preparation of formal nursing classes, but it can also be helpful in the development of nursing care plans during the students' clinical experiences. Only as nursing students become increasingly aware of the many aspects of total patient care and understand the major objectives of this care are they able to develop comprehensive nursing care plans for individual patients. It is only as students develop the many skills and understandings that are involved in providing totality of care that they can come to function in a full nursing capacity. The authors believe that the material in Parts II and III can serve as a guide for students to use while they are developing the many skills and understandings important in nursing.

EVALUATION OF THE ATTAINMENT OF OBJECTIVES

If objectives are well-defined, the development of evaluation tools to measure the attainment of these objectives is markedly facilitated. The type of evaluative method selected will, of course, depend largely upon the kind of behavior that is to be measured. The discussion of general methods of evaluation is not within the scope of this book; however, suggestions are made relative to the possible uses of the science and nursing sections in the development of evaluation tools.

There are a number of criteria to take into consideration when evaluating the nursing care given to patients. Possible criteria include completeness of care, therapeutic effectiveness of care, safety of care for the patient and the staff, and the physical and psychological comfort of the patient. The sections of nursing care included in Parts II and III can be useful in deciding what to look for in relation to criteria such as these while the student's performance is being evaluated.

For paper and pencil tests, test items can be constructed that measure various aspects of the understanding of and the ability to apply scientific knowledge. The material contained in Parts II and III can be of use as a resource for the development of test items concerned with these factors.

Essay-type questions can ask that the student compare and contrast the nursing care of two or three patients with fairly similar physiologic or psychosocial problems, and that she support her answers with scientific facts, principles or hypotheses. The student also might be asked to describe the nursing care of a patient who has a certain kind of physiologic or psychosocial problem and to justify this care on the basis of scientific knowledge. A third type of essay question might ask the student to write possible nursing applications of a particular scientific fact or principle. Still another type would be to describe a certain patient situation and list possible nursing interventions. The student would be asked to select the "best" nursing action and to write her reasons for her choice of that action.

Objective-type questions can be constructed to determine both the student's understanding and her ability to apply scientific knowledge. One type of test experimented with at the University of Washington was called the Application of Sciences Test. Two sets of tests composed of multiple-choice items were constructed, each with a corresponding part for the natural and the social sciences. In one set of tests, the student was asked to select proper courses of action for given situations. In the second set, the student was asked to select science principles that would be the best guides to action in given situations. The items were constructed in such a way that the best answer in an item in the first test was based on the same fact or principle that would be the best guide for action in an item in the second test. Insofar as was possible, the situations in the associated items were sufficiently different to avoid the possibility of choosing the correct answer because of the similarity of items. The second set of tests were given at some time after the first set. Theoretically, such tests can be used to measure not only a student's knowledge but also her ability to apply that knowledge. If she selects the best answers in both associated test items, it may be assumed that she is able to apply the particular science involved.

Tschudin[2], as part of her investigations of students' ability to apply science principles (through the use of the Application of Natural Science Tests) asked that some students, after answering the first test, go back over the test items and state as well as they could the reasons for selecting the answers they chose. The reasons the students gave then were analyzed in terms of whether science principles were utilized, correctly or incorrectly, or whether the answer selected was little more than a guess or based on a rule of thumb.

Construction of any of these kinds of test items can be greatly facilitated by the use of the material in Parts II and III. The material can help in identifying important areas within which questions can be developed, as well as important points to be included. It also provides a good source of ideas for alternative responses in the case of multiple-choice test items.

This chapter was written, not to instruct clinical nursing teachers in the use of the science and nursing sections, but to offer some suggestions as to ways in which it might be helpful. Suggestions have been made relative to the use of the material for defining objectives, planning, selecting and organizing learning experiences, and evaluating the attainment of objectives. It is the hope of the authors that these suggestions will prove to be helpful in the teaching of nursing students and that instructors will find other practical uses for the material.

[2] Tschudin, Mary S.: A Study of the Relationship Between Nursing Students' Knowledge of Scientific Principles and Their Ability to Apply These Principles in Nursing Situations (Unpublished doctoral thesis) Univ. Washington, 1958.

Index

Abdomen
circulatory problems and, 28
distention of, respiration and, 58
incision in, 160
inflammation of nutritional deficiencies
and, 73
lower, cramping in, 28
Abdominal muscles, 157
injury to, 159
weakness in, 160
nursing care in, 162-163
Abortion, 233-234
nursing care in, 238
signs and symptoms of, 231
Abscesses, from pelvic inflammatory
disease, 233
Absorption
abnormal, nursing care in, 82
decrease of, microorganisms and, 76
of food, 69-70
Acceptance, 323, 326
Accidents, prevention of, 152
Accommodation, 200
in presbyopia, 205
Acetone, in breath and urine, 105
Achievement, parental demands for, 296
Acid-base balance, 104-107. See also
Electrolyte balance and *Fluid balance.*
abnormal. See also *Electrolyte
imbalance.*
nursing care in, 106-107
signs and symptoms, 106
anatomy and physiology of, 104
buffering system and, 104
pathology of, 104-106
Acidosis. See *Alkaline reserve,
decrease of.*
Acne vulgaris, 171
Acromegaly, 122
Acoustic nerve, 202, 203
Actinomycosis, 171
Adaptation. See *Adjustment.*
Adaptive mechanism(s). See *Defense
mechanism(s).*
Addisonian crisis, 126
Adenoids, 182
Adipose tissue. See also *Fat(s).*
Adjustment, 279
maternal overprotectiveness and, 295
psychological equilibrium and, 300-301,
317-320
Adolescence. See also *Puberty.*
autonomy in, 278
confusion and contradiction in, 277, 297
conscience development in, 278
ego development during, 277

Adolescence *(Continued)*
nurse-patient relationship in, 302-303
psychological integration in, 280
Adrenal glands
abnormalities of, 124-125
nursing care in, 126-127
anatomy and physiology of, 121-122
cortex of, androgens from, 230
Adrenocortical hormone(s)
action of, 121
fluid loss and, 92
groups of, 121
production of, 120
abnormal, 124
protein metabolism and, 70
reabsorption of ions and, 100
Adrenocorticotrophic hormone,
action of, 120
fluid loss and, 92
Aesthetic appreciation, 312-313
Affection, ego and, 295
Aged. See *Elderly.*
Agglutination, of red blood cells, 20
Aging. See *Elderly.*
Agranulocytosis, 186
Air
chemical makeup of, 50
currents of, in infectious disease, 253
embolus of, 32
Air passage(s)
clear, 58
in unconscious patient, 60
obstruction of, prevention of, 58-60
Air pressure, 50
Albumin, osmotic blood pressure and, 86
Albumin-globulin ratio, 86
Alcohol, evaporation of, 130
Alcoholic beverages, excessive
drinking of, 80
Aldosterone, 121
Alkaline reserve
acid-base balance and, 104
decrease of, 105-106
signs and symptoms of, 104
increase of, 106
signs and symptoms of, 105
Alkalosis. See *Alkaline reserve,
increase of.*
Allergy(ies). See also *Hypersensitivity.*
respiratory tract, 53
to sera or antigen solutions, 35, 41
Alveolus(i)
anatomy and physiology of, 46
inadequate oxygen supply to,
nursing care in, 60
oxygen diffusion from, 48